Advanced Cardiac Care
in the Streets

Advanced Cardiac Care in the Streets

Raymond V. Taylor, BS, EMT-P
Program Director, Emergency Medical Services
Valencia Community College;
Paramedic/Firefighter
City of Orlando Fire Department
Orlando, Florida

Craig B. Key, MD, EMT-P
Associate Medical Director
Houston Fire Department, Emergency Medical Services
Assistant Professor of Medicine
Baylor College of Medicine
Clinical Assistant Professor of Emergency Medicine
University of Texas Medical School at Houston
Houston, Texas

Mark Trach, MD, FACEP
Attending Physician
Department of Emergency Medicine
Florida Hospital Medical Center;
Medical Director, Emergency Medical Services Program
Valencia Community College
Orlando, Florida

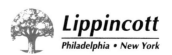
Lippincott
Philadelphia • New York

Acquisitions Editor: Margaret Biblis
Assistant Editor: Patricia Moore
Production Editor: Virginia Barishek
Production Manager: Helen Ewan
Production Service: P.M. Gordon Associates
Compositor: Maryland Composition
Printer/Binder: Courier Book Company/Kendallville
Cover Designer: Christine Cantera
Cover Printer: Lehigh Press

9 8 7 6 5 4 3 2 1

Library of Congress Cataloging-in-Publication Data

Taylor, Raymond V.
    Advanced cardiac care in the streets / Raymond V. Taylor, Craig B.
Key, Mark Trach.
        p.   cm.
    Includes bibliographical references and index
    ISBN 0–7817–1462–1
    1. Cardiovascular emergencies. 2. Electrocardiography.
3. Emergency medical technicians. I. Key, Craig B. II. Trach,
Mark. III. Title.
    [DNLM: 1. Electrocardiography—methods. 2. Heart Diseases—diagnosis.
3. Emergencies. 4. Emergency Medical Services. WG
140 T246a 1998]
RC675.T39 1998
616.1'207547—dc21
DNLM/DLC   97-36819
for Library of Congress   CIP

Care has been taken to confirm the accuracy of the information presented and to describe generally accepted practices. However, the authors, editors, and publisher are not responsible for errors or omissions or for any consequences from application of the information in this book and make no warranty, express or implied, with respect to the contents of the publication.

The authors, editors and publisher have exerted every effort to ensure that drug selection and dosage set forth in this text are in accordance with current recommendations and practice at the time of publication. However, in view of ongoing research, changes in government regulations, and the constant flow of information relating to drug therapy and drug reactions, the reader is urged to check the package insert for each drug for any change in indications and dosage and for added warnings and precautions. This is particularly important when the recommended agent is a new or infrequently employed drug.

Some drugs and medical devices presented in this publication have Food and Drug Administration (FDA) clearance for limited use in restricted research settings. It is the responsibility of the health care provider to ascertain the FDA status of each drug or device planned for use in their clinical practice.

This book is dedicated to my wife Theresa,
daughters Erin and Lindsey, and son Michael.
You have all been a constant source of encouragement
and motivation throughout the many months of writing this text.
I love and cherish you all.

—RVT

CONTRIBUTORS

Philip Dolin, MD, FACEP
  Attending Physician
  Department of Emergency Medicine
  Orlando Regional Medical Center
  Orlando, Florida

Craig B. Key, MD, EMT-P
  Associate Medical Director
  Houston Fire Department, Emergency Medical Services
  Assistant Professor of Medicine
  Baylor College of Medicine
  Clinical Assistant Professor of Emergency Medicine
  University of Texas Medical School at Houston
  Houston, Texas

John F. O'Brien, MD, FACEP
  Assistant Residency Director
  Department of Emergency Medicine
  Orlando Regional Medical Center
  Orlando, Florida
  Clinical Assistant Professor of Medicine
  University of Florida College of Medicine
  Gainesville, Florida

Raymond V. Taylor, BS, EMT-P
  Program Director, Emergency Medical Services
  Valencia Community College;
  Paramedic/Firefighter
  City of Orlando Fire Department
  Orlando, Florida

Mark Trach, MD, FACEP
  Attending Physician
  Department of Emergency Medicine
  Florida Hospital Medical Center;
  Medical Director, Emergency Medical Services Program
  Valencia Community College
  Orlando, Florida

Long gone are the days of simplistic "scoop and run" EMS training consisting of basic CPR and first aid. Today's paramedic has a vast arsenal of advanced medical knowledge and, in the near future, all paramedics will be well versed in the subject of 12-lead ECG interpretation.

For those of us who work in busy emergency departments, recognizing the importance of prehospital ECG interpretation is easy. It is widely known that decreasing the time between the onset of patient symptoms and administration of a thrombolytic agent reduces the morbidity and mortality of patients suffering acute myocardial infarction. The recent "Cardiac Alert" prehospital notification system, patterned after the "Trauma Alert," allows emergency departments to activate resources that provide for personnel, equipment, and the appropriate medication immediately upon the arrival of a patient experiencing an infarct. The paramedic's ability to accurately interpret and act on an abnormal electrocardiogram in the out-of-hospital setting is necessary for this system to work.

Advanced Cardiac Care in the Streets is an excellent text designed to train prehospital professionals in the art of ECG interpretation. It begins by introducing the reader to the basic concepts and components of the electrocardiogram, followed by a detailed discussion of 12-lead ECG interpretation and infarct recognition. Also contained within the text are several chapters dedicated to the treatment and stabilization of cardiac patients. Most important, the information is presented in an easy to understand unintimidating manner. Having worked with the main author/editor of this text along with both his current and former paramedic students, I am familiar with the value of this training within our local EMS system. It is with great confidence that I recommend this book for emergency cardiac care providers and feel that it will soon become the standard of care for paramedics nationwide.

David D. Cassidy, MD, FACEP
Attending Physician
Emergency Medicine Residency Program
Orlando Regional Medical Center
Orlando, Florida

PREFACE

Each year, approximately 1.7 million patients nationwide are admitted to cardiac and other intensive care units for episodes suspected to represent acute myocardial ischemia and infarction. Far more patients yearly are evaluated in the prehospital setting complaining of acute chest pain. Early recognition and management of patients suffering myocardial ischemia and infarction are important paramedic functions. Proficiency not only requires the ability to assess and perform a physical examination, but also the ability to interpret electrocardiograms accurately. For almost three decades, prehospital providers have successfully employed single-lead telemetry for cardiac rhythm analysis and dysrhythmia identification. Today, however, with the growing recognition of the importance for early thrombolysis in evolving myocardial infarction, the out-of-hospital acquisition of 12-lead electrocardiograms has revolutionized the standard of care within advanced life support systems and fueled the demands for the development of this text.

Advanced Cardiac Care in the Streets is designed to provide advanced level emergency medical technicians, paramedics, emergency nurses, and other emergency cardiac care providers with the skills necessary to analyze and identify common dysrhythmias, acquire and interpret diagnostic (12-lead) electrocardiograms, and manage cardiac disorders efficiently and effectively. The information within the text provides the emergency worker with a complete and comprehensive guide to both basic and advanced electrocardiography, cardiac pathophysiology, assessment and evaluation of the patient with chest pain, and the latest therapeutic modalities available for the out-of-hospital treatment of myocardial ischemia and infarction. Most important, *Advanced Cardiac Care in the Streets* is simply written, abundantly illustrated, and presented in an easy to follow step-by-step format that enables the reader to acquire the confidence and knowledge necessary to master the fundamentals of ECG interpretation and optimize patient care.

Chapter 1 begins with a discussion of the historical evolution of the Emergency Medical Services System followed by an overview of the expanding scope of practice for EMS providers and the future role of out-of-hospital cardiology. In Chapter 2, the anatomy, physiology, and electrophysiology of the heart are described in a simplified form, but with sufficient detail to provide a solid basis for the identification and treatment of cardiac dysrhythmias. The concepts and fundamental components of the electrocardiogram are outlined in Chapter 3, along with a detailed description of rhythm strip analysis, interpretation, and dysrhythmia recognition. In Chapter 4, the reader is introduced to the 12-lead electrocardiogram and the different monitoring systems available for use in the out-of-hospital setting. Chapters 5 and 6 are dedicated to the identification, localization, and clinical patterns of acute myocardial ischemia and infarction. Also provided is a systemic analysis of the 12-lead electrocardiogram accompanied by several practice 12-lead ECG recordings of acute myocardial ischemia and infarction. In Chapter 7, a variety of nonischemic conditions that may mimic acute myocardial infarction are presented, followed by a host of additional abnormalities that can substantially alter the electrocardiogram. Again, various practice 12-lead ECG recordings are provided to ensure the reader's ability to differentiate ischemic versus nonischemic electrocardiographic changes. Finally, Chapters 8, 9, and 10 describe the pathophysiology, clinical manifestations, and prehospital evaluation and therapy for acute myocardial ischemia and infarction. As an additional benefit, a key point summary is provided at the end of each chapter for a review of essential information.

Raymond V. Taylor, BS, EMT-P
Craig B. Key, MD, EMT-P
Mark Trach, MD, FACEP

ACKNOWLEDGMENTS

I wish to extend my deepest gratitude to the following individuals for their assistance with the preparation of *Advanced Cardiac Care in the Streets*:

To the entire Lippincott–Raven team, especially Patricia Moore, and editors Rebecca Marnhout and Kristin Odmark (of Little, Brown); through your direction and expertise this book has become a reality. It has been both a pleasure and privilege to have worked with you.

The reviewers, the late Robert Duplis, MD, EMS Medical Director, Orange County, FL; Steve Rudis, MD, FACEP; Matt Hevey, MD, Assistant EMS Medical Director, Valencia Community College, Orlando, FL; Dave Freeman, EMT-P, Manager, Department of Emergency Medical Services, Orange County, FL; Mike Mahoney, BA, EMT-P, Chief of EMS, City of Orlando Fire Department; and my colleagues at Valencia Community College, Orlando, FL, particularly Ruth Webb, RN, EdD; Rob Holborn, Med, EMT-P; Valerie Harris, Med, RN/EMT-P; Rita Schafer, MS; and Lynn Capraun, MS, RRT, who on top of their already busy schedules, spent countless hours editing the manuscript, artwork, and ECG recordings. Your suggestions and tactful criticisms have greatly improved the content of this text.

To my close friend and past partner Ray Alonge, BS, RN/EMT-P, thank you for not only your cautious review of the manuscript, but for your invaluable assistance with the development of Chapter 8, "The Pathophysiology and Clinical Manifestations of Ischemic Heart Disease." Special thanks to Kristine Wanner and Al Hall of Florida Hospital, Orlando, FL, for providing many of the ECG recordings utilized throughout the book. To Chief Robert "Bosco" Logston, Lieutenant Mike Lojko, and all "A" shift personnel at the City of Orlando Fire Department Station Number 1, "The Big House," thank you for your inspiration and many allowances as I often disappeared into the hazardous materials office to work on the manuscript. Furthermore, to the many paramedic students and field practitioners who provided an ongoing evaluation of the manuscript, I will always be grateful.

Finally, the acknowledgments would not be complete without the recognition of my parents, Dr. James A. and Virginia Taylor. Your inspiration, kindness, and direction have instilled in me an invaluable source of confidence and wisdom that has enriched my life.

—RVT

CONTENTS

1

Introduction to Out-of-Hospital Cardiac Care

1. Discuss the historical evolution of modern-day emergency medical services (EMS).

2. Describe the practice of medicine as it relates to EMS personnel.

3. Define on-line and off-line medical direction.

4. Discuss the development and significance of the following out-of-hospital therapeutic interventions: airway management, intravenous access, defibrillation, pharmacotherapy, transcutaneous pacemakers, pulse oximetry, and telemetry.

5. Discuss the importance of the 12-lead ECG for the early recognition and treatment of myocardial ischemia/infarction.

6. Describe the out-of-hospital impact of 12-lead ECG acquisition for early infarct detection.

7. List the benefits of out-of-hospital 12-lead electrocardiography.

INTRODUCTION

Each year in the United States approximately 1 million people die from coronary artery disease. This figure accounts for 25% of all deaths in the United States. In most cases, these deaths occur in the out-of-hospital setting. Recognition of this high mortality rate in the out-of-hospital setting was the stimulus for the development of modern emergency medical services (EMS) systems during the late 1960s.

Today, EMS systems respond to over 25 million incidents each year (more than one call per second in the U.S. alone). Public perception of EMS is that of immediate 9-1-1 access with rapid treatment and transport to high-quality medical facilities anywhere in the country. Popular opinion in the United States holds that EMS systems routinely provide truly lifesaving emergency service in every case.

Despite these commonly held perceptions, many areas of the United States do not have 9-1-1 access. Additionally, paramedics are not universally available in even the largest cities. Although most urban centers do have paramedics, most EMS systems nationwide do not provide paramedic/advanced life-support (ALS) ambulances. Even so, few paramedic-based ALS systems document a significant improvement in patient outcome. In fact, several large urban EMS systems have documented dismal results for out-of-hospital cardiac arrest. Nevertheless, a few communities with well organized EMS systems have documented 10% or greater survival rate from all cases of out-of-hospital cardiac arrest. In fact, these same systems have documented a survival rate in excess of 20% for patients who present in ventricular fibrillation (Blackwell, 1993).

HISTORICAL PERSPECTIVE

European Influence

The roots of modern out-of-hospital care are traced to military field hospitals in the late 18th century. Napoléon's armies used carts, the *ambulance volante* ("flying dressing wagons"), to evacuate wounded soldiers from the battlefield to aid stations. In this country, the practice of evacuating the wounded to aid stations began during the Civil War. In turn, using these same concepts, civilian ambulance services were first established in the United States in the late 1860s in Cincinnati and New York City. These services were hospital-based and limited to the transport of patients to the hospital. Until the 1960s, civilian out-of-hospital care continued to consist of little more than transport of the sick and injured to the hospital. It was in the late 1960s and early 1970s that emergency medical systems developed to provide therapeutic interventions in the out-of-hospital setting.

The city of Belfast, Northern Ireland had the first program cited in the western medical literature to implement advanced out-of-hospital therapeutic intervention. In 1966, Dr. Frank Pantridge of the Royal Victorian Hospital established a mobile coronary care unit (MCCU), which had the ability to monitor patients with chest pain and defibrillate appropriate arrhythmias. Pantridge and colleagues were able to demonstrate the benefits of early intervention during acute myocardial infarction, specifically early defibrillation. Their experience, published in the fall of 1967, caught the imagination of several U.S. investigators who began their own MCCU programs. The American investigators included Keller in Columbus, Ohio; Nagel in Miami, Florida; Graf in Los Angeles, California; Grace in New York; and Cobb in Seattle, Washington. Miami was the first American program to report their experience with out-of-hospital monitoring and intervention in 1970. The other cities soon followed the example of Pantridge.

American Experience

While Pantridge began the MCCU program in Europe, American EMS, as it is known today, saw its roots in the 1966 publication of a white paper from the National Academy of Sciences' National Research Council, titled *Accidental Death and Disability: The Ne-*

glected Disease of Modern Society, addressing not only out-of-hospital emergency care but also emergency department care, particularly trauma care. A brief excerpt reads as follows:

> The available information (regarding ambulance services) shows a diversity of standards, which are often low, frequent use of unnecessarily expensive and usually ill-designed equipment and generally inadequate supplies.
>
> There is no generally accepted standard for the competence or training of ambulance attendants.
>
> Although it is possible to converse with the astronauts in outer space, communication is seldom possible between an ambulance and the emergency department that it is approaching.
>
> For decades, the "emergency" facilities of most hospitals have consisted only of "accident rooms," poorly equipped, inadequately manned, and ordinarily used for limited numbers of seriously ill persons or for charity victims of disease or injury.

Two federal programs were then established to address the problem. First was the National Highway Traffic Safety Administration (NHTSA) in the Department of Transportation, and second, the EMS Systems Act of 1975. Eventually the evolving MCCU programs were expanded to address care of the injured in addition to emergency cardiac care. However, it was the television show *Emergency* that introduced the concept of out-of-hospital care to the public. *Emergency* eventually fostered strong support for the routine institution of EMS systems across the United States.

THERAPEUTIC INTERVENTION IN THE OUT-OF-HOSPITAL SETTING

The Practice of Medicine

It must be kept in mind that EMS is the practice of medicine delegated by the responsible medical director to specially trained EMS personnel. As such, that care is delegated by the medical director (and/or the medical director's representative) in an on-line or off-line manner. On-line medical supervision means direct physician communication for each patient encounter at the time care is rendered. Written protocols are also used in an on-line system to provide some medical direction prior to physician contact or when physician contact is impossible due to technical problems. Off-line medical supervision means that paramedics operate under written protocols alone and do not have direct physician input during the actual patient contact. Some systems use a combination of these two approaches depending on the type of emergency.

Airway Management

In the 1960s, emergency airway management usually consisted of the use of the bag-valve-mask device for assisting ventilation. In 1968, the esophageal obturator airway (EOA) was developed and later a modification of the EOA, called the esophageal gastric tube airway (EGTA), was developed. The tube, inserted into the esophagus, had a balloon tip which upon inflation would theoretically prevent regurgitation and avoid gastric insufflation. However, subsequent studies (Blackwell, 1993; Hauswald et al., 1990 MacLeod et al., 1990) of the EOA/EGTA devices found them to be associated with multiple complications and often inadequate oxygenation of the patient in the hands of EMS personnel.

Later, the need for direct endotracheal intubation was emphasized to improve outcome. Therefore, the current standard for out-of-hospital airway management is endotracheal intubation with the endotracheal tube (ET tube). Recently, the end-tidal CO_2 detector has been employed with endotracheal intubation as an adjunct to confirm correct ET tube placement. New airway tubes, not requiring laryngoscopy for placement, are being investigated (e.g., CombiTube) as an adjunct for basic life-support (BLS) personnel.

Intravenous Access

Intravenous access is one of the basic skills which allows the paramedic to provide drug and fluid therapy for the patient. There is much controversy in the literature regarding the use of intravenous fluid resuscitation in the out-of-hospital setting for cases of uncontrolled hemorrhage (Bickell et al., 1994). Other controversy concerns the time required on-scene to place catheters or even the question of limited therapeutic value for fluids or drugs in the out-of-hospital setting. Additionally, some studies (Blackwell et al., 1993) have demonstrated an increased rate of infection for intravenous lines started in the out-of-hospital setting. Even so, intravenous access continues as an important paramedic invasive skill.

Defibrillation

Defibrillation, without question, makes a positive impact in the outcome of out-of-hospital patients. In the case of adult out-of-hospital cardiac arrest, all other therapies, including drug therapy and airway management, pale in comparison to the significance of early defibrillation. Correctly performed defibrillation, in combination with early basic cardiopulmonary resuscitation (CPR) by bystanders, produces overall community survival rates in excess of 20% for victims of sudden death associated with an ECG presentation of ventricular fibrillation.

In the past, defibrillation was provided by paramedics who interpreted cardiac rhythms and then provided countershock whenever necessary using traditional hard paddles placed across the chest wall. Today, much defibrillation is now first delivered by automated (computerized) defibrillators which are used by basic first responders (e.g., fire apparatus crews or police officers).

Pharmacotherapy

Out-of-hospital pharmacotherapy first began in the 1960s with the use of agents to treat cardiac problems. Today the protocols and agents available most often to the paramedic are those found in the American Heart Association Advanced Cardiac Life Support (ACLS) guidelines. Epinephrine is probably the most commonly and well-studied drug used by paramedics today. Other commonly used pharmacologic agents for cardiac patients include pressor agents (dopamine, Levophed), atropine, and antiarrhythmic agents such as adenosine, lidocaine, and bretylium.

Respiratory distress is most commonly treated with beta-agonists or furosemide, morphine, and nitroglycerin (depending on the etiology of the respiratory distress). Morphine, aspirin, and nitroglycerin, along with oxygen, are typically used to treat chest pain. Naloxone is used to manage respiratory depression resulting from opioid intoxication. Glucose can provide a rather dramatic clinical effect when administered to the hypoglycemic patient. Additionally, analgesic agents are of significant value for the patient who is suffering from a painful condition unless they mask the underlying etiology (e.g., abdominal pathology).

Thrombolytic therapy has recently been studied in the out-of-hospital setting. Although numerous trials have demonstrated the safety of out-of-hospital thrombolysis, evidence for the effectiveness of out-of-hospital thrombolysis (versus brief delays to in-hospital intervention) is still unclear. In addition, only 4 to 5% of patients with chest pain in the out-of-hospital setting meet thrombolytic criteria. Further, the cost of stocking thrombolytic agents and the logistics of delivering the drug are key obstacles to the out-of-hospital use of thrombolytics. Thrombolytic therapy, other than oral aspirin, is uncommon in the out-of-hospital setting in the United States at present.

Transcutaneous Pacemakers

Transcutaneous pacing is most useful for bradycardic patients who are unstable (chest pain, hypotension) and unresponsive to atropine. These bradycardic rhythms especially include third-degree heart block and second-degree heart block (Mobitz II). They may also prove useful for bradyasystolic arrest patients if used immediately. Because of the limited need for and relative expense of transcutaneous pacers, they are not in wide use at present.

Pulse Oximetry

Early hypoxemia or tissue hypoxia may be undetectable by physical examination. Patients may deteriorate significantly before cyanosis, arrhythmias, or shock symptoms manifest themselves. Pulse oximetry provides one adjunct for monitoring the oxygenation status of the patient on a continuous basis. It is important to remember that adequate oxygenation does not necessarily mean adequate ventilation or adequate circulation. That is, the patient on supplemental oxygen may be well oxygenated but not ventilating well enough to blow off carbon dioxide, something undetectable by pulse oximetry. In this instance, the partial pressure of carbon dioxide ($PaCO_2$) may exceed 40 mmHg despite normal circulation and a normal or elevated partial pressure of oxygen (PaO_2). Likewise, a normal PaO_2 does not guarantee tissue oxygenation if circulation or cellular metabolism is compromised.

Telemetry

Transmission of single-lead cardiac rhythm strips via telemetry was commonly used in early modern EMS. It was initially viewed as a significant adjunct to medical supervision. Currently, few EMS systems use telemetry because it rarely adds any useful information beyond the well-trained paramedic's interpretation of the rhythm strip. Recent research (Cayten et al., 1985) has demonstrated no significant improvement in patient outcome with the use of rhythm strip telemetry. It does, however, add to scene time. The primary argument in favor of telemetry is that physicians are significantly more accurate at interpreting rhythm strips than paramedics (demonstrated in several studies). However, most of the arrhythmias that are misinterpreted by paramedics are of a less serious nature. More recently, cellular telephones have provided a method to transmit multi-lead electrocardiographs. As described below, similar debates regarding the need for physician interpretation of multi-lead ECGs have evolved.

EVOLVING ISSUES OF OUT-OF-HOSPITAL CARDIOLOGY

12-Lead Electrocardiography

Recognizing that the earlier the intervention, the better the outcome, numerous researchers in Europe and the United States are interested in the out-of-hospital detection of myocardial infarction and even administration of thrombolytic agents. Out-of-hospital detection of myocardial infarction and thrombolysis offers the opportunity to decrease time delays associated with delivering definitive intervention to the patient. As a result, several centers have studied the impact of rapid identification of myocardial infarction through out-of-hospital 12-lead electrocardiography (e.g., Aufderheide et al., 1990; Karagounis et al., 1990; Weaver et al., 1993; Foster et al., 1994). These studies demonstrated that out-of-hospital 12-lead electrocardiography clearly improves the paramedic's ability to detect and diagnose myocardial ischemia or infarction. In Milwaukee, paramedics are able to obtain a diagnostic quality 12-lead ECG nearly 99% of the time.

Prior to the use of 12-lead ECGs, researchers (Aufderheide et al., 1990; Aufderheide et al., 1991) found that only 62% of patients having cardiac chest pain were suspected of having cardiac chest pain by paramedics. Therefore, 38% of patients with cardiac chest pain were being misassessed by paramedics (i.e., patients were suspected of having chest pain of noncardiac origin). When paramedic suspicion of cardiac chest pain was combined with the 12-lead ECG, 90% of the patients with cardiac chest pain were detected in the field. This demonstrates an improved sensitivity for detecting chest pain of cardiac origin, thus expediting interventions when necessary (Table 1–1).

Further, only 71% of patients suspected of having cardiac chest pain by paramedics were actually experiencing chest pain of cardiac etiology. That is, 29% of patients that paramedics suspected of having cardiac chest pain had noncardiac chest pain. Again, when paramedic suspicion of cardiac chest pain was combined with 12-lead electrocardiography, an appropriate identification of cardiac chest pain was demonstrated in 99% of cases. Therefore, the specificity for paramedic identification was improved.

The most significant benefit realized from out-of-hospital 12-lead electrocardiography is that of early warning for the receiving hospital. Early warning via a cardiac alert allows the receiving facility to prepare in advance for possible thrombolysis or rapid transfer to the cardiac catheterization lab. For many years, Level I trauma centers have had well-organized trauma teams to respond to trauma alerts from paramedics at the scene. A well-organized CLOT (coronary lysis on time) team activated by EMS providers would allow for rapid diagnosis and treatment of myocardial infarction in a similar manner. Multiple studies have demonstrated a 40- to 70-minute decrease in the time required to provide thrombolysis for the acute myocardial infarction patient because of early warning. This decreased delay in treatment was realized even without the existence of a CLOT team in each study.

Several additional sources offer further benefits for out-of-hospital 12-lead electrocardiography. The 12-lead ECG allows localization of the area of ischemia. Localization of the infarct is important in the presence of inferior infarction. Inferior myocardial infarction is frequently associated with right ventricular infarction. Right ventricular infarction occurs because, in most patients, the right coronary artery supplies the inferior left ventricle and the entire right ventricle. With right ventricular infarction, left ventricular filling is decreased (due to decreased left ventricular preload) and hypotension results. The treatment for hypotension from right ventricular infarction is judicious fluid administration to increase filling pressure (preload).

The right coronary artery also supplies the AV node. If AV nodal infarction occurs, the patient may develop a complete heart block. Diagnosis of inferior infarction, therefore, allows the paramedic to be alert for both hypotension and complete heart block.

The 12-lead ECG also assists the identification of left ventricular injury. Anterior myocardial infarction often involves a large percentage of the myocardium. Cardiogenic shock, commonly associated with anterior left ventricular infarction, results when a large percentage of the myocardium is dysfunctional (due to infarction). These patients

TABLE 1–1   •   **Paramedic Diagnosis of Cardiac Pain**

	MEDIC	MEDIC + 12-LEAD
Sensitivity	62%	90%
Specificity	71%	99%

TABLE 1–2 • **Benefits of Out-of-Hospital 12-Lead Electrocardiography**

Improved paramedic identification of cardiac-related chest pain
Early warning for receiving hospitals
Reduced in-hospital delay for thrombolysis via cardiac alert
Inferior myocardial infarction diagnosis
  right ventricular infarction and hypotension
  AV nodal infarction and heart block
  anterior infarction and cardiogenic shock
Detection of ischemia that resolves prior to hospital arrival
Diagnosis of wide-complex tachycardia
Allows possible out-of-hospital thrombolysis

will usually require inotropic support from pressor agents such as dopamine and nore-pinephrine (Levophed). Again, localization of the infarction to the anterior left ventricular myocardium allows the paramedic to prepare for cardiogenic shock.

Occasionally, patients suffer from an ischemic event which resolves either spontaneously or as a result of treatment (e.g., oxygen, nitroglycerin, aspirin, etc.) prior to arrival at the hospital. In these cases, the hospital 12-lead ECG will not demonstrate the acute ischemic event. An out-of-hospital 12-lead ECG would, however, document ischemia prior to intervention and resolution of the ischemia.

Wide-complex tachycardias present an additional diagnostic challenge for the paramedic. The question always arises: Is this ventricular tachycardia or supraventricular tachycardia with an aberrant conduction (such as a bundle branch block)? With the availability of more leads, the 12-lead ECG can provide clues for the diagnosis of wide-complex tachycardias (Table 1–2).

There are several criticisms of the out-of-hospital 12-lead ECG concept. The most serious concern is that paramedics may not entertain the diagnosis of acute myocardial infarction if the 12-lead ECG is nondiagnostic. The 12-lead ECG does not detect all acute myocardial infarctions. A negative 12-lead ECG does not exclude the diagnosis of acute myocardial infarction. Care must be taken not to minimize the patients' complaints in light of a negative 12-lead ECG. Triage of the patient to BLS transport based on 12-lead ECG cannot be done on a routine basis. These patients need the continued care of paramedics in the out-of-hospital phase of their treatment.

Likewise, a negative 12-lead ECG in the out-of-hospital setting may also cause emergency department delays for those who are actually having acute myocardial infarction. Emergency department personnel may also minimize the patient's complaints if the ECG is normal. Lastly, performing 12-lead electrocardiography in the field adds, on average, 5.2 minutes to the out-of-hospital phase of the patient's emergency care. It is unknown what effect this delay may have in the ultimate outcome for the patient.

Future Possibilities for Out-of-Hospital Cardiac Treatment

The cardiac alert mentioned previously has the most immediate potential to improve the out-of-hospital management of acute myocardial infarction. There is a nationwide movement to reduce the delays associated with delivery of thrombolytic therapy in emergency departments. Early warning from EMS providers is one modality that offers an important method to effect more efficient delivery of emergency department therapy. Therefore, EMS providers will likely play a more significant role in the overall management of acute myocardial infarction.

Out-of-hospital thrombolytic therapy is currently an unproven treatment option. Should out-of-hospital thrombolysis ever become a practical therapy, 12-lead electrocardiography will be an essential component. While transmission of 12-lead ECGs is possible via cellular phone, future investigations may find transmission of 12-lead ECGs no more necessary than single-lead telemetry.

SUMMARY

Out-of-hospital therapy has advanced considerably since the days of horse-drawn hospital transport in the 1860s. A wide variety of therapeutic modalities are now available to the modern rescuer in the out-of-hospital setting. Lifesaving interventions such as early defibrillation of the patient in ventricular tachycardia or fibrillation produce improved survival rates for the out-of-hospital patient. Even so, many out-of-hospital therapies remain to be proven.

Indeed, some devices and therapies previously used by the paramedic are of no value or have fallen out of favor with out-of-hospital providers. The EOA/EGTA devices, anti-shock garments, and telemetry of single-lead rhythm strips are just a few examples of methods which have been critically evaluated and now called into question. The evolving fuel for EMS systems is research, not as an adjunct, but as an intrinsic element of EMS systems.

KEY POINTS SUMMARY

Historical Perspective

1. The historical evolution of modern out-of-hospital care is often traced to military field hospitals used by Napoléon's armies. In the United States, the practice of evacuating wounded soldiers to medical aid stations principally began during the Civil War.
2. Civilian ambulance services were first established in the United States in the late 1860s in Cincinnati and New York City. These services were hospital-based and limited only to the transport of patients.
3. In the late 1960s and early 1970s, emergency medical services, as we know them today, formally developed providing therapeutic interventions in the out-of-hospital setting.
4. The city of Belfast, Northern Ireland had the first program cited in western medical literature to implement advanced out-of-hospital emergency care. In 1966 Frank Pantridge of the Royal Victorian Hospital in Belfast, established the first mobile coronary care unit designed for the early recognition and treatment of acute cardiac disorders.

Therapeutic Intervention in the Out-of-Hospital Setting

5. Emergency medical services is the practice of medicine which is delegated by a medical director or directors to specially trained EMS personnel. Emergency care is delegated in either an on-line (direct physician communication) or off-line (written protocol) manner.
6. Advanced out-of-hospital emergency care includes the delivery of such interventions as airway management (endotracheal intubation), intravenous therapy, cardiac monitoring and defibrillation, pharmacotherapy, transcutaneous pacing, oximetric monitoring, and diagnostic 12-lead electrocardiography.

Prehospital 12-Lead Electrocardiography

7. Diagnostic 12-lead electrocardiography has revolutionized the out-of-hospital care for the patient experiencing myocardial ischemia/infarction. Early prehospital detection of myocardial infarction offers the ability to decrease time delays associated with delivering definitive intervention to such patients (i.e., thrombolytic therapy).
8. Research has demonstrated the ability of paramedics to acquire a diagnostic-quality 12-lead ECG in over 95% of cases, as well as improved sensitivity for detecting chest pain of cardiac origin.

Benefits of Out-of-Hospital 12-Lead Electrocardiography

9. The most significant benefit of out-of-hospital 12-lead electrocardiography is early warning for the receiving hospital, which allows the receiving facility to prepare in advance for possible thrombolysis or rapid transfer to the cardiac catheterization lab. Additional benefits of out-of-hospital 12-lead electrocardiography include localization of the area of ischemia/infarction, improved treatment plans regarding atrioventricular block and hypotension, identification of prehospital ischemia that resolves prior to hospital arrival, and the differentiation of wide-complex tachycardias.

BIBLIOGRAPHY

American Heart Association Emergency Care Committee Subcommittee on ACLS. Guidelines for cardiopulmonary resuscitation and emergency cardiac care. *Journal of the American Medical Association.* 1992;268:2171–2302.

Aufderheide TP, Hendley GE, Thakur RK, et al. The diagnostic impact of prehospital 12-lead electrocardiography. *Annals of Emergency Medicine.* 1990;19:1280–1287.

Aufderheide TP, Hendley GE, Woo J, et al. A prospective evaluation of prehospital 12-lead ECG application in chest pain patients. *Journal of Electrocardiology.* 1991;24(suppl.):8–13.

Becker LB, Ostrander MP, Barrett J, Kondos GT. Outcome of CPR in a large metropolitan area—Where are the survivors? *Annals of Emergency Medicine.* 1991;20:355–361.

Bertazzoni G, Aguglia F. Cardiophone. *RAYS.* 1991;16:463–471.

Bickell WH, Wall MJ, Pepe PE, et al. Immediate versus delayed fluid resuscitation for hypotensive patients with penetrating torso injuries. *New England Journal of Medicine.* 1994;331:1105–1109.

Blackwell TH. Prehospital care. *Emergency Medicine Clinics of North America.* 1993;11(1):1–14.

Braun O, McCallion R, Fazackerley J. Characteristics of midsized urban EMS systems. *Annals of Emergency Medicine.* 1990;19:536–546.

Cayten CG, Oler J, Walker K, et al. The effect of telemetry on urban prehospital cardiac care. *Annals of Emergency Medicine.* 1985;14:976–981.

Committee on Trauma and Committee on Shock, Division of Medical Sciences, National Academy of Sciences, National Research Council. Accidental death and disability: The neglected disease of modern society. U.S. Department of Health, Education, and Welfare, Public Health Service, Health Services and Mental Health Administration, Division of Emergency Health Services, Rockville, MD, 1966:1–38.

Cummins RO, Eisenberg MS. From pain to reperfusion: What role for the prehospital 12-lead ECG? *Annals of Emergency Medicine.* 1990;19:1343–1346.

Falk JL. Medical direction of emergency medical service systems: A full-time commitment whose time has come. *Critical Care Medicine.* 1993;21:1259–1260.

Foster BD, Dufendach JH, Barkdoll CM, Mitchell BK. Prehospital recognition of AMI using independent nurse/paramedic 12-lead ECG evaluation: Impact on in-hospital times to thrombolysis in a rural community hospital. *American Journal of Emergency Medicine.* 1994;12:25–31.

Gokli AR, Kovar JL, Kowalenko T, Nowak RM. Prehospital care of acute myocardial infarction: A review. *Henry Ford Hospital Medical Journal.* 1991;39:170–175.

Grim P, Feldman T, Martin M, et al. Cellular telephone transmission of 12-lead electrocardiograms from ambulance to hospital. *The American Journal of Cardiology.* 1987;60:715–720.

Hargarten KM, Aprahamian C, Stueven H, et al. Limitations of prehospital predictors of acute myocardial infarction and unstable angina. *Annals of Emergency Medicine.* 1987;1325–1329.

Hauswald M, Drake C. Innovations in emergency medical services systems. *Emergency Medicine Clinics of North America.* 1990;8(1):135–144.

Hunt RC, McCabe JB, Hamilton GC, Krohmer JR. Influence of emergency medical services systems and prehospital defibrillation on survival of sudden cardiac death victims. *American Journal of Emergency Medicine.* 1989;7:68–82.

Jones SE. Prehospital 12-lead ECGs. *Annals of Emergency Medicine.* 1991;20:942–943.

Karagounis L, Ipsen SK, Jessop MR, et al. Impact of field-transmitted electrocardiography on time to in-hospital thrombolytic therapy in acute myocardial infarction. *The American Journal of Cardiology.* 1990;66:786–791.

Kowalenko T, Kereiakes DJ, Gibler WB. Prehospital diagnosis and treatment of acute myocardial infarction: A critical review. *American Heart Journal*. 1992;123:181–190.

MacLeod BA, Seaberg DC, Paris PM. Prehospital therapy past, present, and future. *Emergency Medicine Clinics of North America*. 1990;8(1):57–74.

Narad RA. Emergency medical services system design. *Emergency Medicine Clinics of North America*. 1990;8(1):1–14.

National Heart Attack Alert Program Coordinating Committee 60 Minutes to Treatment Working Group. Emergency Department: Rapid Identification and Treatment of Patients with Acute Myocardial Infarction. Bethesda, MD: U.S. Department of Health and Human Services, Public Health Service, National Institutes of Health, National Heart, Lung, and Blood Institute, 1993:1–37.

Otto LA, Aufderheide TP. Evaluation of ST segment criteria for the prehospital electrocardiographic diagnosis of acute myocardial infarction. *Annals of Emergency Medicine*. 1994;23:17–24.

Pantridge JF, Geddes JS. A mobile intensive-care unit in the management of myocardial infarction. *Lancet*. 1967;ii:271–273.

Pepe PE. Emergency medical services. *Academic Emergency Medicine*. 1994;1:131–133.

Pepe PE, Mattox KL, Duke JH, et al. Effect of full-time, specialized physician supervision on the success of a large, urban emergency medical services system. *Critical Care Medicine*. 1993;21:1279–1286.

Weaver WD, Cerqueira M, Hallstrom AP, et al. Prehospital-initiated vs hospital-initiated thrombolytic therapy: The myocardial infarction triage and intervention trial. *Journal of the American Medical Association*. 1993;270:1211–1216.

White RD. Prehospital 12-lead ECG. *Annals of Emergency Medicine*. 1992;21:586.

OUTLINE

Cardiac Anatomy, Physiology, and Electrophysiology

1. Describe the location, size, and position of the heart within the thoracic cavity.

2. Name the coverings of the heart and describe their importance to mechanical action.

3. Describe the structure and function of the three tissue layers of the heart.

4. Name and describe the chambers of the heart and the blood vessels that enter or leave each.

5. Name the valves of the heart and describe their location and functions.

6. Explain what causes the two heart sounds heard on auscultation.

7. Describe the importance of coronary circulation, naming the major branches and their distribution.

8. Discuss the cardiac conduction system: its inherent characteristics, its normal sequence of activation of the heart, and its relationship to pump action.

9. Describe the events of the cardiac cycle.

10. Explain stroke volume, Starling's law of the heart, and cardiac output.

11. Describe the effects of the relationship between stroke volume and Starling's law on cardiac output.

12. Describe the anatomical and physiological characteristics of the autonomic nervous system and explain its regulation of cardiac output.

13. Identify the structural and functional characteristics of cardiac electrophysiology.

14. Describe the resting membrane potential and its importance to both electrical and mechanical action.

15. Discuss the role of the sodium-potassium exchange pump as it relates to electrolytic concentrations.

16. Describe the phases of depolarization and repolarization in relationship to ionic channels and electrolyte movement.

17. Discuss the phases of the action potential and explain their relationship to the cardiac cycle and the ECG.

18. Define the refractory period and describe its appearance on the ECG.

INTRODUCTION

Emergency medical providers are often responsible for treating and stabilizing individuals suffering from a broad variety of acute cardiovascular emergencies. To diagnose and treat these problems effectively, familiarity with normal as well as abnormal cardiac function is necessary. The electrical, mechanical, and metabolic functions of the heart are all interrelated and must be understood to treat cardiac disorders efficiently and effectively. Often, individuals experiencing myocardial infarction develop structural changes within the heart muscle. These abnormalities are the result of inadequate blood supply and oxygen delivery to the cardiac tissues. Because of this, changes in cardiac function result. Clinically, these problems are expressed as disturbances in cardiac rate and rhythm, as well as an overall reduction in the pumping abilities of the heart. Identification of these problems, followed by the aggressive prehospital administration of oxygen, pharmacological therapy, and appropriate cardiac monitoring, is vital to the restoration of normal cardiac function. Therefore, through an adequate understanding of cardiac and circulatory anatomy, paramedics can enhance their diagnostic skills and better anticipate potential complications associated with coronary atherosclerosis and cardiovascular crisis.

LOCATION, SIZE, AND ORIENTATION OF THE HEART

The heart is a hollow, cone-shaped muscular organ possessing four chambers: two atria superiorly and two ventricles inferiorly. It is located within the thoracic cavity in the lower portion of the mediastinum (Figure 2–1). Approximately two-thirds of the mass of the heart is located to the left of the midline sternum and the remaining one-third is located to the right. The heart lies anterior to the vertebral column and posterior to the sternum. The lungs flank the heart laterally and partially conceal it. The size of the heart varies with the size of an individual. Very approximately, it is the size of a closed adult fist. The blunt, rounded point of the heart is called the apex. The apex is directed anteriorly and extends downward and to the left. It rests on the diaphragm at the level of the fifth intercostal space. The larger opposite end of the heart is called the base. The base is directed posteriorly and superiorly projects toward the right shoulder just beneath the second rib. It is through the base that the great vessels enter the heart.

TISSUE LAYERS OF THE HEART

The heart is enclosed by a double-layered fibroserous membranous sac known as the pericardium. The pericardium has two layers: a thin inner-serous membrane layer and an outer fibrous membrane (Figure 2–2). The inner layer of the pericardium is called the visceral pericardium, which is closely applied to the surface of the heart like a tight-fitting glove. The outer layer of the pericardium is known as the parietal pericardium. It is composed chiefly of tough connective tissue and is applied loosely to the surface of the heart, allowing movement within. Both pericardial layers lie in close proximity to one another and are separated by a small amount of serous fluid. The serous fluid (pericardial fluid) serves to reduce friction during cardiac contraction. Located between the parietal pericardium and visceral pericardium is a potential space, the pericardial cavity. The cavity is a potential space because there is not enough serous fluid to separate

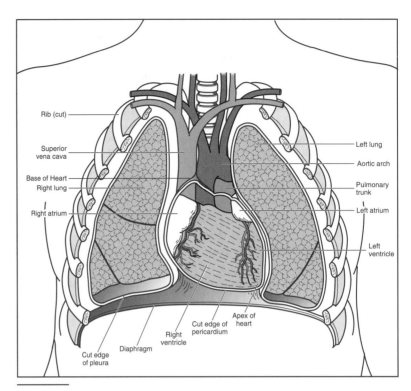

Figure 2–1.

Location of the heart within the chest.

Modified from G. Tortora, *Introduction to the Human Body*, 3rd ed. New York: HarperCollins, 1994.

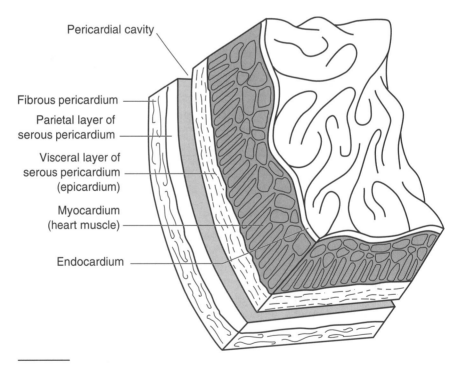

Figure 2–2.

Structure of the pericardium and heart wall.

Modified from G. Tortora and T. Anagostakos, *Principles of Anatomy and Physiology*, 6th ed. New York: HarperCollins, 1990.

the layers to any significant degree. However, certain inflammatory disease processes and injuries can cause the pericardial sac to fill with blood or fluid, compressing the heart and limiting its ability to pump blood.

The heart wall itself is composed of three distinct layers of tissue, all richly supplied with blood vessels. The outermost layer is the epicardium. The epicardium is contiguous with the visceral pericardium and contains the vessels that nourish the heart wall. The thick middle layer of the heart wall is the myocardium. The myocardium forms the bulk of the heart and is composed chiefly of cardiac muscle tissue. This layer performs the work of the heart, contracting to force blood into the vascular system. The cells of the myocardium anatomically connect into a network that provides a common linkage to all components of the muscle. Electrical stimulation of any portion of this network spreads to all of its parts, resulting in simultaneous contraction of the entire myocardium. Specialized myocardial fibers promote the rapid distribution of electrical impulses from one cell to another.

The innermost layer of the heart wall is the endocardium. This tissue layer lines the cardiac chambers and valves, and provides a smooth surface permitting blood to move easily through the heart. Located within the endocardium are specialized muscle fibers known as the Purkinje network. These fibers which conduct the electrical impulses that activate myocardial muscular contraction.

CHAMBERS OF THE HEART

The heart contains four chambers that are responsible for receiving and discharging blood (Figure 2–3). The two superior chambers are called the atria and the two inferior chambers are called the ventricles. Internally, the chambers are supported and anchored by the heart's fibrous skeleton. The fibrous skeleton consists of a group of connective tissue fibers arranged in ropelike rings that surround the chambers and their valves. These fibers provide firm attachments for the chambers and valves, as well as for various muscle fibers. In addition, both the thin-walled atria and the thick-walled ventricles are separated by the septum, an internal partition that divides the heart longitudinally. This partition can be further divided into the interatrial septum and the interventricular septum.

Functionally, the atria are the receiving chambers of the heart. The right atrium receives oxygen-poor blood returning from the peripheral circulation via the superior vena cava, inferior vena cava, and coronary sinus. The superior vena cava returns venous blood from above the level of the diaphragm and the inferior vena cava from levels below the diaphragm. The coronary sinus collects venous blood draining from the myocardium. The left atrium receives oxygenated blood from the lungs by way of the four pulmonary veins. The right and left atria pump the blood they receive into the ventricles. Little force is required to do this, so the walls to the atria are thin (i.e., contain little myocardium) and their force of contraction is minimal compared to the ventricles.

The ventricles are the discharging chambers of the heart. The right ventricle forms most of the anterior surface of the heart and is responsible for pumping blood through the pulmonary arteries into the lungs for gas exchange. The left ventricle forms the heart's apex and the majority of the heart's inferior surface. It ejects blood into the aorta, the largest artery in the systemic circulation. The myocardial layer is thick in the ventricles, especially the left ventricle, therefore they can contract with great force. This greater muscular strength is necessary because the ventricles must eject blood into arteries, which present some resistance to the outflow of blood. The aorta presents much more resistance than the pulmonary arteries, so the left ventricle has a thicker myocardial layer than the right ventricle.

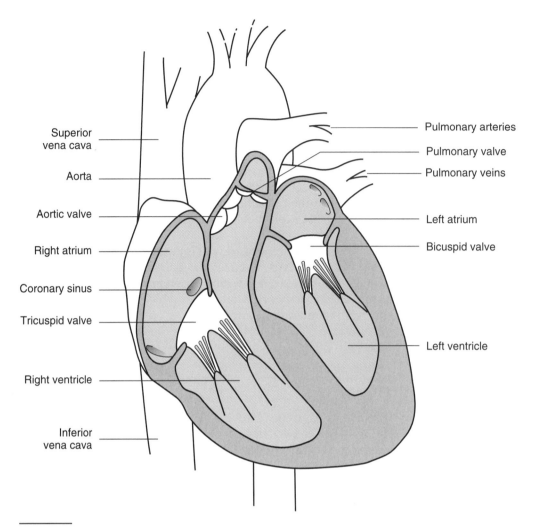

Figure 2–3.
The chambers and valves of the heart.

Modified from B. Bledsoe, R. Porter, and B. Shade, *Paramedic Emergency Care*, 2nd ed. Englewood Cliffs, NJ: Brady, 1994.

CARDIAC VALVES

The chambers of the heart are separated by two sets of valves that ensure that blood flows through the heart in one direction (Figure 2–4). This process is necessary to prevent the backflow of blood through the heart which can reduce the volume available to the circulation. Both sets of valves operate on the same principle of unidirectional movement. This means that the valves open in only a single direction due to the pressure exerted by the blood on their respective sides.

The two atrioventricular valves are located at the junction of the atria and the ventricles. The right atrioventricular valve is termed the tricuspid valve because it has three flexible leaflets (cusps). The left atrioventricular valve is termed the bicuspid (or mitral) valve because it has only two leaflets. Located in the ventricles and attached to each of the atrioventricular valves are columns of specialized tissue known as the papillary muscles. Fibrous strands called the chordae tendinae extend from the papillary muscles to the flaps of the atrioventricular valves. The chordae tendinae tether the edges of the

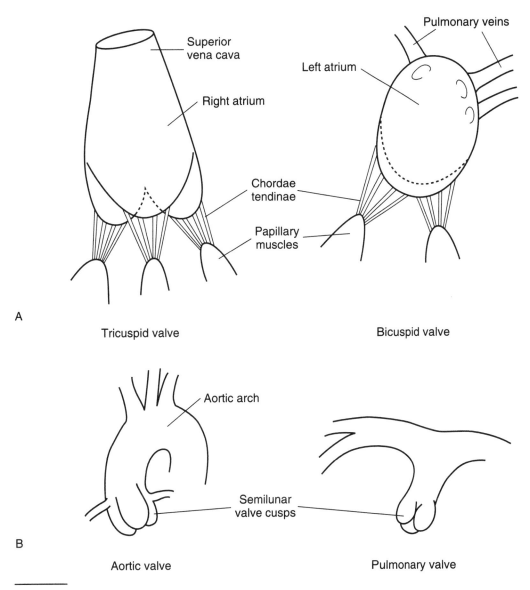

Figure 2–4.
The valves of the heart.
(A) The tricuspid valve has three flexible flaps, and the bicuspid valve has two. The chordae tendinae of the uppermost bicuspid valve are not depicted to simplify the figure. (B) The aortic and pulmonary valves each have three flaps. The flaps are called "semilunar" because their circular shape resembles a half moon.
Modified from R. Seeley, T. Stevens, and P. Tate, *Anatomy and Physiology*. St. Louis: Mosby, 1989.

flaps to prevent valve leaflet eversion, or prolapse, into the atria during ventricular contraction. During right and left ventricular contraction the papillary muscles contract, tightening the chordae tendinae and preventing the prolapse of the atrioventricular valves (Figure 2–5).

The semilunar valves are located at the junction of the ventricles and the bases of the arteries into which they empty. The pulmonary semilunar valve is located between the right ventricle and pulmonary artery. The aortic semilunar valve is located between the left ventricle and the aorta. Both valves operate on the same principles as the atrioventricular valves, preventing the backflow of blood into their respective ventricles.

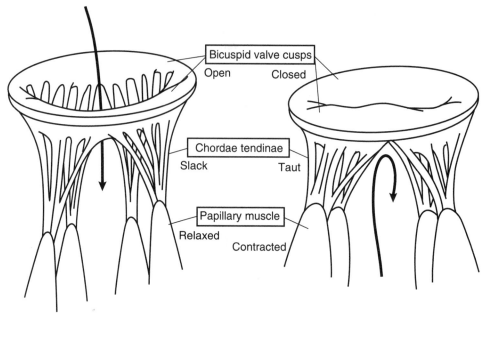

A   Bicuspid valve open

B   Bicuspid valve closed

Figure 2–5.
Atrioventricular (AV) valves.
(A) Bicuspid valve open. (B) Bicuspid valve closed.
Modified from G. Tortora, *Principles of Human Anatomy*, 6th ed. New York: HarperCollins, 1992.

HEART SOUNDS

There are two distinguishing heart sounds that can be heard during auscultation of the thorax. Both sounds are rhythmical and repetitive and are due to vibrations in the cardiac tissues caused by the closing of the valves. These sounds are commonly described as "lub-dup".

The first heart sound (lub), referred to as S_1, is produced by the closure of the atrioventricular valves at the beginning of ventricular contraction (Table 2–1). The second heart sound (dup), or S_2, is produced by closure of the semilunar valves when the ventricles begin to relax. It has a higher pitch, but is of shorter duration than the first heart sound. The time between the first and second heart sounds represents the period of ventricular contraction. The time between the second heart sound and the first heart sound of the next beat represents the period of ventricular relaxation. Because relaxation lasts

TABLE 2–1 • **Heart Sounds**

S1—Closure of the atrioventricular valves (tricuspid and mitral)
S2—Closure of the semilunar valves (pulmonary and aortic)
Extra Heart Sounds
S3—Produced by rapid ventricular filling (congestive heart failure)
S4—Produced by forceful atrial contraction into a noncompliant ventricle (hypertension)
Murmur—turbulent blood flow through incompetent valves

longer than contraction, the pause between the first heart sound and the second sound is shorter than that following the second sound preceding the next cycle. Both S_1 and S_2 are normal findings.

The assessment of heart sounds is of particular interest because it provides information concerning the condition of heart valves. Abnormal heart sounds are caused by defective valves and commonly present as murmurs, audible vibrations that occur because of turbulent blood flow through a partially closed valve. This results in blood leaking back through the valve, producing a hissing wavelike sound. Furthermore, the identification of certain cardiac pathologies (diseases) can be determined with the auscultation of heart sounds. For example, a third heart sound, or S_3, is produced by rapid ventricular filling and is frequently a sign of congestive heart failure. A fourth heart sound, or S_4, is due to a forceful atrial contraction in the presence of reduced ventricular compliance. This sound is often identified in patients with acute myocardial infarctions and coronary artery disease.

CORONARY ARTERY CIRCULATION AND DISTRIBUTION

Although the heart is continuously filled with blood, cardiac cells do not exchange nutrients and metabolic waste products with the blood inside the chambers. Instead, the coronary arteries supply blood to all structures in the heart (Figure 2–6 on p. 22).

The coronary arteries originate from the base of the aorta. This origination site ensures that the coronary arteries are continuously supplied with oxygen-rich blood under the greatest amount of pressure. Blood flows through the coronary arteries only when the heart is relaxed. Ventricular contraction compresses the coronary arteries, shutting off flow. Many anastomoses exist within the coronary arterial branches, providing abundant collateral pathways of circulation. The collateral circulation enables the heart to establish alternative routes of blood distribution in the event that one of its coronary arteries becomes blocked.

The coronary arteries are divided into the left main coronary artery and the right coronary artery. The left coronary artery provides approximately 75% of the blood supply to the myocardial muscle, and the right coronary artery supplies the remaining 25% in individuals with dominant left systems. However, approximately 25–30% of the population have dominant right circulation in which the right coronary artery provides the majority of myocardial circulation.

The left coronary artery subdivides into two major branches, the left anterior descending and circumflex arteries. The left anterior descending artery supplies blood to the left anterior wall of the ventricular myocardium and the intraventricular septum. The circumflex artery supplies blood to the left atrium, lateral walls of the left ventricle, and to portions of the right ventricle and posterior left ventricle. The right coronary artery (RCA) courses around the right side of the heart, supplying most of the right atrium, right ventricle, and the inferior aspect of the left ventricle. In approximately 60% of the population the right coronary artery provides the usual blood supply for the sinoatrial and atrioventricular nodes. It also subdivides into two major branches, the marginal and posterior descending arteries. The marginal artery perfuses the lateral portion of the myocardium's right side and the posterior descending artery perfuses the posterior ventricular walls.

Knowledge of coronary artery distribution is essential to identify the damaged cardiac tissues that result from coronary artery occlusion (Table 2–2 on p. 23). Identification of the artery involved in infarction enables the clinician to better anticipate potential problems that may occur. Review both the diagram and table of coronary anatomy and the tissues supplied. A detailed discussion concerning this topic, as well as the evolution of myocardial infarction, will follow in Chapters 6 and 8.

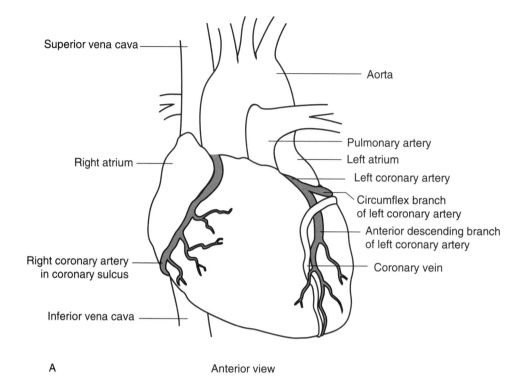

Superior vena cava

Aorta

Pulmonary artery

Left atrium

Left coronary artery

Right atrium

Circumflex branch
of left coronary artery

Anterior descending branch
of left coronary artery

Right coronary artery
in coronary sulcus

Coronary vein

Inferior vena cava

A   Anterior view

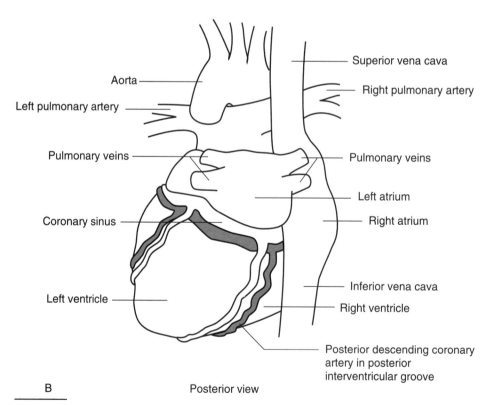

Aorta

Superior vena cava

Left pulmonary artery

Right pulmonary artery

Pulmonary veins

Pulmonary veins

Coronary sinus

Left atrium

Right atrium

Left ventricle

Inferior vena cava

Right ventricle

Posterior descending coronary
artery in posterior
interventricular groove

B   Posterior view

Figure 2–6.
Coronary arteries.
(A) Anterior view, showing the takeoff point of left and right coronary arteries from the aorta. (B) View from below and behind, showing the coronary sinus.

Modified from N. Caroline, *Emergency Care in the Streets*, 5th ed. Boston: Little, Brown, and Company, 1995.

TABLE 2–2 • **Anatomical Coronary Artery Supply**

RIGHT CORONARY ARTERY
Sinoatrial and atrioventricular nodes
Right ventricle
Inferior wall of the left ventricle
Posterior wall of the left ventricle (posterior descending)

LEFT CORONARY ARTERY
Bundle branches
Interventricular septum
Anterior wall of the left ventricle (left anterior descending)
Lateral wall of the left ventricle (circumflex)

THE ELECTRICAL CONDUCTION SYSTEM OF THE HEART

The electrical tissues of the heart (1) initiate the electrical impulse that leads to myocardial contraction and (2) conduct that impulse to all parts of the heart. Two different types of cells perform these two jobs: pacemaker cells and conduction fibers. Pacemaker cells possess the property of self-excitation (also termed automaticity). This means that they spontaneously generate electrical impulses. Pacemaker cells can be found in many parts of the heart, but are mainly concentrated in the sinoatrial node and atrioventricular junction. The conduction fibers of cardiac tissue possess properties similar to those of an electrical cable. They function as the hard wiring of the heart, spreading the electrical impulse throughout the atria and ventricles. The complete electrical conduction system of the heart consists of the following structures: sinoatrial node, internodal and interatrial tracts, atrioventricular node, bundle of His, right and left bundle branches, and Purkinje network fibers (Figure 2–7).

Normally, the heart's electrical impulse originates in the sinoatrial (SA) node. The SA node is located in the upper portion of the right atrium at the junction with the superior vena cava. The pacemaker cells of the sinoatrial node spontaneously generate impulses at a rate faster than that of other pacemaker sites (Table 2–3). Because of the SA node's rapid rate of intrinsic discharge it is considered the heart's dominant pacemaker. The sinoatrial node is capable of electrically discharging between **60 to 100 times per minute.**

NOTE: All electrocardiographic rhythms originating in the sinoatrial node are termed sinus rhythms. Normal sinus rhythm produces an electrical rate between 60 to 100 times per minute.

From the sinoatrial node, the electrical excitation wave travels through three conducting pathways and an interatrial tract to stimulate the contractile cells of the atrial muscle. The three conducting pathways, known as internodal tracts, transmit the impulse from the SA node to the atrioventricular (AV) node. The interatrial tract, referred to as Bachman's bundle serves to conduct the electrical current from the SA node across to the left atrium. Following the distribution of electricity, the atrial muscle cells are activated in an organized manner resulting in simultaneous atrial contraction.

The three internodal conducting pathways meet in an area referred to as the atrioventricular junction. The junctional region is the anatomical site where the atrial and ventricular tissues merge. Located within the atrioventricular junction is the AV node. The AV node is positioned in the right atrial wall above the tricuspid valve, anterior to the coronary sinus. Because of this location the AV node is well situated for mediating conduction between the atria and ventricles. Within the AV node are pacemaker cells that possess an intrinsic firing rate of **40 to 60 times per minute.** Should the SA node fail

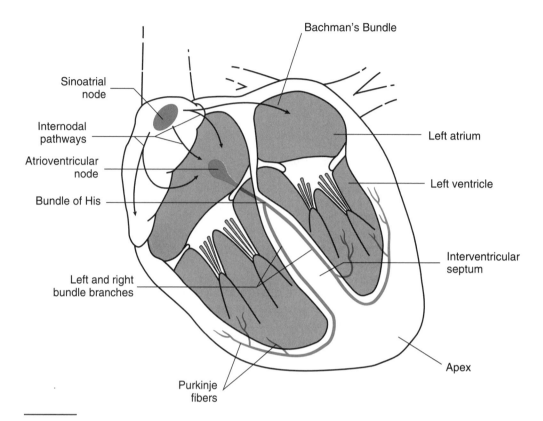

Figure 2–7.
Electrical conduction system of the heart.
Modified from R. Seeley, T. Stevens, and P. Tate, *Anatomy and Physiology.* St. Louis: Mosby, 1989.

to discharge, or if the rate of the SA node decreases below that of the junctional tissues, these cells can take over and stimulate the heartbeat, though at a much slower rate. The primary function of the AV node, though, is to relay electrical impulses from the atria to the ventricles in a timely and orderly fashion. The impulse travel time through the AV node is the slowest within the conduction system. This reduction in electrical velocity provides a brief delay during which the atria are able to contract and fill the ventricles prior to ventricular stimulation. Without a delay in atrioventricular conduction, the ventricles would not receive adequate blood volume prior to contracting. In addition, the conduction delay across the AV node exerts a protective effect during rapid atrial dysrhythmias (disturbance in the discharge rate of the atria).

After transversing the atrioventricular node, the impulse descends down to the bundle of His. The bundle of His begins anatomically as the tail of the AV node and lies on the right side of the interventricular septum. The His bundle is a short, thick cable of electrical fibers that forms the electrical connection between the atria and the ventricles.

The fibers of the bundle of His bifurcate into the right and left bundle branches. The right bundle branch extends down the right side of the interventricular septum to the

TABLE 2–3 • **Electrical Conduction System Activation Rates**
Sinoatrial node: 60–100 per minute
Atrioventricular node: 40–60 per minute
Purkinje network: 20–40 per minute

right ventricle where it merges with the Purkinje network. The left bundle branch divides into an anterior and posterior division referred to as fascicles. The anterior fascicle extends anteriorly down the left side of the interventricular septum to reach the anterior papillary muscle. The posterior fascicle is a short thick branch, extending downward to the posterior papillary muscle of the left ventricle. Both fascicles interconnect with the Purkinje fiber system and equally share in the spread of electrical impulses to the left ventricle.

The Purkinje system is a network of twiglike fibers on the endocardial surface of the heart that penetrates the myocardium of both ventricles. The Purkinje network is responsible for the rapid transmission of electrical impulses to the myocytes (myocardial cells) of both ventricular walls, stimulating contraction. Ventricular activation and contraction occur in sequential phases, beginning with the septum. Septal activation is the result of stimulation by the bundle branches and occurs in a left-to-right direction. Activation of the ventricular muscle begins from the apex and spreads toward the base. Ventricular contraction proceeds from the endocardium to the epicardium. In addition, the Purkinje system also contains specialized pacemaker cells capable of self-excitation. These cells possess an intrinsic rate of discharge range of **20 to 40 times per minute** and function as a safety mechanism should other pacemaking sites fail.

PATHWAY OF BLOOD FLOW THROUGH THE HEART

Blood returning from the body, which is oxygen-poor and carbon dioxide-rich, enters the right atrium from the superior and inferior vena cava, and from the heart via the coronary sinus (Figure 2–8). During right atrial contraction, the majority of the blood passes through the tricuspid valve into the right ventricle as the right ventricle is relaxed. Once filled, intraventricular pressure rises and contraction of the right ventricle forces blood against the tricuspid valve, compressing it closed while opening the pulmonary semilunar valve. Blood now flows into the pulmonary trunk, dividing into a right and left pulmonary artery responsible for carrying blood to the lungs. Once in the lungs, blood offloads its carbon dioxide and takes on oxygen via diffusion and pressure gradients.

The freshly oxygenated blood from the lungs is transported by the four pulmonary veins back to the left atrium. Left atrial contraction results in the opening of the mitral valve and completes the filling of the left ventricle. Contraction, and a rise in the intraventricular pressure of the left ventricle, forces the opening of the aortic semilunar valve and the closing of the mitral valve. Blood under great pressure enters the aorta and is distributed via smaller systemic arteries to the body tissues where the exchange of gases and nutrients occur.

CARDIAC CYCLE

The cardiac cycle includes all of the events associated with the flow of blood through the heart. This cycle is based upon rhythmic contractions of the myocardial muscle, forcing blood out of the heart chambers, followed by brief periods of relaxation allowing the chambers to refill. The cardiac cycle is divided into a contraction phase and a relaxation phase. The contraction phase of the heart muscle is known as systole, and includes both atrial and ventricular systole. The relaxation phase of both atrial and ventricular muscle is known as diastole. Pressure changes within the cardiac chambers occurring during the cycle of contraction and relaxation determines the movement of blood through the heart, according to the principle that any fluid will move from areas of higher pressure to areas of lower pressure. Contraction and relaxation continuously range between 60 to 100 times per minute in the average adult at rest. The entire cardiac cycle is coordinated by the electrical events of the conduction system.

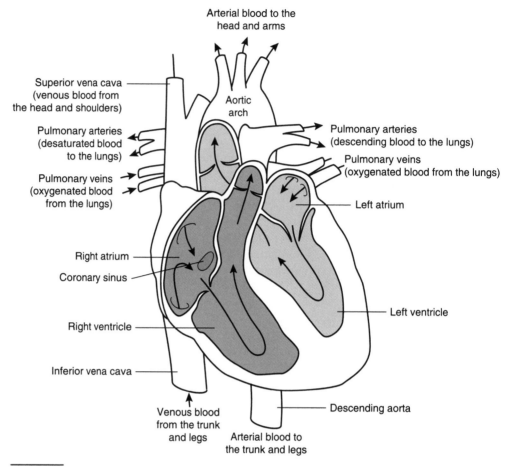

Figure 2–8.

Blood flow through the heart.
Desaturated blood enters the right atrium from the venae, proceeds into the right ventricle, and thence out the pulmonary arteries to the lungs. Oxygenated blood enters the left atrium from the pulmonary veins, proceeds to the left ventricle, and thence to the body via the aorta.

Modified from N. Caroline, *Emergency Care in the Streets*, 5th ed. Boston: Little, Brown, and Company, 1995.

The events of the cardiac cycle occur sequentially. The atria contract while the ventricles relax and the ventricles contract while the atria relax. During atrial systole the ventricles are in a period of diastole and during ventricular systole the atria are in a period of diastole. This alternating process ensures the proper filling of both the atrial and ventricular chambers prior to the ejection of blood. The cardiac cycle is usually described in terms of the events that occur during ventricular diastole and systole.

Ventricular Diastole

At the beginning of ventricular diastole, pressure in the ventricles is relatively low but still high enough to keep the atrioventricular valves closed (Figure 2–9). Because these valves are closed, a large amount of blood collects in the atria. As the ventricles relax, the pressure within them falls. At the moment when the pressure in the ventricles is lower than the pressure in the atria, the higher atrial pressure pushes open the tricuspid and mitral valves and blood flows passively into the ventricular cavity. The majority of ventricular filling (70%) occurs during this period of time when both the atria and ven-

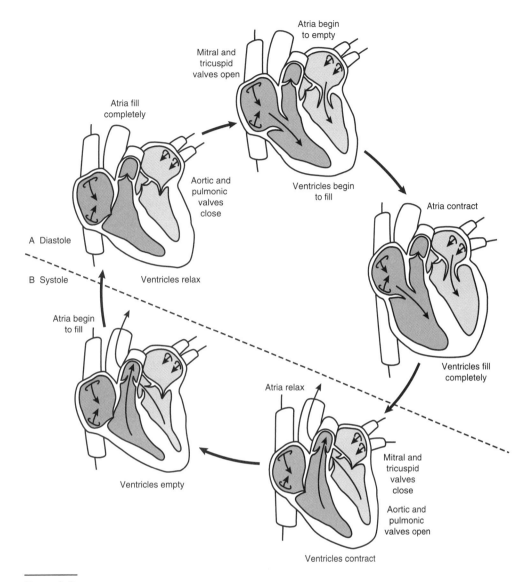

Figure 2–9.
(A) Ventricular diastole. (B) Ventricular systole.
Modified from R. Huszar, *Basic Dysrhythmias Interpretation and Management*, 2nd ed. St. Louis: Mosby, 1994.

tricles are relaxed. Toward the end of ventricular diastole the atria contract, propelling the residual blood remaining in its chambers into the ventricles. This phase of atrial systole, referred to as the atrial kick, provides the remaining 30% of ventricular filling volume.

Ventricular Systole

As the atria relax, the ventricular myocardium begins to contract. During the first part of ventricular systole, intraventricular pressure rises and then exceeds the atrial pressure, resulting in closure of the atrioventricular valves. The aortic valve remains closed at this point. Once the blood that was ejected into the aorta during the preceding ventricular systole moves through the aortic arch, the back pressure of blood on the aortic valve lessens. When ventricular pressure exceeds this back pressure, the aortic valve opens. When this occurs, blood from the ventricles is pumped into the pulmonary and systemic circuits. Ventricular ejection is fast at first, reflecting the great muscular power of the ventricles. As ejection slows, minimal amounts of blood are moving from the ventricle into the aorta. At some point pressure in the first part of the aorta exceeds ventricular pressure, and the semilunar valves shut. With the onset of ventricular relaxation, ventricular pressure rapidly decreases. Eventually atrial pressure exceeds ventricular pressure, and the tricuspid and mitral valves open, preparing the ventricles for the next cardiac cycle.

STROKE VOLUME

The amount of blood ejected from either ventricle during a single cardiac contraction is termed the stroke volume. At the end of ventricular diastole each ventricle contains 120 mL of blood. Under normal conditions, the ventricles eject approximately two-thirds of their volume, producing an average stroke volume of 70 mL for each ventricle. The portion of blood that is ejected is crucial in maintaining adequate circulatory volume and tissue perfusion. The stroke volume is influenced by three physiological parameters: preload, afterload, and cardiac contractility.

Preload is directly related to the volume of blood distending the ventricles at the end of diastole. It is the amount of blood within the ventricles at the end of diastole. Preload is an important determinant of ventricular function, according to Starling's law of the heart. Starling's law states that up to a point, the more myocardial muscle fibers are stretched by chamber filling, the greater will be its force of contraction. The more blood that returns, the more blood there will be within the ventricles at the onset of ventricular systole, so the greater the stretch on the ventricular muscle fibers and the stronger their force of contraction. Starling's law explains how ventricular pumping is matched to the amount of blood entering the heart, so that the ventricles basically empty with each ventricular systole and the output of the right side of the heart matches the output of the left side. Unfortunately, Starling's law only works up to a point. If one side of the heart or the other weakens, blood will accumulate in the ventricles. Eventually the accumulated blood distends the walls of the ventricles so much that the myocardial fibers are stretched beyond Starling's limit, and contractile force weakens.

The second physiological mechanism involved in the regulation of stroke volume is *afterload*. Afterload is the amount of tension that the left ventricle must overcome in order to eject blood into the aorta for systemic distribution. It is the resistance to blood flow produced by the vascular system that the ventricle must overcome to empty its contents. Afterload is thus a direct reflection of peripheral vascular resistance. An increase in the afterload results in an increase in myocardial workload which increases myocardial oxygen requirements. When conditions such as hypertension and vasoconstriction increase peripheral vascular resistance, aortic pressure and thus afterload increase, and stroke volume decreases. The degree of afterload greatly influences myocardial tension and the volume of ventricular ejection.

The final component influencing the regulation of stroke volume is *myocardial contractility*. Contractility, or inotropy, is the degree to which the heart muscle contracts. Changes in contractility are expressed in terms of positive or negative inotropy. Positive inotropy means a change in direction of stronger contraction, and negative inotropy a change in the direction of weaker contraction. Contractility is mainly influenced by Starling's law and the sympathetic nervous system (discussed below). In addition, certain drugs affect contractility; some increase it (sympathomimetics and digitalis) and some decrease it (beta adrenergic blockers). Finally, coronary blood supply is a factor. Coronary artery insufficiency reduces oxygen supply to the myocardium, greatly reducing the contractility of the myocardium.

CARDIAC OUTPUT

Cardiac output is defined as the amount of blood ejected by the ventricles over one minute. Although the right and left ventricles pump equivalent volumes of blood into their respective circulatory pathways, cardiac output is calculated based on the flow of blood out of the left ventricle into the aorta each minute. The measurement of cardiac output is equivalent to the stroke volume in milliliters (volume of blood ejected from the left ventricle during each contraction) times the heart rate (number of cardiac contractions per minute). The equation is calculated as follows:

$$\text{cardiac output} = \text{stroke volume} \times \text{heart rate}$$

Cardiac output is commonly expressed in liters per minute. The average adult value is 6 liters.

Cardiac output varies with changes in stroke volume or heart rate. Under normal conditions, changes in one variable are compensated by reciprocal changes in the other variable. If heart rate decreases, stroke volume increases because the slower heartbeat lengthens the period of diastole, thus allowing greater ventricular filling time (Starling's law). Conversely, if the stroke volume decreases, heart rate increases to compensate for the reduced amount of blood ejected. Effective cardiac output is the product of adequate stroke volume, cardiac rate, and a vascular system capable of reflexive adjustments based on the body's physiological needs.

Autonomic Nervous System Control of the Heart

Heart rate and myocardial contractility are influenced by the autonomic nervous system. The autonomic nervous system is a division of the peripheral nervous system that functions without conscious awareness (i.e., it is involuntary). The autonomic nervous system has two divisions, the sympathetic and parasympathetic nervous systems. Both systems regulate cardiac function by producing equal but opposite effects on the heart, thereby maintaining a delicate balance between increases in cardiac activity and decreases in cardiac activity based on the body's changing physiological needs. Normal cardiac function is attained through the continuous interaction among these two systems.

The sympathetic and parasympathetic nervous systems exert their regulatory effects of cardiac action via the release of neurotransmitters. Neurotransmitters are specialized chemicals used to convey electrical impulses between nerve cells or between a nerve cell and its target organ. Neurotransmitters of both systems are released at the synapse (Figure 2–10). The synapse is the space that exists between two nerve cells or between a nerve cell and the organ that it innervates. Neurotransmitters are released by the nerve endings and travel across the synapse, activating receptors (attachment sites) on the adjoining nerve or target tissue. Once attachment to and activation of the receptors has occurred, the impulse either continues along the neural pathway or a physiological response is produced within the target organ.

The sympathetic (adrenergic) division of the autonomic nervous system is predominantly concerned with preparing the body for emergency situations (Table 2–4). It is often referred to as the "fight or flight" system because it allows the body to function under stress. Nerve fibers of the sympathetic nervous system originate from the thoracic and lumbar segments of the spinal cord. These nerves exit the spinal cord and lie in chains running parallel to the vertebral column. Sympathetic control of myocardial function is achieved through a group of nerves known as the cardiac plexus. The cardiac plexus originates from ganglia within the sympathetic chain and its nerve fibers extend into the atria, ventricles, and the sinoatrial and atrioventricular nodes. At their terminal

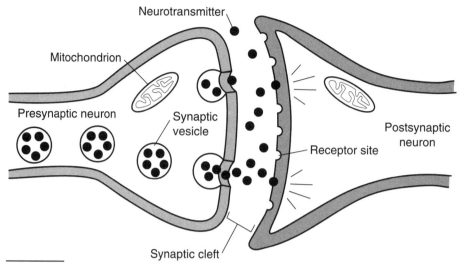

Figure 2–10.
Nerve cell synapse.

Modified from G. Tortora and T. Anagostakos, *Principles of Anatomy and Physiology*, 6th ed. New York: HarperCollins, 1990.

ends, these fibers release norepinephrine. Norepinephrine is the primary neurotransmitter of the sympathetic nervous system. Its release from sympathetic ganglia into the heart results in an increase in rate and stronger myocardial contraction. Additionally, sympathetic stimulation promotes the secretion of epinephrine from the adrenal medulla. Epinephrine reacts with specific receptors within the heart, potentiating the effects of sympathetic stimulation, as well as prolonging sympathetic action.

The physiological effects created from the release of norepinephrine and epinephrine are the direct result to stimulation of receptors (Table 2–5). The two sympathetic receptors are the adrenergic and dopaminergic receptors. Adrenergic receptors are referred to as alpha and beta. Both alpha and beta receptors are subdivided into alpha 1, alpha 2, beta 1, and beta 2. Alpha 1 receptors are located in the circulatory smooth muscle. Their stimulation promotes contraction of the muscle and the subsequent vasoconstriction of the vessel. Alpha 2 receptors are located on the surface membranes of presynaptic neurons, and prevent the oversecretion of norepinephrine into the synapse. Therefore, when alpha 2 receptors are activated the release of norepinephrine is inhibited. Beta 1 receptors are located in the myocardial muscle. Their stimulation results in an increase in heart rate, an increase in myocardial contractile force, enhancement of au-

TABLE 2–4 • **Differences Between the Two Divisions of the Autonomic Nervous System**	
SYMPATHETIC ("FIGHT OR FLIGHT")	**PARASYMPATHETIC ("FEED OR BREED")**
Nerve fibers originate in thoracic and lumbar spinal cord	Nerve fibers originate in cervical and sacral spinal cord
Neurotransmitter is norepinephrine	Neurotransmitter is acetylcholine
Target organs are cardiac muscle and vascular muscle	Target organs are cardiac muscle and SA and AV nodes
Leads to cardiac stimulation	Leads to cardiac suppression

TABLE 2–5 • **Sympathetic Receptors**

TYPE	LOCATION	PHYSIOLOGICAL ACTION
Alpha 1	Vascular smooth muscle	Vasoconstriction
Alpha 2	Presynaptic neuron Neuroeffector junction	Inhibition of norepinephrine
Beta 1	Myocardial muscle	Increase heart rate Increase stroke volume Increase automaticity Increase conduction
Beta 2	Bronchopulmonary smooth muscle Vascular smooth muscle	Bronchodilation Vasodilation
Dopaminergic	Coronary arteries Renal arteries Mesentery arteries	Vasodilation Vasodilation Vasodilation

tomaticity and conduction, and an increase of myocardial oxygen demand. Beta 2 receptors are located within the bronchopulmonary and circulatory smooth muscle, causing bronchodilation and vasodilation upon stimulation. Dopaminergic receptors are located in the coronary, renal, and mesenteric arteries. Activation of dopaminergic receptors results in dilation of these vessels.

The parasympathetic (cholinergic) division of the autonomic nervous system is most active under restful conditions. It is concerned with the restoration and conservation of bodily functions. Its influence on myocardial function is opposite that of the sympathetic nervous system (Table 2–6). Nerve fibers of the parasympathetic nervous system originate in the cervical and sacral segments of the spinal cord. Transmission of the parasympathetic stimulus which influences the action of cardiac muscle occurs through the vagus nerve, which innervates the atrial muscle, sinoatrial and atrioventricular nodes, and a small portion of the ventricles. The neurotransmitter of the parasympathetic nervous system is acetylcholine. The release of acetylcholine from vagal nerve endings decreases heart rate, reduces atrioventricular conduction, and decreases the force of atrial contraction and possibly ventricular contraction. In theory, it is thought that the parasympathetic nervous system provides the dominant control of cardiac rate, thus maintaining a resting pulse of approximately 70 beats per minute.

NOTE: Vagal maneuvers or the stimulation of the vagus nerve is often used to assist in the control of rapid atrial dysrhythmias. Methods of vagal stimulation include the Valsalva maneuver (straining against a closed glottis), carotid sinus massage, coughing, and the application of ice to the facial structures (mammalian diving reflex).

TABLE 2–6 • **Sympathetic and Parasympathetic Effects on the Heart**

FUNCTION	SYMPATHETIC	PARASYMPATHETIC
Automaticity	Increase	Decrease
Conductivity	Increase	Decrease
Contractility	Increase	Decrease
Heart rate	Increase	Decrease

CARDIAC ELECTROPHYSIOLOGY

Cardiac electrophysiology includes all of the biochemical and physiological processes necessary for electrical formation and distribution, and the mechanical contraction of myocardial muscle. Two cell types perform these functions: the electrical (pacemaker) cells described earlier and the myocardial working cells. The working cells contract in response to electrical stimulation from the pacemaker cells. Knowledge of the electrophysiological events of cardiac cells is crucial because they comprise the cardiac cycle and produce the waveforms recorded on the electrocardiogram (ECG).

Structure and Organization of Cardiac Cell Fibers

Cardiac muscle tissue is composed of striated cells that are cylindrical in shape and are attached both laterally and end to end to other adjacent cells. Each cell consists of a single nucleus and numerous filaments of actin and myosin that aid in myocardial contraction. The fibers of cardiac cells are all interconnected, forming a longitudinal network that branches into a three-dimensional arrangement. Located at the junction where the branching cells join together with their neighboring cells are specialized structures known as intercalated disks (Figure 2–11). Intercalated disks help to hold adjacent cells together and transmit the force of contraction from cell to cell. Because the disks interconnect the myocardial fibers, electrical activation of the myocardial cells results in simultaneous contraction of the entire muscle.

The ability of myocardial muscle cells to function as a single coordinated unit is based on the principle of syncytium. Cardiac muscle tissue consists of a mass of merging cells that are tightly bound together as an individual unit. Because of this special characteristic, the heart functions in an all-or-nothing manner. That is, when one cell becomes excited, the action potential (electrical events of a cell) spreads rapidly throughout all of the cardiac cells, resulting in contraction of the muscle as a whole. The heart has two separate functional syncytia, the atrial wall syncytium and the ventricular wall syncytium. The atrial syncytium contracts in a superior-to-inferior direction while the ventricular syncytium contracts inferiorly to superiorly.

As previously noted, each cardiac cell contains two types of intracellular contractile proteins, actin and myosin. These proteins are arranged in a lengthwise configuration

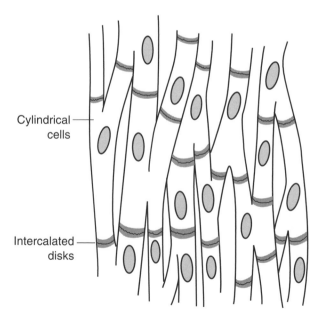

Cylindrical cells

Intercalated disks

Figure 2–11.
Cardiac cells.

Modified from R. Huszar, *Basic Dysrhythmias Interpretation and Management*, 2nd ed. St. Louis: Mosby, 1994.

forming units known as sarcomeres. The sarcomere is a portion of the muscle fiber located between the two interacting ends of the actin and myosin filaments. The sarcomere allows for the actin and myosin proteins to overlap one another at each end, forming crossbridges that are interlaced. The interconnection between the actin and myosin myofilaments provides the myocardial cells with the property of contractility. Contraction of the myocardial muscle occurs from the movement of electrolytes into and out of the cell, causing a change in the electrical charge across the cell membrane. The net result of electrolytic movement is the activation of muscular contraction. In addition to the myofibrils, another important intracellular structure needed for myocardial contraction is the sarcoplasmic reticulum. Calcium ions that are necessary for the binding between the actin and myosin filaments are stored and released from the sarcoplasmic reticulum.

Cardiac cells also contain two other structures that are essential for maintaining normal cardiac contraction. The first, known as transverse tubules, are an extension of the cell membrane which function to convey calcium and conduct the depolarization wave to structures deep inside the cell. This process allows for the release of large quantities of calcium ions into the cell, making it possible for the myocardial muscle to maintain contraction for a sustained period of time. Mitochondria are the second constituent of the myocardial cells, necessary for maintaining aerobic metabolism during cellular energy production. Within the mitochondria are the specialized respiratory enzymes that enable the cardiac cells to keep up with the immense energy requirements produced from continuous contraction.

Resting Membrane Potential

Electrical activation and deactivation of the heart are the result of physical changes in the permeability of the cardiac cell membranes. Alterations in membrane permeability permit the movement of electrically charged ions across the intracellular and extracellular spaces. Ions are believed to flow through ion-specific channels located along the membrane. These channels are designated as slow channels or fast channels, determined by the rate of ionic movement. Those ions transversing the channels that are responsible for initiating, conducting, and maintaining the electrical charge needed to ensure normal cardiac function are potassium, sodium, and calcium (Table 2–7). Their movement into and out of the cell creates an electrical (voltage) difference across the cell membrane referred to as the transmembrane potential. The transmembrane potential is the electrical difference between the interior of the cell and the exterior of the cell, formulating the basis of impulse conduction and muscular contraction.

TABLE 2–7 • **Role of Electrolytes in Cardiac Function**

ELECTROLYTE	ROLE IN CARDIAC FUNCTION
Sodium (Na$^+$)	Flows into cell to initiate depolarization
Potassium (K$^+$)	Flows out of cell to initiate repolarization
	*hypo*kalemia → increased myocardial irritability
	*hyper*kalemia → decreased automaticity/conduction
Calcium (Ca^{++})	Major role in depolarization of pacemaker cells and in myocardial contractility
	*hypo*calcemia → decreased contractility and increased myocardial irritability
	*hyper*calcemia → increased contractility

From Caroline, N. *Emergency Care in the Streets*, 5th ed. Boston: Little, Brown, and Company, 1995, p. 449.

The resting membrane potential is the electrical potential that exists across cardiac cell membranes when the cells are at rest. In myocardial cells, the normal resting membrane potential is −90 millivolts (mV), whereas that of the pacemaker cells of the sinoatrial and atrioventricular nodes is −60 mV. The electrical potential (voltage) that is created between the interior and the exterior of the cell is derived from the unequal distribution of positively charged ions and negatively charged ions. During cellular inactivity, there are more positive ions outside of the cell in comparison to those located inside. Specifically, a high concentration of positively charged sodium and calcium ions are present outside the cell, whereas a large concentration of potassium and negatively charged phosphate ions are located intracellulary. Due to the difference in the electrical charges of these ions across the cell membrane, a negative electrical potential exists. That is, the interior of the cell is electrically negative in comparison to the outside of the cell. This negative potential is made possible by the cell's impermeability to sodium, as well as the active removal of intracellular sodium ions by the sodium-potassium pump. The maintenance of the normal resting membrane potential of −90 mV in myocardial cells is established by the electrogenic negativity produced by the sodium-potassium exchange pump and the diffusion of electrolytes across cell membranes.

Sodium-Potassium Exchange Pump

The sodium pump is a specialized ionic transporter located in the cardiac sarcolemma. Its primary responsibility is to restore and maintain the normal resting membrane potential. The pump functions by generating large sodium and potassium gradients across the cell membrane by actively pumping sodium ions out of the cell in exchange for potassium ions. The sodium-potassium pump normally transports three sodium ions out of the cell in exchange for two potassium ions that are brought into the cell. Consequently, a greater number of charged ions are transferred outward than inward, creating an unequal distribution of ions across cell membranes. This process creates a net positive charge on the outside of the cell, producing the normal negativity of the intracellular resting membrane potential. The energy needed for the active transport of sodium and potassium ions through cellular membranes is derived from adenosine triphosphate (ATP).

Depolarization and Repolarization

The initiation of a cardiac impulse, followed by the activation of myocardial cells, begins with the phase of depolarization. Depolarization is the process by which muscle fibers are stimulated to contract due to the rapid reversal of their resting membrane potential. This is accomplished by changes in the concentration of intracellular and extracellular electrolytes (Figure 2–12). Upon electrical stimulation of the myocardial cells, a rapid sequence of events occurs that enables the heart muscle to contract. The sequence begins with the temporary inactivation of the sodium-potassium pump. This results in an increase in the cell membrane's permeability to sodium ions, allowing extracellular sodium to enter the cell. As the intracellular movement of positively charged sodium ions continues, the cell's internal negativity is changed. The normal resting membrane potential of −90 mV becomes less negative (i.e., more positive). When the membrane potential drops to −60 mV, the fast sodium channels open momentarily, facilitating the positive influx of sodium ions. This now results in the interior of the cell assuming a positive charge in comparison to the negatively charged exterior. The rapid egress of sodium through the fast channel gating mechanism enables the cardiac cell to reach threshold potential (electrical activation), or the voltage to which the cell must be reduced before a reversal in electrical polarity can occur. Cardiac cells cannot become electrically active or contract until they have reached their threshold potential. For this to oc-

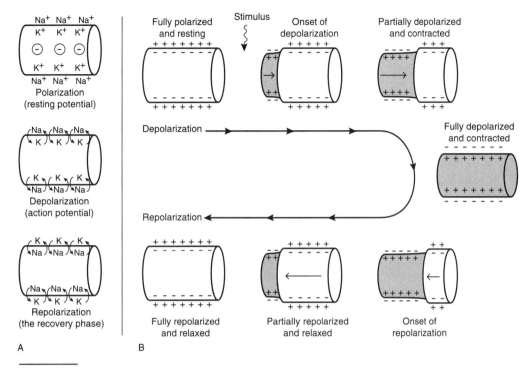

Figure 2-12.
(A) Schematic of ion shifts during depolarization and repolarization. (B) Reversal of electrical charges across the cell during depolarization and repolarization.

Modified from B. Bledsoe, R. Porter, and B. Shade, *Paramedic Emergency Care*, 2nd ed. New Jersey: 1994. R. Huszar, *Basic Dysrhythmias Interpretation and Management*, 2nd ed. St. Louis: Mosby, 1994.

cur, the cells must be electrically converted from a negative internal state to a positive internal state.

An interesting difference in depolarization exists between the mechanical cells of the myocardium and the specialized pacemaker cells of the electrical conduction system. The mechanical cells of myocardial tissue, which are ultimately responsible for uniform contraction and the adequate ejection of blood, contain both fast sodium and slow calcium channels. The pacemaker cells of the sinoatrial and atrioventricular nodes do not possess fast sodium channels, but instead contain only slow calcium-sodium channels. The slow channels of the pacemaker cells open when the cell's membrane potential reaches approximately −50 mV. Because of the difference in the membrane potential of the pacemaking cells, they depolarize at a much slower rate due to the sluggish intracellular movement of positively charged calcium and sodium ions.

Following the immediate depolarization of cardiac cells, positively charged potassium ions rapidly escape from the cell, initiating the phase of repolarization. Repolarization is the process by which the cardiac cells return to their resting state. This phase reestablishes the cell's internal negativity (−90 mV) in preparation for the next wave of electrical stimulation. Repolarization is accomplished by a sequence of events that are almost the opposite of depolarization. Repolarization begins with the cell decreasing its membrane permeability to sodium ions, thereby restricting sodium's entry into the cell. Furthermore, sodium ions are removed from the cell and potassium ions returned through an active ion transport system. Both the phases of depolarization and repolarization constitute the electrical waveforms seen on the electrocardiogram.

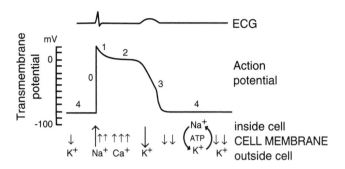

Figure 2–13.
Schematic representation of ventricular myocardial working cell action potential.
Arrows indicate times of major ionic movement across the cell membrane.

Modified from American Heart Association, *Textbook of Advanced Cardiac Life Support*, Dallas: TX, 1994.

Electrical Cardiac Cycle and the Action Potential

The action potential is an electrical process that precedes mechanical contraction of muscle cells. It is defined as the sequence of electrical events that occur inside the cell during depolarization and repolarization. The action potential is composed of five phases which correspond to the electrophysiological events that result from changes in the normal resting membrane potential (Figure 2–13). These phases are referred to as 0 through 4 and correlate with the waveforms recorded on the ECG (Figure 2–14). The following information describes the action potential of a typical myocardial working cell.

Phase 4 (resting phase). During the resting state, the cardiac cell maintains a difference in the electrical potential (voltage) across the cell membrane. The inside of the cell is electrically negative and the outside of the cell is positive. This difference results from the relative permeability of the cell membrane to the surrounding sodium and potassium ions. At the onset of phase 4 sodium ions are found in high concentrations outside the cell and potassium ions are found in high concentrations inside the cell. The resting ionic distribution that exists between sodium and potassium is the direct result of continuous action by the sodium-potassium pump. This pump is responsible for establishing the electrolytic environment necessary for normal cardiac cellular electrical physiology. In the resting cardiac state the cell membrane is more permeable to intracellular potassium than to extracellular sodium. This enables small amounts of potassium ions to diffuse out of the cell from areas of higher concentration into the lower concentrated extracel-

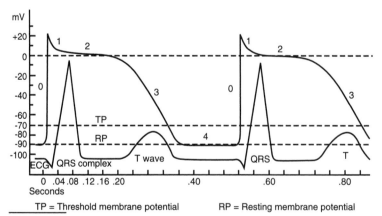

TP = Threshold membrane potential   RP = Resting membrane potential

Figure 2–14.
Cardiac action potential of myocardial cells and their representation on the ECG.

Modified from R. Huszar, *Basic Dysrhythmias: Interpretation and Management*, 2nd ed. St. Louis: Mosby, 1994.

lular fluid. The net result is the greater extraction of positive charges from the intracellular compartment, creating a maximal negative resting membrane potential. The intracellular loss of potassium leaves the inside of the cell electrically negative (−90 mV). Therefore, phase 4 of the working cell action potential is dependent upon the potassium gradient across the cell membrane. Phase 4 is representative of electrical diastole and constitutes the isoelectric (baseline) on the ECG.

Phase 0 (rapid depolarization). Depolarization of the cell is the result of an increase in the membrane permeability to sodium. Extracellular sodium ions rush into the cell through the rapid opening and abrupt closing of fast channels. The influx of positive sodium ions reverses the electrical charge across the cell membrane to where the interior of the cell becomes positively charged (20 mV) and the exterior becomes electrically negative. Phase 0 is schematically identified as the sharp, tall upstroke of the action potential. During this period of time the cell membrane reaches its threshold potential and myocardial contraction begins. On the ECG phase 0 is represented as the QRS complex (ventricular depolarization and contraction).

Phase 1 (early repolarization). Phase 1 is the rapid, brief beginning of repolarization immediately following atrial and ventricular contraction. This phase reflects the inactivation or closing of the sodium channels, terminating the rapid flow of sodium ions into the cell. The net result is an increase in the intracellular negativity, leaving the inside of the cell slightly less positive (0 mV). Phase 1 ends in the plateau of the action potential.

Phase 2 (plateau). During this period of the action potential no net change in the electrical charge across the cell occurs. Electrical neutrality is maintained between the influx and efflux of positively charged ions. The slow inward movement of calcium ions through the calcium specific channels, accompanied by the outward movement of potassium, is responsible for the sustained plateau of the cell's action potential. This phase is referred to as a period of slow repolarization, allowing the myocardial cells to complete their contraction and begin relaxing. Phase 2 represents the ST segment (period between ventricular depolarization and repolarization) on the ECG.

Phase 3 (rapid repolarization). During rapid repolarization, the slow inward currents of calcium and sodium are inactivated and the inside of the cell once again becomes electrically negative (−90 mV). Additionally, the sodium pump actively removes intracellular sodium ions, restoring the cell to its maximal diastolic negativity. The entire process results in a reduction of the positive charges inside the cell. Phase 3 is represented as the schematic downslope of the action potential and corresponds to the T wave (ventricular repolarization) on the ECG.

The action potential of the pacemaker cell differs from that of the previously described myocardial working cell (Figure 2–15). The pacemaker cells of the sinoatrial and atrioventricular nodes possess the property of automaticity (self-excitation). Their electrical events occur through a slow response mechanism. Depolarization of the pacemaker cells is attributed to the slow inward currents of calcium and sodium ions in com-

---

Figure 2–15.
Schematic representation of pacemaker cell action potential.
Modified from American Heart Association, *Textbook of Advanced Cardiac Life Support*, Dallas: 1994.

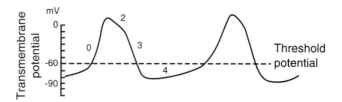

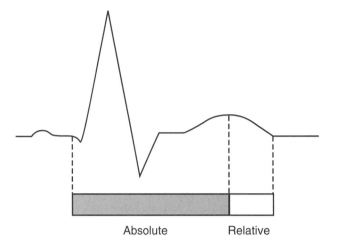

Figure 2–16.
Relationship of refractory period to electrocardiogram.
Modified from American Heart Association, *Textbook of Advanced Cardiac Life Support*, Dallas: 1994.

Absolute   Relative

parison to the rapid sodium channel entry of myocardial cells. Therefore, during phase 4 of the action potential calcium and sodium ions gradually enter the cell, reducing its negative charge until spontaneous depolarization occurs. Following electrical formation and activation, the impulse is distributed via the conduction system to the atrial and ventricular myocardium.

Refractory Periods

The onset of time between ventricular depolarization and the end of repolarization is known as the refractory period (Figure 2–16). The refractory period is the interval in which a cardiac cell or fiber is unable to respond to an electrical stimulus because it has already been activated by a previous impulse. It is the time frame in which the cardiac cells are unable to depolarize and remain unresponsive. The refractory period of myocardial cells begins with the onset of phase 0 of the action potential and terminates at the end of phase 3. On the electrocardiogram, the refractory period originates at the beginning of the QRS complex and extends to the end of the T wave. It is commonly divided into two portions, absolute and relative refractory periods.

The absolute refractory period begins with the onset of phase 0 and ends midway through phase 3. On the ECG, this is portrayed as the beginning of the QRS complex to the apex of the T wave. During this period, the cardiac cells have depolarized and are currently repolarizing. Because the cell is not fully repolarized it is incapable of generating or conducting electricity. Therefore, during the absolute refractory period the myocardial muscle is unable to be stimulated.

The relative refractory period extends through the remaining portion of phase 3. It corresponds to the downslope of the T wave on the ECG. Because the relative refractory period represents the end of repolarization just prior to depolarization, a strong stimulus may generate a normal or abnormal electrical cycle.

KEY POINTS SUMMARY

Location, Size, and Orientation of the Heart

1. The heart is a triangular shaped organ located in the mediastinum with two-thirds of the mass to the left of the body midline and one-third to the right. The apex rests on the diaphragm and the base lies at the level of the second rib. The size of the heart varies with the size of an individual, but it usually approximates the size of a closed fist.

Anatomy

2. Tissue Layers: The heart is enclosed in a two-layered fibrous sac called the pericardium. The inner layer is the visceral pericardium and the outer layer is the parietal pericardium. Both layers are separated by a small amount of serous fluid that serves to reduce friction. The heart wall is composed of three distinct tissue layers: endocardium (innermost layer), myocardium (cardiac muscle), and epicardium (outermost surface).

3. Chambers: The two upper chambers are called the atria and the two lower chambers are called the ventricles. The atria (right and left) are receiving chambers and the ventricles are discharging chambers.

4. Valves: Four valves (two atrioventricular and two semilunar) keep blood flowing through the heart in one continuous direction. The atrioventricular valves are located at the junction of the atria and ventricles. The right atrioventricular valve is the tricuspid valve and the left atrioventricular valve is the mitral valve. The semilunar valves are located at the junction of the ventricles and the bases of the arteries into which they empty. The right semilunar valve is the pulmonary valve and the left is the aortic valve.

5. Heart Sounds: Heart sounds are two distinct sounds heard in every heartbeat on auscultation. The first heart sound (lub) is caused by the vibration and closure of the atrioventricular valves during contraction of the ventricles. The second heart sound (dup) is caused by the closure of the semilunar valves during relaxation of the ventricles.

6. Coronary Artery Distribution: Blood, which supplies oxygen and nutrients to the myocardium of the heart, flows through the right and left coronary arteries. The right coronary artery supplies the right atrium and ventricle and the inferoposterior aspects of the left ventricle. The left coronary artery divides into two main branches, the left anterior descending artery and the circumflex artery. The left anterior descending artery supplies the anterior wall of the left ventricle, while the circumflex artery supplies the lateral aspects of the left ventricle.

7. Conduction System: The heart's normal electrical impulse originates in the sinoatrial node (SA node) located in the wall of the right atrium near the opening of the superior vena cava. The impulse then travels through three internodal tracts to the atrioventricular node (AV node). The AV node is located in the right atrium along the lower part of the interatrial septum. The AV node holds the impulse momentarily before sending it to the bundle of His located in the septum of the ventricles. Following activation of the septum, the impulse travels rapidly down two bundle branches (right and left) to the Purkinje fibers located in the walls of the ventricles.

Cardiac Cycle

8. Blood Flow Through the Heart: Venous blood enters the right atrium through the superior and inferior vena cava. From the right atrium blood passes through the tricuspid valve into the right ventricle. Blood then continues through the pulmonary semilunar valve to the pulmonary artery and into the lungs. From the lungs, blood enters the left atrium, passing through the mitral valve to the left ventricle. Blood in the left ventricle is pumped through the aortic semilunar valve into the aorta and is distributed to the body.

9. The cardiac cycle includes all of the events associated with the flow of blood through the heart. It is divided into a contraction phase and a relaxation phase. The contraction phase of the heart is referred to as systole and the relaxation phase is referred to as diastole.

10. Stroke Volume: Stroke volume is the amount of blood ejected from either ventricle during a single cardiac contraction. The average stroke volume is approximately 70 mL.

11. Preload: Preload is the volume and pressure available to the ventricles for cardiac pumping. It is directly related to the amount of blood within the ventricles at the

end of diastole (relaxation). Starling's law states that, up to a point, the more myocardial muscle fibers are stretched by chamber filling, the greater will be its force of contraction.

12. Cardiac Output: Cardiac output is the amount of blood ejected by the ventricles over one minute. It is equivalent to the stroke volume times the heart rate.

Autonomic Nervous System Control of the Heart

13. The autonomic nervous system is composed of two divisions, the sympathetic and parasympathetic nervous systems. Both systems regulate cardiac action via the release of neurotransmitters (chemical mediators).

14. Sympathetic Nervous System: Sympathetic control of myocardial function is achieved through the release of norepinephrine and epinephrine (catecholamine neurotransmitters). Both norepinephrine and epinephrine directly stimulate adenergic receptor sites (alpha and beta), causing vascular constriction, increased heart rate, and myocardial contractility, and enhanced automaticity and conductivity.

15. Parasympathetic Nervous System: Parasympathetic influence on myocardial function is opposite that of the sympathetic nervous system. Transmission of parasympathetic stimuli occurs through the vagus nerve and the release of acetylcholine (neurotransmitter). The release of acetylcholine decreases heart rate, reduces atrioventricular conduction, and decreases the force of atrial and possibly ventricular contractions.

Cardiac Electrophysiology

16. Cardiac electrophysiology includes all of the biochemical and physiological processes necessary for electrical formation and distribution and the mechanical contraction of myocardial muscle. Two cells perform these functions: electrical (pacemaker) cells and myocardial (working) cells.

Resting Membrane Potential

17. The resting membrane potential (voltage) is the electrical potential that exists across cardiac cell membranes when the cells are at rest. In myocardial (working) cells, the normal resting membrane potential is -90 mV, whereas that of pacemaker cells is -60 mV. The electrical potential of both cell types is created from the unequal distribution of positively charged ions and negatively charged ions on each side of the cell membrane.

Sodium-Potassium Pump

18. The sodium-potassium pump is a specialized ionic transporter that functions to restore and maintain the normal resting membrane potential. The pump operates by transporting additional sodium ions out of the cell in comparison to the number of potassium ions transferred inward. This process creates a net positive charge on the outside of the cell and a negative charge (-90 mV) inside the cell.

Depolarization and Repolarization

19. Depolarization: The process by which cardiac muscle fibers are stimulated to contract due to the rapid reversal of their resting membrane potential. This is accomplished through the influx of sodium ions into the cell.

20. Repolarization: The process by which cardiac cells return to their resting state in preparation for the next wave of electrical stimulation. This phase is accomplished through the removal of intracellular sodium ions.

Action Potential

21. The action potential is the electrical process that precedes mechanical contraction of cardiac muscle cells. It is defined as the sequence of electrical events that occur inside the cell during depolarization and repolarization and consists of the following five phases:

    Phase 4: Resting cardiac cell state

    Phase 0: Rapid depolarization

    Phase 1: Early repolarization

    Phase 2: Electrical neutrality

    Phase 3: Rapid repolarization

Refractory Period

22. The refractory period is the onset of time between ventricular depolarization and the end of repolarization. It represents the period in which cardiac cells remain unresponsive to additional electrical impulses. On the ECG, the refractory period originates at the start of the QRS complex and extends to the end of the T wave.

BIBLIOGRAPHY

American Heart Association. *Textbook of Advanced Cardiac Life Support.* Dallas, TX; 1987, 1992.

Applegate EJ. *The Anatomy & Physiology Learning System Textbook.* Philadelphia, PA: WB Saunders; 1995.

Bledsoe BE, Porter RS, Shade BK. *Paramedic Emergency Care.* 2nd ed. Englewood Cliffs, NJ: Brady; 1994.

Caroline NL. *Emergency Care in the Streets.* 5th ed. Boston, MA: Little, Brown, & Company; 1995.

Conover MB. *Understanding Electrocardiography Arrhythmias and the 12-Lead ECG.* St. Louis, MD: Mosby; 1992.

Huszar RJ. *Basic Dysrhythmias Interpretation and Management.* St. Louis, MO: Mosby; 1994.

Langer F. *EKG 2 and 3.* Orlando, FL: Florida Hospital Orlando; 1992.

Marieb EN. *Human Anatomy and Physiology.* 3rd ed. Redwood City, CA: The Benjamin/Cummings Publishing Company, Inc.; 1995.

McCance KL, Huether SE. *Pathophysiology—The Biological Basis for Disease.* St. Louis, MO: Mosby; 1994.

Price SA, Wilson LM. *Pathophysiology: Clinical Concepts of Disease Procedures.* 4th ed. St. Louis, MO: Mosby; 1992.

Sanders MJ. *Mosby's Paramedic Textbook.* St. Louis, MO: Mosby; 1994.

Scanlon VC, Sanders T. *Essentials of Anatomy & Physiology.* Philadelphia, PA: FA Davis Company; 1991.

Thelen LA, Davie, JK, Urder, LD. *Textbook of Critical Care Nursing.* St. Louis, MO: Mosby; 1990.

Thibodeau GA. *Structure and Function of the Body.* St. Louis, MO: Mosby; 1992.

Tortora GJ. *Introduction to the Human Body/The Essentials of Anatomy and Physiology.* New York, NY: HarperCollins; 1994.

3

The Electrocardiogram: Monitoring, Analysis, and Dysrhythmia Recognition

1. Describe the basic concepts of the electrocardiogram.

2. Describe unipolar and bipolar leads and identify their anatomical placement.

3. Discuss routine ECG monitoring and explain what information can and cannot be obtained from a monitoring lead.

4. Describe the application of monitoring electrodes and list the guidelines for their use.

5. Describe the grids and markings on the ECG graph paper.

6. Describe the measurements of voltage and time as they relate to the ECG.

7. Describe the normal sequence of electrical conduction through the heart.

8. Describe the relationship between ECG waveforms and intervals with the process of depolarization and repolarization.

9. Define the following terms or phrases and describe their ECG characteristics: isoelectric line, P wave, QRS complex, T wave, U wave, PR interval, ST segment, QT interval, R–R interval, and electrical artifact.

10. List and describe the seven steps for systematic ECG analysis.

11. Discuss the analysis of normal sinus rhythm and list its rules for interpretation.

12. Define the term dysrhythmia and name ten causes.

13. Discuss the origin of dysrhythmias and describe the following pathological mechanisms: disturbances in automaticity, disturbances in conductivity, and reentry.

14. Describe the etiology, ECG characteristics, clinical implications, and prehospital management for the following dysrhythmias: sinus bradycardia, sinus tachycardia, sinus dysrhythmia, sinus arrest, wandering atrial pacemaker, premature atrial complexes, paroxysmal supraventricular tachycardia, atrial flutter, atrial fibrillation, premature junctional complexes, junctional rhythm, accelerated junctional rhythm, paroxysmal junctional tachycardia, ventricular escape complexes and rhythms, premature ventricular complexes, ventricular tachycardia, ventricular fibrillation, asystole, artificial pacemaker rhythms, first-degree atrioventricular block, second-degree atrioventricular block (Type I), second-degree atrioventricular block (Type II), and third-degree atrioventricular block.

INTRODUCTION

The electrocardiogram is a record of the electrical forces generated by the heart. Its history dates back to the early 1900s, when Willem Einthoven recorded an electrical current from the human heart using an instrument called a galvanator. Since this time, the electrocardiogram has evolved into a tool of remarkable clinical power, remarkable both for the ease at which it can be mastered and for the extraordinary range of situations in which it can provide helpful and even vital information. One glance at the electrocardiogram can identify a potentially life-threatening dysrhythmia, diagnose an evolving myocardial infarction, and pinpoint the adverse effects of drugs and electrolytes. Its use is essential to the delivery of effective prehospital emergency cardiac care. This chapter will address the basic principles of cardiac monitoring and introduce techniques necessary to analyze, identify, and treat abnormalities of cardiac rhythm, all of which are fundamental to the emergency care worker.

BASIC CONCEPTS OF THE ELECTROCARDIOGRAM

The electrocardiogram (ECG) is a graphic display of electrical forces generated by depolarization and repolarization of the atria and ventricles. These forces (voltage) are readily detected as they spread from the heart through the body to surface electrodes. Once detected, the voltage is input to an ECG machine, amplified, and displayed visually on the oscilloscope (screen) and/or graphically onto ECG paper. Voltage may be positive (seen as an upward deflection on the ECG), negative (seen as a downward deflection on the ECG), or isoelectric (seen as a straight line on the ECG).

Information about the mechanical events of myocardial muscle do not appear on the electrocardiogram. Neither the force of contraction nor volume of ventricular ejection are measured by the ECG. Therefore, the evaluation of vital signs and a patient's clinical presentation must accompany its use. Remember that the ECG is only a tool, and like any tool is only as capable as its user.

ECG LEADS

An ECG machine can provide many views of the heart's electrical field by monitoring voltage changes through electrodes placed on the body surface. Each pair of electrodes is referred to as a lead and each lead provides a slightly different view of the heart's electrical field. Generally, three leads are employed in the field for cardiac rhythm analysis and dysrhythmia (abnormal rhythm) recognition. One lead is all that is necessary for detecting life-threatening dysrhythmias. However, with the advent of thrombolytic therapy and the importance of early infarct detection, the use of 12-lead ECGs in the prehospital phase of emergency medicine is revolutionizing the standard of care within advanced life support systems. A detailed discussion of 12-lead ECGs will follow in subsequent chapters.

ECG leads are of two types, bipolar and unipolar (Figure 3–1). Bipolar leads measure electrical potential between a negative electrode and positive electrode. Unipolar leads use a single positive electrode and an indifferent reference point created by using all four limb leads as "negatives," thus creating a *central terminal* in the body's center mass.

Bipolar Leads

Bipolar leads are leads I, II, and III. They are traditionally placed on the extremity, but are often placed at the root of the limb for practical purposes. Each is obtained by attaching a positive electrode to the left arm or left leg and a single negative electrode to either the right or left arm.

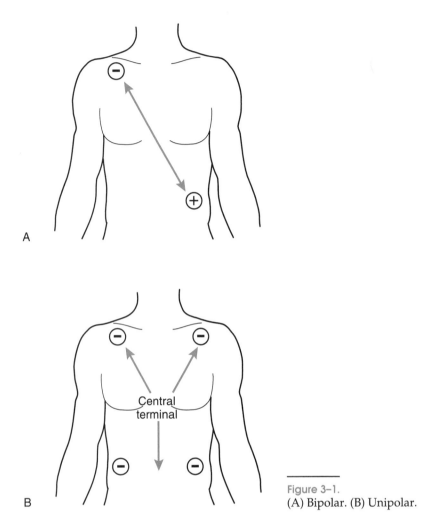

Figure 3–1.
(A) Bipolar. (B) Unipolar.

Bipolar leads measure electrical forces recorded between two extremities at one time. The direction from the negative to the positive electrode determines the axis of each lead. This means that if an imaginary line were drawn between the positive and negative electrode, it would represent the direction of electricity to or from the electrode. For example, lead I uses the right arm for the negative pole and the left arm for the positive. Therefore, the axis of lead I runs from shoulder to shoulder (Figure 3–2). Lead II uses the right arm for the negative pole and the left leg for the positive. The axis of lead II runs from right shoulder to left leg. Lead III uses the left arm as the negative pole and the left leg for the positive. The axis of lead III runs from left shoulder to left leg. All three leads surround the heart on the frontal plane (i.e., toward the head or feet or toward the right or left side of the body) in what is known as Einthoven's triangle.

Unipolar Limb Leads

Leads aVR, aVL, and aVF are augmented unipolar limb leads. These leads record the difference in electrical potential between extremity lead sites and a reference point (center of the heart). They utilize the central terminal as "negative" with positive electrodes placed on the right arm (aVR), left arm (aVL), and left leg or foot (aVF) (Figure 3–3). Electrical forces are then recorded from one extremity at a time in relation to the central terminal. Augmented leads are also traditionally placed on the extremities, but can be moved toward the root of the limb for practical purposes.

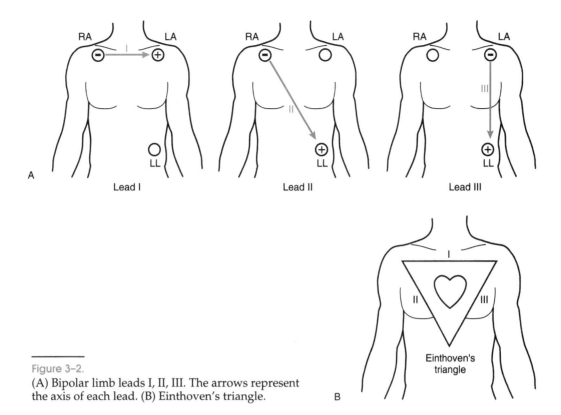

Figure 3–2.
(A) Bipolar limb leads I, II, III. The arrows represent the axis of each lead. (B) Einthoven's triangle.

Unipolar Chest Leads

Leads V_1 through V_6 are unipolar chest leads. They utilize the negative central terminal created by the limb electrodes, allowing the positive as the sole influence on the recording. These leads are placed across the precordium to measure the heart's electrical activity in the horizontal plane (i.e., toward or away from the anterior and left surface of the chest) (Figure 3–4). Chest leads are necessary for identifying electrical forces within the anterior septum and lateral walls of the left ventricle. Their proper placement is crucial for the diagnosis of certain cardiac disorders (e.g., myocardial ischemia). A **greater** discussion of unipolar limb and chest leads will follow in Chapter 4.

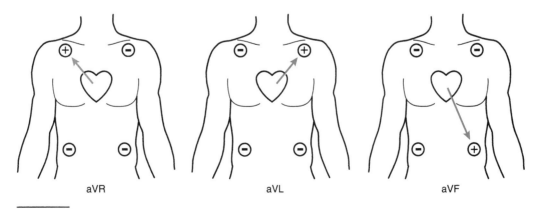

Figure 3–3.
Unipolar limb leads aVR, aVL, aVF.
The arrows represent the axis of each lead.

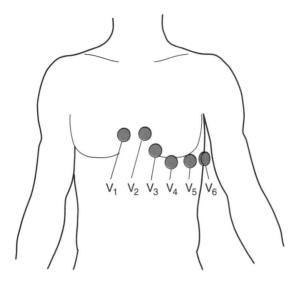

Figure 3–4.
Placement of the six chest electrodes across the anterior and left lateral precordium.

ROUTINE ECG MONITORING

Routine ECG monitoring in the out-of-hospital setting, emergency department, or critical care unit is performed with a single monitoring lead. The most common are lead II and the modified chest lead (MCL$_1$). Lead II is most frequently used because of the location of its positive pole (i.e., left lower chest wall or left leg). As you recall from Chapter 2, the general flow of depolarization moves from the SA node in the right atrium toward the apex of the heart. This is directly toward the positive pole of lead II. Therefore, lead II is an excellent lead for creating large waveforms. MCL$_1$ on the other hand is a special monitoring lead that is useful for determining the origin of abnormal complexes. It may also be beneficial for distinguishing between wide-complex tachycardias and aid in the diagnosis of conduction blocks occurring within the bundle branches. (See Chapters 4 and 7 for placement and use of the MCL leads.) Considerable information can be obtained from a single monitoring lead and in the majority of patients, a single lead is all that is necessary. The following information can be obtained from a single monitoring lead:

- How fast the heart is beating
- The regularity of the heartbeat
- The length of time required to conduct electrical impulses through various regions of the heart

Information that cannot be obtained from a single monitoring lead:

- Presence or location of an infarct (requires multilead)
- Axis deviation and chamber enlargement
- Right to left differences in conduction or impulse formation
- Presence or quality of mechanical pumping action

APPLICATION OF MONITORING ELECTRODES

Effective contact between the electrode and skin surface is essential to inhibit unnecessary interference within an ECG tracing. Electrodes used for prehospital monitoring are pregelled, stick-on disks (dots) that are easily applied to the chest. Contained within the electrode is an abrasive that reduces the superficial waterproof layer of the skin. This enhances the skin surface as an electrical conductor. When applying electrodes, the following guidelines should be considered to minimize the many technical problems that may interfere with uniform monitoring.

1. Identify the correct anatomical landmarks on the chest where the electrodes are to be applied.
2. Avoid placing electrodes over large muscle masses, over large quantities of hair, or any position that prohibits the electrode from lying flat against the skin. Electrodes should always be placed over intercostal spaces, not over bony structures.
3. Cleanse the selection site with alcohol to remove any dirt or body oils, improving adhesion and electrode-to-skin contact.
4. Attach ECG lead wires to the electrodes. Most ECG cables are identified based on their color and are labeled for appropriate application. For example, the white cable commonly represents the negative lead, whereas the red and black cables signify the positive and ground leads respectively.
5. Attach the preconnected electrodes to the prepared site. If the patient is sweating profusely, tincture of benzoin or extra dry deodorant spray applied to the skin may aid in securing the electrode.
6. Activate the ECG monitor and select the desired monitoring lead.

ECG GRAPH PAPER

ECG graph paper is used to record the sequence of electrical events as they occur through the conduction system. ECG paper is divided into a standardized grid of small squares and large boxes, with light and dark lines running vertically and horizontally. Horizontal lines measure time in seconds and distance in millimeters (mm). Vertical lines measure voltage in millimeters. Dark lines are spaced 5 mm apart and lighter lines are spaced 1 mm apart (Figure 3–5).

Voltage

The sensitivity of the ECG machine is standardized (calibrated) at 1 millivolt (mV) equaling 10 mm. Each small square (1 mm) equals 0.1 mV and each large box (5 mm) equals 0.5 mV. A standard calibration pulse is 10 mm (two large boxes) high and should be placed at the beginning of the first ECG tracing. Calibration is necessary for accurate measurement of voltage in the vertical direction.

Time

Standard printer speed is 25 mm/second. At that speed each 1 mm (small square) represents **0.04 seconds**. Each 5 mm (large box) is five times greater or equals **0.20 seconds**. Time marks are printed in the ECG paper's margin as short vertical lines or small triangles every 75 mm. At standard paper speed (25 mm/second), these lines represent a 3-second period; for instance, 150 mm will equal 6 seconds. These increments are used to measure the duration of ECG complexes and intervals.

ECG Graph Paper Summary

- Horizontal lines measure time in seconds and distance in millimeters
- Vertical lines measure voltage in millimeters

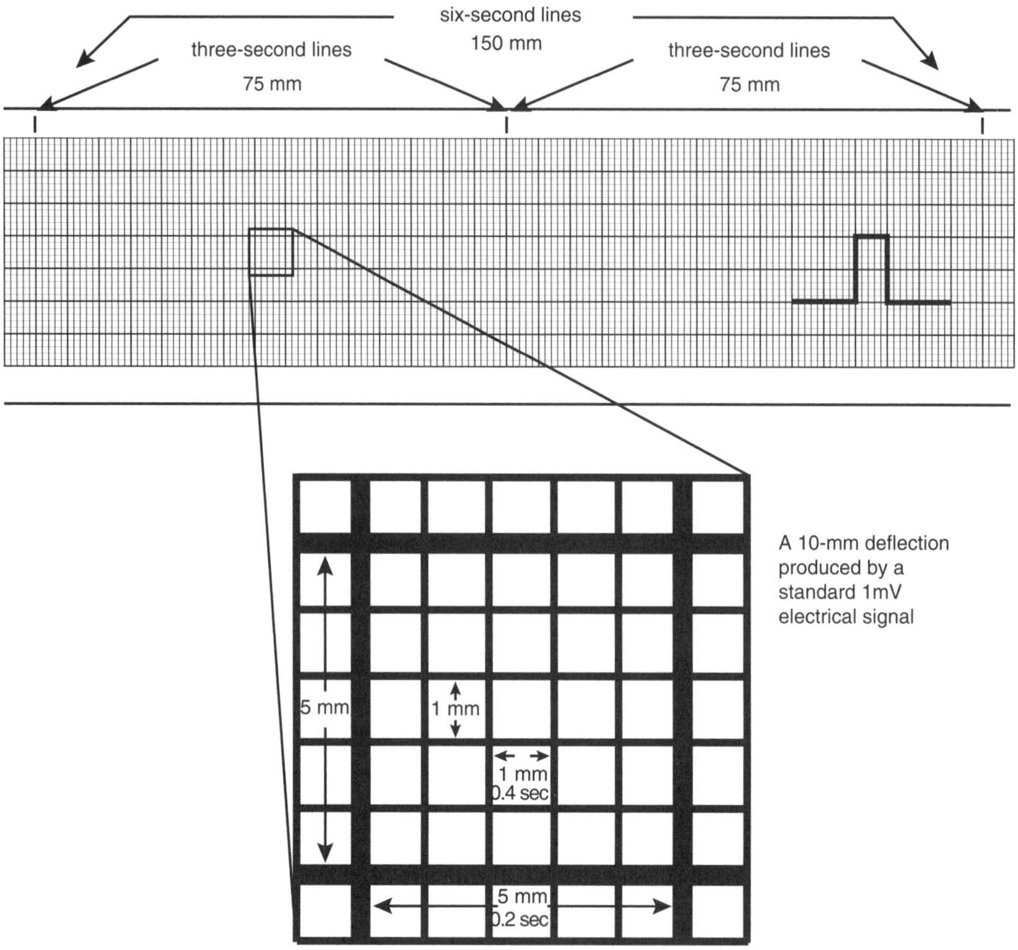

Figure 3–5.
ECG graph paper.

Modified from R. Huszar, *Basic Dysrhythmias Interpretation and Management*. St Louis: Mosby, 1994.

- Each small square equals 0.04 seconds
- Each large box equals 0.20 seconds

BASIC ECG PRINCIPLES

When the ECG machine is not connected to a patient, a straight line will be displayed. This is called the baseline or isoelectric line. Once the patient is connected to the machine, electrical forces will rouse deflections along this line. Forces moving toward a positive electrode will cause a positive (upward) deflection from the baseline (Figure 3–6). Forces moving away from a positive electrode will cause a negative (downward) deflection. The absence of deflection indicates there is no electrical impulse (isoelectric line), or the impulse is moving perpendicular to the lead, producing an equiphasic (equally positive and negative) deflection.

Depolarization and Repolarization as Seen on the ECG

Normal conduction through the heart is as follows. The SA node discharges, followed by depolarization of the atria. This creates a small rounded wave called the P wave. The impulse is then delayed as it passes through the resistant AV node. This delay is

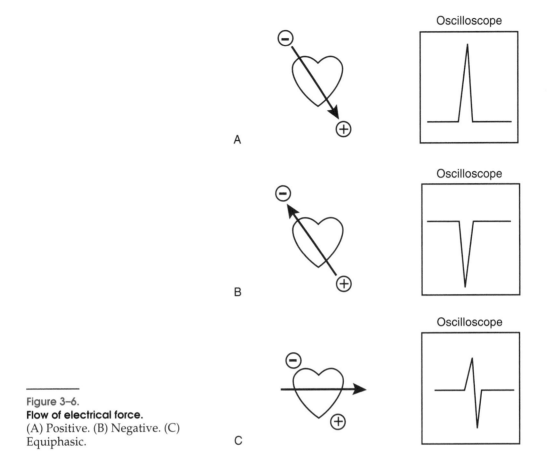

Figure 3–6.
Flow of electrical force.
(A) Positive. (B) Negative. (C)
Equiphasic.

recorded as the isoelectric PR segment. Once past the AV node and His bundle, the impulse races down the rapidly conducting bundle branches to the Purkinje fibers, depolarizing the ventricular myocardium. This creates a group of waves called the QRS complex. Typically, repolarization of the atria does not create enough energy to be seen on the ECG. Repolarization of the larger ventricles, however, inscribes an upright rounded wave called the T wave. On occasion, a small rounded U wave may be seen following the T wave (Figure 3–7).

ELECTROCARDIOGRAPHIC WAVEFORMS (refer to Figure 3–7)

P Wave

The P wave represents depolarization of the atrial muscle from start to finish. Because the sinus node is located in the right atrium, the right atrium begins to depolarize before the left and finishes earlier as well. Therefore, the first half of the P wave represents right atrial depolarization and the second half left atrial depolarization. Furthermore, because there is relatively little atrial muscle mass, only low voltages are produced. The amplitude of the P wave should not exceed 3 mm, and its duration not more than 0.11 seconds. Greater amplitude or duration may indicate enlargement of the atria (see Chapter 7). Normal P wave morphology is round, not notched or peaked.

P Wave Summary

- Mechanism: Right and left atrial depolarization
- Duration: Not broader than 0.11 sec
- Amplitude: Not taller than 3 mm
- Shape: Small and round

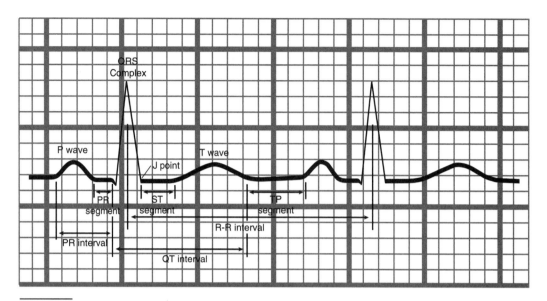

Figure 3–7.
Components of the ECG.

QRS Complex

The QRS complex represents ventricular depolarization. It is naturally the largest complex on the ECG because the ventricles are so much larger than the atria. In fact, QRS amplitude may reach 25 mm (5 large boxes) or more. The QRS complex consists of several distinct waves. It begins at a point where the first wave of deflection deviates from the baseline and terminates where the last wave returns to the baseline. Because the precise configuration of the QRS complex may vary so greatly (i.e., positive, negative, or both), a standard format for naming each component has been devised (Figure 3–8):

Q wave: The first deflection of the complex is called a Q wave if it is negative. Q waves represent depolarization of the interventricular septum and when present are narrow and small (< 25% of the succeeding R wave).

R wave: The first positive deflection of the complex is called an R

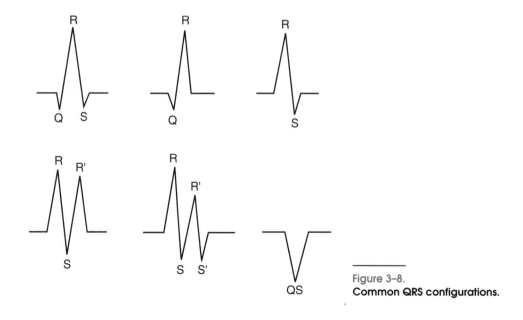

Figure 3–8.
Common QRS configurations.

wave. It may or may not be preceded by a Q wave. R waves represent the majority of ventricular depolarization. Positive deflections following the first R wave are labeled R prime (R′), R double prime (R″), and so forth.

S wave: The first negative wave following the R wave is an S wave. S waves represent the final stages of ventricular depolarization. Negative deflections following the first S wave are labeled S prime (S′), S double prime (S″), and so forth.

When conduction through the ventricles is normal, the duration of the QRS complex should be between **0.04 to 0.12** seconds (1–3 small squares). Durations of 0.12 seconds and greater indicate an intraventricular conduction delay. QRS width is measured from the onset of the complex to its end.

QRS Summary

- Mechanism: Depolarization of the ventricles
- Duration: 0.04 sec to 0.12 sec
- Components
  Q wave: First negative deflection following the P wave
  R wave: First positive deflection following the P wave
  S wave: First negative wave following the R wave

T Wave

The T wave corresponds to repolarization of the ventricles. It is identified as the first slightly rounded and asymmetrical wave following the QRS complex. The T wave is normally inscribed in the same direction as the QRS, but with less amplitude. Abnormalities of the T wave usually take the form of inversion (inscribed in the opposite direction to the QRS), as seen with myocardial ischemia (see Chapter 5). They may also become excessively tall or peaked, as seen with potassium intoxication (hyperkalemia).

T Wave Summary

- Mechanism: Ventricular repolarization
- Shape: Rounded and asymmetrical
- Deflection: Same as the QRS

U Wave

The U wave is a small, rounded wave of low voltage occasionally seen following the T wave. Its inscription is usually the same as that of the T wave. The origin of the U wave is unknown, but it is suggested to either represent repolarization of the papillary muscles or Purkinje fibers.

U Wave Summary

- Mechanism: Repolarization of the papillary muscles or Purkinje fibers
- Shape: Small, with the same deflection as the T wave
- ECG representation: Follows the T wave

SEGMENTS AND INTERVALS

Segments and intervals are the different straight lines connecting the various waves on the ECG. A segment is a straight line connecting two waves, whereas an interval encompasses at least one wave plus the connecting straight line (refer to Figure 3–7). These include the PR interval, ST segment, and QT interval.

PR Interval

The PR interval corresponds to the time required for an impulse to travel from the SA node through the conduction system to the first muscle fibers stimulated in the ventricles. It is measured from the onset of the P wave to the onset of the QRS complex (refer to Figure 3–7). Normal PR interval duration is from 0.12 to 0.20 seconds (3 to 5 small squares). Shorter intervals indicate accelerated conduction from the atria to the ventricles, while longer intervals indicate a delay in conduction somewhere between the AV node and His bundle.

PR Interval Summary

- Mechanism: Atrial depolarization and a delay at the AV junction
- Duration: 0.12 sec to 0.20 sec
- Shortened: Accelerated conduction through the AV node
- Prolonged: Delayed conduction through the AV node

ST Segment

The ST segment is the straight line connecting the end of the QRS complex with the beginning of the T wave (refer to Figure 3–7). It measures the time from the end of ventricular depolarization to the onset of ventricular repolarization. The ST segment is normally isoelectric and gradually blends into the upslope of the T wave. The point at which the ST segment takes off from the QRS is the J point.

The duration of the ST segment is not important. However, in diagnostic electrocardiography (i.e., 12-lead ECGs), the position of the ST segment relative to the baseline is important. Dramatic ST segment elevation is one of the hallmarks of acute myocardial infarction, while depression is highly suggestive of myocardial ischemia. These and other causes of ST segment shifts will be discussed in later chapters.

ST Segment Summary

- Mechanism: Early repolarization of the ventricles
- Shape: Gradual upward slope, not sharp or horizontal
- Evaluation: Position relative to the baseline
    Elevated ST: Suggestive of myocardial infarction
    Depressed ST: Suggestive of myocardial ischemia

QT Interval

The QT interval represents the repolarization duration of the ventricles. It is measured from the onset of the QRS complex to the end of the T wave. Normal intervals vary with heart rate (shortening as the rate increases and lengthening as the rate decreases), sex, and age, making it difficult to identify an absolute value. At normal rates the QT interval is less than 0.44 seconds (< 11 small squares). The use of a QT interval chart that plots normal intervals against heart rate and sex is an invaluable tool (Table 3–1.)

QT Interval Summary

- Mechanism: Duration of ventricular repolarization
- Duration: 0.36 to 0.44 sec
- ECG representation: Onset of the QRS complex through the T wave

TABLE 3–1   •   **QT Interval Chart**

HEART RATE PER MINUTE	MEN AND CHILDREN (SEC)	WOMEN (SEC)
40	0.49	0.50
45	0.47	0.48
50	0.45	0.46
55	0.43	0.44
60	0.42	0.43
65	0.40	0.42
70	0.39	0.41
75	0.38	0.39
80	0.37	0.38
85	0.36	0.37
90	0.35	0.36
95	0.35	0.36
100	0.34	0.35

R–R Interval

The R–R interval is the distance between two consecutive R waves (refer to Figure 3–7). It is measured from the beginning of the R wave in one complete cycle to the onset of the R wave in the next cycle. The R–R interval is used to calculate ventricular rate and regularity.

ARTIFACTS

Artifacts are deflections on the ECG produced by factors other than the heart's electrical activity. They are classified as either internal or external, occurring naturally or from outside influences. Internal artifacts include muscle tremors, shivering, and patient movement, all of which can cause a grossly uneven wandering baseline, which prohibits accurate ST segment analysis. External artifacts include machine malfunction, 60 cycle interference, and a loose or dislodged electrode. These can mimic certain life-threatening dysrhythmias, prompting erroneous evaluation of the patient's clinical condition.

ECG INTERPRETATION

ECG interpretation requires a systematic approach. Attempts to examine the ECG in a fortuitous manner can lead to an incorrect interpretation. Paramedics are encouraged to use the following criteria when evaluating the ECG.

- Always use a consistent approach
- Memorize the rules for each dysrhythmia
- Analyze a given rhythm tracing according to a specific format
- Compare your analysis to the rules for each dysrhythmia
- Identify the dysrhythmia based on similarity to established rules

Rhythm Analysis

There are several standard formats for ECG analysis. The following steps will provide the basic information needed to analyze dysrhythmias (Table 3–2).

Step 1: Obtain a Rhythm Strip

The tracing should be at least 6 seconds (150 mm) in length. Note the lead in which the tracing is recorded and discard if artifact or interference is present. Include a calibration pulse. This will inscribe a 1 mV signal into the recording that is 10 mm high. Standard-

TABLE 3–2 • **Steps for Rhythm Analysis**

Step 1: Obtain a rhythm strip (6 sec)
Step 2: Determine cardiac rate (no. heartbeats/min)
Step 3: Analyze the rhythm (regular or irregular)
Step 4: Analyze the P wave (presence, regularity, shape)
Step 5: Measure the PR interval (0.12 to 0.20 sec/duration)
Step 6: Analyze and measure the QRS complex (0.04 to 0.12 sec/duration)
Step 7: Measure the QT interval (0.36 to 0.44 sec/duration)

ization is adjusted to increase or decrease the size of the QRS waveforms in order to make ECG interpretation easier.

Step 2: Determine the Rate

Heart rate is calculated as the number of heartbeats per minute. In most cases this means ventricular rate (number of QRS complexes per minute), but it can also refer to atrial rate (number of P waves per minute). If atrial and ventricular rates differ, they should be calculated separately. In both cases, one of four methods may be used (three are shown in Figure 3–9). For instructional purposes, ventricular rate will be calculated.

- Six second method: This method is the easiest to use, but the least accurate. It provides an estimate of heart rate and is useful when the rhythm is irregular. Note the short vertical lines or triangular figures at the top or bottom of the ECG graph paper. They usually represent 3-second intervals (75 mm). Count the number of QRS complexes in a 6-second interval and multiply by 10 (6 sec × 10 = 60 sec) to obtain the ventricular rate.
- R–R interval method: The R–R interval method may be used in several different ways. For it to be accurate the cardiac rhythm must be regular. It can be calculated by the following methods.
  Method 1: Measure the duration in seconds between the peaks of two consecutive R waves. Divide this number by 60 to obtain the rate. Example: 60 ÷ 0.60 = 100 beats/min.
  Method 2: Count the number of large boxes between consecutive R waves. Divide this number into 300 to obtain the rate (300 divisions = 1 minute). Example: 300 ÷ 4 large boxes = 75 beats/min.
  Method 3: Count the number of small squares between two consecutive R waves. Divide this number into 1500 to obtain the rate. Example: 1500 ÷ 20 small squares = 75 beats/min. This method is the most precise.
- Triplicate method: This method requires memorizing two sets of numbers: 300-150-100 and 75-60-50. These numbers represent the heart rate for consecutive large boxes (i.e., 1 large box gives a heart rate of 300 beats/min, 2 give 150 beats/min, and so on). Using the method of triplicates, calculate as follows.
  1. Select an R wave that falls on a heavy dark line.
  2. Number the next six dark vertical lines consecutively from left to right as 300-150-100-75-60-50.
  3. Identify where the next R wave falls with reference to the six dark vertical lines. Example: If the R wave falls on 75, the rate is 75 beats/min. If the R wave falls halfway between 100 and 150, the rate is estimated at 125 beats/min. (Figure 3–9C)

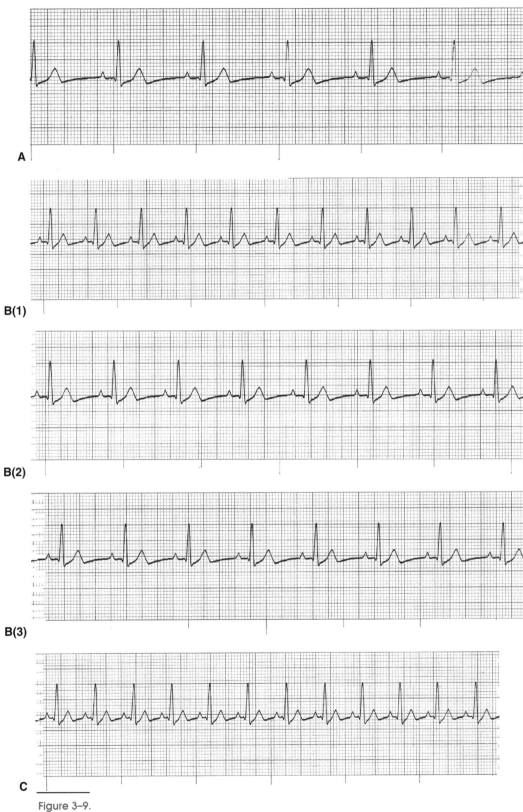

A

B(1)

B(2)

B(3)

C

Figure 3–9.
Methods of determining heart rate.
(A) Six second method. The heart rate is approximately 60 beats/min. (B)
R–R interval methods 1, 2, and 3. (C) Triplicate method.

- Heart rate calculator rulers: Commercially available heart rate calculators are reasonably accurate only if the rhythm is regular. Because they may not always be readily available, mechanical devices should not be relied upon to determine rate.

Step 3: Analyze the Rhythm

Measure the R–R intervals for equality across the ECG tracing from left to right. If the distances between R waves are equal or vary by less than 0.16 seconds (4 small squares), the rhythm is regular. If the shortest and longest R–R intervals vary by more than 0.16 seconds, the rhythm is irregular. Determine if irregular rhythms fit into one of the following patterns.

- Occasionally irregular (only 1 or 2 R–R intervals are unequal)
- Regularly irregular (patterned irregularity or group beating)
- Irregularly irregular (no relationship between R–R intervals)

Step 4: Analyze the P Waves

The normal P wave in lead II is positive and gently rounded, preceding each QRS complex. This indicates that the pacemaker originates from the SA node. Evaluation of P waves include the following five criteria.

- Are P waves present?
- Are P waves regular (Can the P–P interval be plotted similar to R–R intervals)?
- Is there one P wave for each QRS complex?
- Are P waves upright or inverted (compared to the QRS)?
- Do all P waves have the same morphology (shape)?

Step 5: Analyze the PR Interval

The PR interval should be constant across the ECG tracing. The normal PR interval is 0.12 to 0.20 seconds. Any deviation is an abnormal finding. A prolonged PR interval (> 0.20 sec) indicates a delay of conduction through the AV node (AV block). A short PR interval (< 0.12 sec) indicates that the impulse progressed from the atria to the ventricles through pathways other than the AV node.

Step 6: Analyze the QRS Complex

Examine the QRS complex for regularity and width. Normal QRS duration is 0.04 to 0.12 seconds. Complexes equal to or greater than 0.12 seconds indicate a conduction abnormality in the ventricles.

Step 7: Measure the QT Interval

The normal QT interval is 0.36 to 0.44 seconds. A prolonged QT interval predisposes a patient to ventricular dysrhythmias.

ANALYSIS OF NORMAL SINUS RHYTHM

Normal sinus rhythm (NSR) originates in the SA node and progresses through a normal conducting system, resulting in sequential depolarization and repolarization of the atria and ventricles. In the healthy heart, this results in optimal mechanical function, producing normal cardiac output. ECG characteristics of normal sinus rhythm are as follows (Figure 3–10).

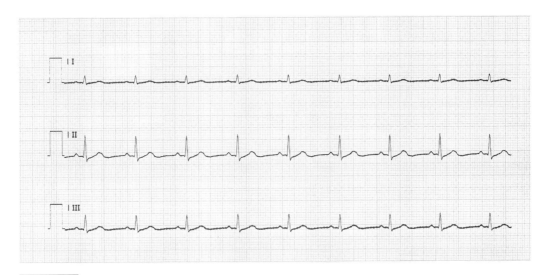

Figure 3–10.
Normal sinus rhythm.

- Rate: 60 to 100 beats/min
- Rhythm: Regular (both atrial P–P and ventricular R–R intervals)
- P wave: Normal, upright, and appear before each QRS complex
- PR interval: 0.12 to 0.20 sec and constant
- QRS complex: 0.04 to 0.12 sec with normal morphology
- QT interval: 0.36 to 0.44 sec and constant

DYSRHYTHMOGENESIS

Any disturbance in the heart's normal electrical rate or rhythm is a dysrhythmia. The term arrhythmia (absence of cardiac electrical activity) is often used, but the authors have chosen to use the more precise term. Factors that influence the development of dysrhythmias are numerous and include ischemia of the myocardium, hypoxemia, hypertension, electrolyte disturbances, autonomic nervous stimulation or blocking, hypothermia, drug effects or toxicity, direct trauma to the myocardium, electrical shock, chemical inhalants, and a host of other causes. All of these cause dysrhythmias by disturbing automaticity and/or conductivity.

Ectopic Impulses

An ectopic (out of sequence) impulse results when the pacemaker function is assumed by cells other than those in the SA node. Depolarizations that occur from ectopic cells may be intermittent or sustained and are often seen as premature (early) beats because they occur before the SA node is scheduled to fire. Depending on the location of the ectopic focus, the premature impulses may be atrial, junctional, or of ventricular origin. Ectopic impulse formation and conduction are the principal mechanisms of dysrhythmia development.

Disturbances in Automaticity

Each cell in the conduction system capable of producing a spontaneous impulse has a rate of discharge relative to its position. Overall, the more proximal the cell, the faster is its rate of spontaneous discharge. Cells distal to the dominant pacemaker are normally latent. When influenced, normal inherent rates can be altered, changing pacemaker rates and locations. For example, excessive vagal (parasympathetic) tone will slow the discharge rate of the SA node causing sinus bradycardia, while local ischemia may greatly accelerate the autonomic rate of a His bundle cell, causing it to take over as the dominant pacer. This would result in an accelerated junctional rhythm. When other automatic cells completely assume the sinus node's function, they are referred to as secondary or latent pacemakers. These are just two of a multitude of situations where disturbances in automaticity cause dysrhythmias.

Disturbances in Conductivity

Alterations in conduction velocity and resultant changes in refractoriness (responsiveness) frequently cause dysrhythmias. Most occur from decreased (slowing of impulse transmission) versus increased conductivity. Decreased conductivity can range from a

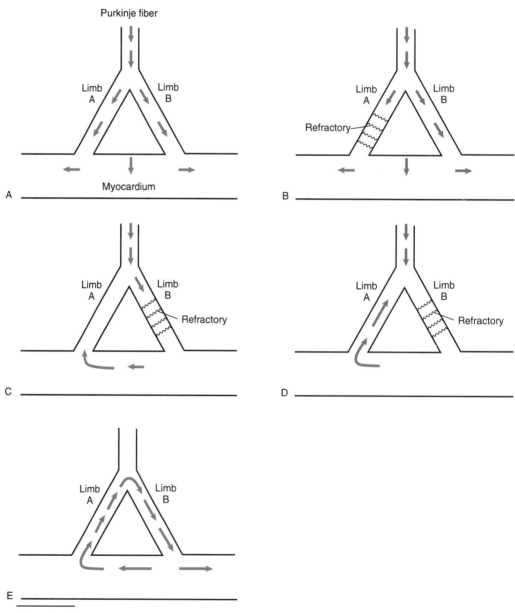

Figure 3–11.
Reentry mechanism.

simple slowing of conduction to a complete block of impulse transmission. A simple example would be infarction (death) of the bundle branches as often occurs with septal infarct. If both bundle branches suffer tissue death they cannot conduct supraventricular (above the ventricles) impulses into the ventricles. This would result in complete electrical block.

Decreased conductivity in the sinus node or atria may impair sinus impulses from spreading throughout the heart. This may produce long pauses in the cardiac rhythm that encourages secondary pacemaker formation. Decreased conduction through the AV node impairs the relationship between atrial and ventricular contractions. This can result in very slow rhythms that inhibit cardiac output. Ventricular conduction disturbances may impair ventricular contraction, thus decreasing cardiac output. Furthermore, changes in conductivity can also lead to the formation of dysrhythmias caused by *reentry*.

Reentry

Reentry is the phenomenon in which a stimulus reexcites a conduction pathway through which it has already passed. For reentry to develop, two limbs of a conduction pathway must have differing conduction velocities and refractory periods. This setup can occur in almost any portion of the conduction system. We will use the example of a Purkinje fiber that branches into two limbs as it reaches a section of myocardium.

Normally, the conduction down both limbs is equal and refractory periods are equivalent. This results in uncomplicated delivery of the impulse to the myocardium (Figure 3–11A). If one limb of the fiber changes conduction velocity and refractoriness (e.g., from ischemia) then the mechanism for reentry exists. In this scenario, the impulse travels down the Purkinje fiber and finds limb *A* refractory to the impulse due to slower repolarization than limb *B* (Figure 3–11B). As the impulse moves across the myocardium between limbs, limb *A* has time to recover while limb *B* is now refractory, due to its recent stimulation (Figure 3–11C). As the impulse reaches limb *A*, it finds it ready to conduct and proceeds up the limb (Figure 3–11D). By this time, limb *B* has now recovered and is ready to accept an impulse. It then carries the impulse back to the myocardium and a continuous circle of depolarization has begun (the impulse chases its refractory tail) (Figure 3–11E). This will result in ventricular tachycardia. Remember, reentry can occur virtually anywhere along the conduction pathways and is the primary cause of supraventricular and ventricular tachydysrhythmias.

DYSRHYTHMIA INTERPRETATION

Classifications

Cardiac dysrhythmias can be classified in a number of different ways. Examples of classification methods include:

- Changes in automaticity versus disturbances in conduction
- Major dysrhythmias versus minor dysrhythmias
- Life-threatening dysrhythmias versus non-life-threatening dysrhythmias
- Tachydysrhythmias versus bradydysrhythmias
- Site of origin or site of the conduction disturbance

This text classifies dysrhythmias according to the location of their origin. Such an anatomical approach is the easiest to understand. The dysrhythmias addressed utilizing this method include the following categories:

- Dysrhythmias originating in the SA node
- Dysrhythmias originating in the atria

- Dysrhythmias originating in the AV junction
- Dysrhythmias originating in the ventricles
- Artificial pacemaker rhythms
- Dysrhythmias resulting from disorders of conduction

Disorders of conduction constitute a separate division of dysrhythmia classification. Conduction disturbances will be classified according to the degree of block versus their site of origin.

Important Points

Two important points exist when evaluating and treating dysrhythmias. (1) When interpreting the ECG, never leave anything to chance. Describe the basic, underlying rhythm first, then add any additional components present within the tracing (i.e., sinus bradycardia with PVCs or sinus rhythm with a first-degree AV block). (2) Dysrhythmias can result from a number of causes, but regardless of the cause or type of dysrhythmia, the patient and his or her symptoms are treated, not merely the dysrhythmia. Emergency therapy should only be considered if clinical evidence indicates that the dysrhythmia has produced serious side effects or the dysrhythmia is likely to degenerate into a much more serious dysrhythmia.

Because lead II is the most common prehospital monitoring lead, each dysrhythmia presented in this chapter appears in that form. For comparison, many of the same dysrhythmias are also shown in leads I and III.

DYSRHYTHMIAS ORIGINATING IN THE SINUS NODE

Dysrhythmias originating in the SA node are designated as such because the rate is too slow or too fast, the rhythm is irregular, or a sinus node impulse either does not form within the sinus node or fails to exit from the sinus node. The majority of these dysrhythmias result from changes in autonomic tone. Sinus dysrhythmias include sinus bradycardia, sinus tachycardia, sinus dysrhythmia, and sinus arrest.

Sinus Bradycardia

Description. Sinus bradycardia is characterized by a decrease in the rate of atrial depolarization due to slowing of the sinus node.

Etiology. Sinus bradycardia may occur from any of the following conditions.

- Intrinsic sinus node disease
- Increased parasympathetic (vagal) tone or decreased sympathetic tone
- Drug effects (digitalis, propranolol, quinidine)
- Normal finding in well-conditioned individuals (athletes)
- Normal variant

ECG Characteristics. (Figure 3–12.)

- Rate: Less than 60/min
- Rhythm: Regular
- P waves: Upright and normal morphology with one P wave preceding each QRS complex
- PR interval: 0.12 to 0.20 sec and constant
- QRS complex: 0.04 to 0.12 sec (normal)

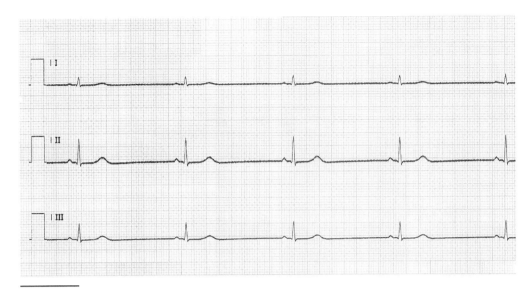

Figure 3–12.
Sinus bradycardia.

Clinical Implication. The decreased heart rate may compromise cardiac output and result in hypotension, angina, or central nervous system symptoms (dizziness, weakness, and/or syncope). This is especially true for rates less than 50 per minute. When sinus bradycardia is profound and occurs in the setting of acute myocardial infarction, the prognosis is poor (see Chapter 6). Because of the slow heart rate, ectopic atrial and ventricular rhythms may also occur.

Prehospital Management. Treatment is unnecessary unless hypotension or ventricular irritability (PVCs) are present. If treatment is required, administer 0.5 to 1.0 mg of atropine every three to five minutes until a satisfactory rate (60 to 100 per minute) has been achieved or a total of 3 mg has been given. If atropine fails to accelerate the rate, immediate application of transcutaneous cardiac pacing (TCP) is necessary. An intravenous infusion of either dopamine or epinephrine may be useful if atropine and/or external pacing are ineffective. Isoproterenol is rarely required, but may be beneficial in certain atropine refractory bradycardias. It should be emphasized that many individuals have heart rates well below 60 beats per minute. Treatment is guided by evaluation of the underlying cause and the presence or absence of clinical symptoms.

NOTE: By definition, any rhythm with a rate less than 60 beats per minute is classified as a bradycardia.

Sinus Tachycardia

Description. Sinus tachycardia results from an increase in the rate of sinus node discharge. It often reflects situations of increased physiologic demand for oxygen (e.g., stress, fever, pain, etc.). The sinus node gradually increases its rate in response to the needs of the body. When those needs no longer exist, the rate of sinus node discharge gradually decreases.

Etiology. Sinus tachycardia may result from any of the following conditions.

- Exercise
- Fever
- Anxiety
- Hypovolemia
- Anemia
- Congestive heart failure
- Cardiogenic shock (pump failure)
- Increased sympathetic tone

ECG Characteristics. (Figure 3–13.)

- Rate: Greater than 100/min, rarely exceeding 180/min
- Rhythm: Regular
- P waves: Upright and normal morphology with one P wave preceding each QRS complex
- PR interval: 0.12 to 0.20 sec and constant
- QRS complex: 0.04 to 0.12 sec (normal)

Clinical Implication. Sinus tachycardia is often a benign process. In some cases, it may be a compensatory mechanism for decreased stroke volume. If the rate is in excess of 140 beats per minute, cardiac output may decrease because of a reduction in ventricular filling time. Very rapid rates may increase myocardial oxygen consumption and precipitate or worsen myocardial ischemia and infarction. Prolonged sinus tachycardia in the presence of infarction is highly suggestive of cardiogenic shock (pump failure).

Prehospital Management. Treatment is directed at the underlying cause. If the tachycardia is inappropriate (hypovolemia, congestive heart failure, etc.), or if the patient is symptomatic, the cause is identified and corrected.

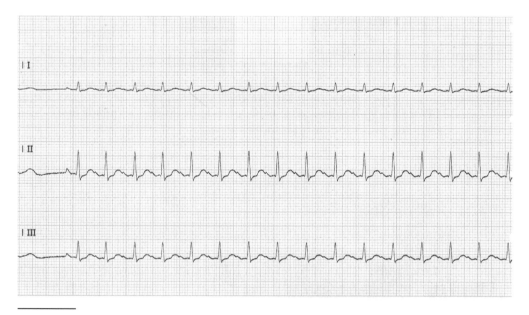

Figure 3–13.
Sinus tachycardia.

NOTE: By definition, any rhythm with a rate greater than 100 beats per minute is classified as a tachycardia.

Sinus Dysrhythmia

Description. Sinus dysrhythmia is characterized by a phasic variation of the R–R interval greater than 0.16 seconds. It is usually a sinus rhythm with a rate that varies with respiration.

Etiology. Sinus dysrhythmia is often a normal finding and is sometimes related to the respiratory cycle and changes in intrathoracic pressure. It is most pronounced in the young and becomes less marked as the child grows older. When related to the respiratory cycle, sinus dysrhythmia is synchronized with breathing, slowing with expiration and speeding up with inspiration. Pathologically, sinus dysrhythmia can be caused by enhanced vagal tone.

ECG Characteristics. (Figure 3–14.)

* Rate: Usually 60 to 100/min (varies with respiration); slow phase may be less than 60/min
* Rhythm: Irregular (slows with expiration and accelerates with inspiration)
* P waves: Upright and normal morphology with one P wave preceding each QRS complex
* PR interval: 0.12 to 0.20 sec and constant
* QRS complex: 0.04 to 0.12 sec (normal)

Clinical Implication. Sinus dysrhythmia is a normal phenomena, particularly in the young and aged.

Prehospital Management. Typically, no treatment is required unless the bradycardic phase of the dysrhythmia is prolonged, causing symptoms. If this occurs, atropine is the agent of choice to accelerate the heart rate.

Sinus Arrest

Description. Sinus arrest is a failure of impulse formation in the sinus node, resulting in short periods of cardiac standstill. Cardiac standstill persists until lower latent pacemakers discharge (escape beats) or the sinus node resumes its discharge.

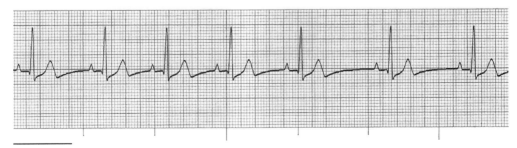

Figure 3–14.
Sinus dysrhythmia.

Etiology. Sinus arrest can result from any of the following conditions.

- Sinus node ischemia
- Digitalis toxicity
- Excessive vagal tone
- Degenerative fibrotic disease
- Myocardial infarction
- Potassium imbalance

ECG Characteristics. (Figure 3–15.)
- Rate: Normal to slow, depending on the frequency and duration of the arrest
- Rhythm: Irregular, with pauses that have no relationship to the underlying cardiac cycle
- P waves: Upright and normal morphology when preceding the QRS complex
- PR interval: 0.12 to 0.20 sec and constant
- QRS complex: 0.04 to 0.12 sec (normal)

Clinical Implication. Frequent and prolonged episodes may compromise cardiac output by decreasing the heart rate, resulting in hypotension, syncope, and other symptoms. The greatest danger is complete cessation of sinus node activity, occasionally resulting in cardiac standstill.

Prehospital Management. If the patient is asymptomatic, observation is all that is necessary. However, if the patient is extremely bradycardic and symptomatic, administer 0.5 to 1.0 mg of atropine and continue with 0.5 mg increments every three to five minutes until a satisfactory rate has been obtained or the maximum dosage has been delivered (3 mg). If atropine is ineffective, consider immediate transcutaneous cardiac pacing.

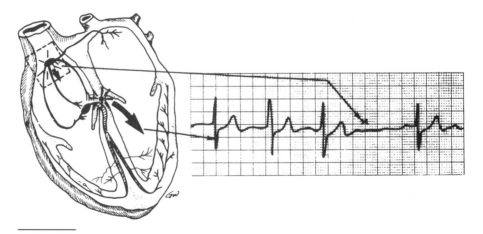

Figure 3–15.
Sinus arrest.

Reproduced with permission from Caroline, N.L., *Emergency Care in the Streets*, 5th ed. Boston: Little, Brown and Co., 1995. p. 536.

DYSRHYTHMIAS ORIGINATING IN THE ATRIA

Atrial dysrhythmias are those rhythms that originate outside the SA node in the tissue of the atria. Ischemia, hypoxia, atrial dilation, and other factors can cause atrial dysrhythmias. The atrial rhythms covered in this section are a wandering atrial pacemaker, premature atrial complexes (PACs), atrial tachycardia, atrial flutter, and atrial fibrillation, all of which are grouped under the broad category of supraventricular, which refers to the area above the branching portion of the bundle of His. Therefore, supraventricular dysrhythmias are rhythm disturbances that originate above the ventricles. Several ECG features are common to all atrial dysrhythmias.

- P waves differ in appearance from sinus P waves
- The PR interval may be normal, shortened, or prolonged
- QRS complexes are of normal duration (less than 0.12 sec)

Wandering Atrial Pacemaker

Description. Wandering atrial pacemaker is the passive transfer of pacemaker sites from the sinus node to other latent pacemakers in the atria or AV junction. Often more than one pacemaker site exists, causing variation in R–R intervals and P wave morphology.

Etiology. Wandering atrial pacemaker can result from any of the following conditions.

- A variant of sinus dysrhythmia
- Normal phenomenon in the very young or the elderly
- Ischemic heart disease
- Chronic lung disease
- Valvular (mitral and tricuspid) heart disease

ECG Characteristics. (Figure 3–16.)

- Rate: 60 to 100/min
- Rhythm: Slightly irregular (P–P and R–R intervals) because each
  impulse travels through the atria via a different route

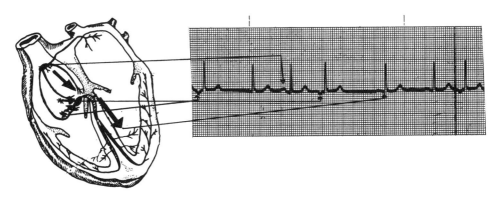

Figure 3–16.
Wandering atrial pacemaker.

Reproduced with permission from Caroline, N.L., *Emergency Care in the Streets*, 5th ed. Boston: Little, Brown and Co., 1995. p. 538.

- P waves: Morphology varies from beat to beat and may disappear completely
- PR interval: Varies and may become less than 0.12 sec or greater than 0.20 sec
- QRS complex: 0.04 to 0.12 sec (normal)

Clinical Implication. Wandering atrial pacemaker usually has no detrimental effects. Occasionally, it may precipitate other atrial dysrhythmias.

Prehospital Management. Treatment is geared toward resolving the underlying cause. Observation is all that is required in the out-of-hospital setting.

Premature Atrial Complexes (Contractions)

Description. Premature atrial complexes (PACs) result from a single electrical impulse originating in the atria outside the SA node, which causes an early depolarization of the heart before the next expected sinus beat. Because the PAC results in depolarization of the atria, this impulse also depolarizes the SA node, interrupting its regular cadence. This creates a noncompensatory pause in the underlying rhythm as the sinus node continues to fire at its inherent rate. Therefore, the next expected P wave of the underlying rhythm appears earlier than it would have if the SA node had not been disturbed. Electrically, this means that the duration of two cycles, including the premature complex, is less than the sum of two normal cycles.

Etiology. A premature atrial complex can result from any of the following conditions.

- Stress, caffeine, tobacco, or alcohol
- Sympathomimetic drugs
- Heart failure, myocardial ischemia
- Digitalis toxicity
- Chronic obstructive pulmonary disease (COPD)
- Normal finding

ECG Characteristics. (Figure 3–17.)

- Rate: Depends on the underlying rhythm
- Rhythm: Irregular; the R–R interval is irregular; the premature complex interrupts the regularity of the underlying rhythm.
- P wave: The shape of the P wave of the PAC differs from the P wave of the underlying rhythm. The location of the ectopic impulse in the atria determines the morphology of the P wave. If the focus is in the vicinity of the sinus node, the closer will be its resemblance. The more distal the focus, the greater the difference of P wave morphology. Additionally, the P wave of the PAC occurs earlier than the next expected P wave and may be hidden within the preceding T wave.
- PR interval: The PR interval may be normal, short, prolonged, or absent. The length of the PR interval depends on the origin of the PAC and the ability of the AV node to conduct the early impulse to the ventricles.
- QRS complex: Normal (0.04 to 0.12 sec) if conduction in the ventricles is undisturbed. However, if the AV node conducts the premature impulse into partially refractory (repolarized) ventricles, the resulting QRS complex will appear wide and abnormally

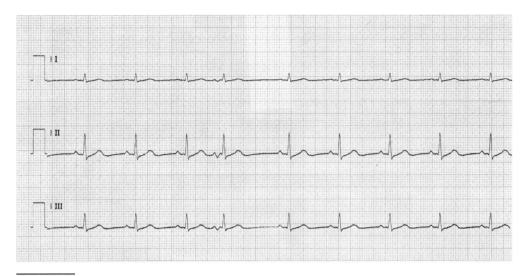

Figure 3–17.
Premature atrial complexes.

shaped. This is known as a PAC with aberration. When a PAC occurs so early that it is unable to penetrate the unresponsive ventricles (absolute refractory), the premature P wave will not be followed by a QRS complex. This is known as a nonconducted PAC.

Clinical Implication. Isolated PACs are of minimal significance. Frequent PACs may suggest organic heart disease and may precipitate other atrial dysrhythmias.

Prehospital Management. Treatment of PACs is usually not indicated unless untoward clinical signs and symptoms are present. Attention is directed to determining the underlying cause. Observation is all that is required in the out-of-hospital setting.

Paroxysmal Supraventricular Tachycardia

Description. Paroxysmal supraventricular tachycardia (PSVT) is a rhythm originating in the atria outside the SA node. It results when rapid atrial depolarization overrides the SA node. PSVT often occurs in paroxysm with sudden onset, lasts minutes to hours, and terminates abruptly.

Etiology. The hallmark of PSVT is abnormal conduction through a reentry circuit, resulting in a rapid supraventricular dysrhythmia. A reentry is formed by two pathways that are connected at their upper and lower ends, providing an uninterrupted circuit for impulse conduction. Most PSVTs are due to AV nodal reentry tachycardia. This involves two pathways within the AV junction in which an impulse is conducted slowly down one pathway toward the ventricles and is then conducted rapidly back into the atria along the second. Thus, the atria and ventricles are depolarized almost simultaneously. PSVT may occur at any age, unassociated with heart disease. Frequently, PSVT may be precipitated by stress, overexertion, smoking, and/or the ingestion of caffeine. PSVT is often associated with underlying atherosclerotic and rheumatic heart disease. Furthermore, it may be the result of an accessory conduction pathway such as Wolff-Parkinson-White syndrome (WPW) (see Chapter 7).

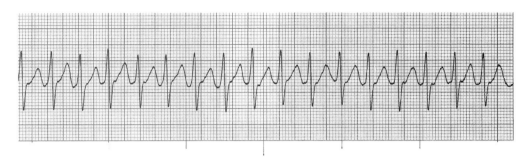

Figure 3–18.
Paroxysmal supraventricular tachycardia.

ECG Characteristics. (Figure 3–18.)

- Rate: 160 to 240/min
- Rhythm: Characteristically regular except at its onset and termination. The atrial rhythm is regular and the ventricular rhythm is most often regular with 1:1 conduction (one atrial depolarization preceding each ventricular depolarization).
- P waves: Atrial P waves differ in morphology from the sinus P waves. Often, the P wave is buried within the preceding T wave, making it impossible to observe.
- PR interval: Usually normal. May be short (< 0.12 sec) when the ectopic pacemaker site is near the AV node or when the speed of conduction through the AV node accelerates.
- QRS complex: 0.04 to 0.12 sec (normal). Once the impulse reaches the AV node its path of conduction through the ventricles generally remains undisturbed.

Clinical Implication. Young patients with good cardiac reserve may tolerate PSVT for short periods of time. However, rapid rates can significantly compromise cardiac output in patients with underlying heart disease because of inadequate ventricular filling time. Coronary artery perfusion may also be compromised since the diastolic phase of the cardiac cycle is reduced. PSVT is often sensed by the patient as palpitations and can precipitate angina, hypotension, or congestive heart failure.

Prehospital Management. Prehospital therapy is directed at slowing the ventricular rate. Intervention is contingent with the stability or hemodynamic instability as evidenced by the patient. The stable patient is first treated with vagal maneuvers, followed by pharmacological management, concluding with electrical therapy. The unstable patient is treated with immediate synchronized cardioversion. The following interventions describe the order of appropriate care.

- Vagal maneuvers. Valsalva maneuver (forced expiration against a closed glottis), application of ice to the face, or carotid sinus massage may be performed.
- Pharmacological therapy. Adenosine (Adenocard) is the drug of choice to terminate PSVT (see Chapter 9). It is highly effective if the etiology of the dysrhythmia is of reentry origin. Rapidly administer 6 mg of Adenocard IV through a proximal injection port. Immediately follow the administration with a 30 to 50 cc fluid bolus to ensure its onloading into the central circulation. If the patient does not convert after 1 to 2 minutes, administer a

second bolus of 12 mg in the same fashion. If this fails, and the patient is normotensive, consider verapamil, diltiazem, or beta blockers (see Chapter 9).

• Electrical therapy. If the ventricular rate is greater than 150 beats per minute, or if the patient is hemodynamically unstable, synchronized cardioversion should be utilized. If time allows and the patient is conscious, sedate the patient with 5 to 10 mg of diazepam (Valium) or 2.5 to 5 mg of midazolam (Versed). Begin synchronized countershock at 50 joules and if unsuccessful, repeat a second shock at 100 joules, the third at 200 joules, the fourth at 300 joules and the fifth at 360 joules.

Atrial Flutter

Description. Atrial flutter is a rhythm resulting from a rapid atrial reentry circuit and an AV node which physiologically is unable to conduct all impulses to the ventricles. Instead, the AV junction allows impulse transmission in a 1:1 (rare), 2:1, 3:1, 4:1 ratio or greater, resulting in a discrepancy between atrial and ventricular rates. The ratio of atrioventricular block (P waves to QRS complexes) may remain constant or vary.

Etiology. Atrial flutter may occur in normal hearts, but is usually associated with organic heart disease. It rarely occurs as a direct result of infarction, but is seen in patients over 40 years of age with ischemic heart disease. Damage to the SA node, mitral or tricuspid valve disorders, and corpulmonale (right heart failure) are also contributing factors.

ECG Characteristics. (Figure 3–19.)

• Rate: Atrial rate is between 240 to 350/min. Ventricular rate varies with the ratio of AV conduction. Ventricular rate is usually slower than the atrial rate.
• Rhythm: Atrial rhythm is regular. Ventricular rhythm is regular

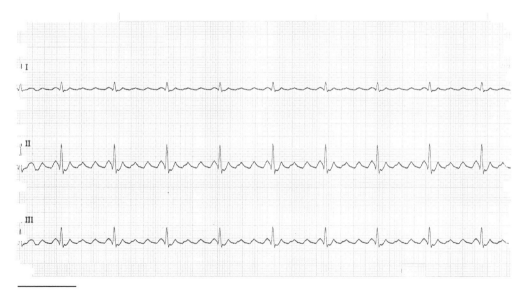

Figure 3–19.
Atrial flutter.

if the conduction ratio is even (i.e., 2:1, 3:1, etc.); it is irregular if the conduction ratio is variable.

- P waves: P waves are absent. Instead, flutter waves (F waves) are present, resembling a sawtooth or picket fence shape. This pattern may be difficult to identify in a 2:1 flutter. Suspect 2:1 flutter when the rhythm is regular and the ventricular rate is greater than 150.
- PR interval: The PR or FR interval is usually constant, but may vary.
- QRS complex: 0.04 to 0.12 sec (normal)

Clinical Implication. Atrial flutter with normal ventricular rates is usually well tolerated. Rapid ventricular rates may compromise cardiac output and precipitate associated symptoms.

Prehospital Management. The goal of therapy is aimed at converting atrial flutter to sinus rhythm or to maintain control of the ventricular response. Treatment in the field is indicated for rapid ventricular rates (> 150 beats per minute) with hemodynamic compromise. In the unstable patient (e.g., chest pain, dyspnea, hypotension, and/or decreased mentation) deliver one or more synchronized countershocks of 50-100-200-300-360 joules. If time permits, sedate the patient with 5 to 10 mg of diazepam prior to cardioversion. In the stable patient, the administration of calcium channel blockers (diltiazem or verapamil), digoxin, beta blockers, and procainamide should precede electrical therapy (see Chapter 9).

Atrial Fibrillation

Description. Atrial fibrillation is a supraventricular dysrhythmia that results from multiple areas of reentry within the atria or from multiple ectopic atrial foci bombarding an AV node which physiologically cannot handle all of the impulses. The AV node, faced with this extraordinary blitz of atrial impulses, allows only occasional impulses to pass through at variable intervals. Therefore, AV conduction is random and ventricular response highly irregular.

Etiology. Atrial fibrillation is often a chronic dysrhythmia commonly associated with underlying cardiac pathology. Conditions such as congestive heart failure, atherosclerotic heart disease, valvular disease (especially mitral stenosis and mitral regurgitation), and rheumatic heart disease are common causes.

ECG Characteristics. (Figure 3–20.)

- Rate: Atrial rate is 350 to 700/min and cannot be calculated. Ventricular rate varies greatly and can be classified as controlled (60 to 100/min), rapid (> 100/min), or slow (< 60/min).
- Rhythm: Irregularly irregular as the transmission of multiple atrial impulses occurs randomly through the AV node.
- P waves: No discernible P waves are present. Instead, fibrillatory (F) waves are present that indicate chaotic electrical activity within the atria. F waves are small, poorly defined, irregularly shaped waves that distort the baseline.
- PR interval: None
- QRS complex: Usually normal (0.04 to 0.12 sec) unless aberrant ventricular conduction or a preexisting intraventricular conduction disturbance is present.

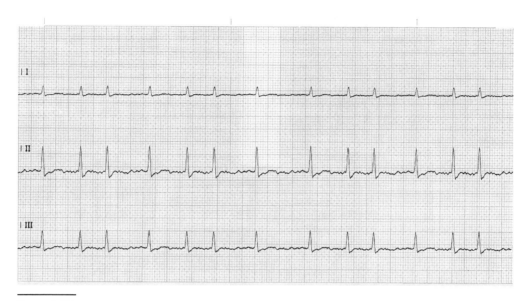

Figure 3–20.
Atrial fibrillation.

NOTE: The irregularly irregular appearance of QRS complexes in the absence of discrete P waves is the key to identifying atrial fibrillation.

Clinical Implication. Chaotic atrial depolarization results in uncoordinated mechanical contraction and loss of the atrial kick, thus reducing forward stroke volume by 20 to 25%. If the rate of ventricular response is normal, as often occurs in patients on digitalis, the rhythm is usually well tolerated. When the ventricular rate is less than 60, cardiac output may decrease. If the ventricular response is rapid, coupled by the loss of the atrial kick, cardiovascular decompensation may occur, resulting in angina, infarction, congestive heart failure, or shock. In addition, atrial fibrillation predisposes patients to peripheral and pulmonary emboli as clots may form within the atria because of stagnant blood flow.

Prehospital Management. Treatment of atrial fibrillation is the same as that for atrial flutter. Control of rapid ventricular rates with pharmacologic and/or electrical intervention is the goal of therapy.

DYSRHYTHMIAS ORIGINATING IN THE AV JUNCTION

Junctional or nodal dysrhythmias are those rhythms that originate within or around the AV node. As you recall from Chapter 2, the AV junction has the potential of assuming the pacemaker role should the SA node fail to discharge or the impulse is delayed in reaching the AV node. Ischemia, hypoxia, and increased vagal tone are primary causes of junctional dysrhythmias. Several common ECG features exist among dysrhythmias originating in the AV junction. These include:

- Inverted P waves in leads II and III. The ectopic impulse emerging from the AV junction travels in a retrograde (backward) direction to depolarize the atria and in an antegrade (forward) direction to depolarize the ventricles. The relationship of the P wave to QRS depolarization is dependent on the timing of atrial and ventricular depolarization. If the P wave appears before the

QRS complex, the atria were depolarized first as the impulse spreads through the atria before it has time to reach the ventricles. If the P wave occurs immediately following the QRS complex, the atria were depolarized after the ventricles. Finally, if the P wave is buried within the QRS complex, it is assumed that the atria and ventricles were depolarized simultaneously.

- PR interval will frequently be less than 0.12 sec.
- QRS complexes are of normal duration.

Premature Junctional Complexes (PJCs)

Description. Premature junctional complexes result from a single electrical impulse originating from the area in and around the AV node that occurs before the next expected beat of the underlying rhythm.

Etiology. Premature junctional complexes result from those same causes outlined for PACs.

ECG Characteristics/Lead II Monitoring. (Figure 3–21.)

- Rate: Depends on the underlying rhythm along with the number of PJCs.
- Rhythm: Depends on the underlying rhythm, usually regular except for the PJC.
- P waves: Inverted; may appear before or after the QRS complex or be absent. If present, they usually differ from sinus P waves in morphology and direction.
- PR interval: If the P wave precedes the QRS complex, the PR interval will be less than 0.12 sec. If the P wave follows the QRS complex, it is termed an RP interval and is less than 0.20 sec.
- QRS complex: 0.04 to 0.12 sec (normal). However, it can be greater than 0.12 sec if the PJC is abnormally conducted through partially refractory ventricles.

Clinical Implication. Isolated PJCs are of minimal significance. Frequent PJCs often indicate organic heart disease and may be forerunners to other junctional dysrhythmias.

Prehospital Management. Specific therapy for PJCs is usually not indicated. Clinically, PJCs are observed much less frequently than PACs and observation is all that is necessary in the field.

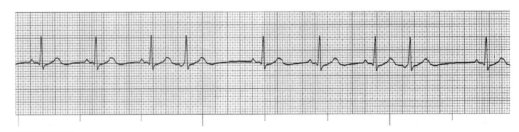

Figure 3–21.
Premature junctional complex.

Junctional Rhythm

Description. A junctional rhythm is a passive escape dysrhythmia that usually results secondary to depression of the primary pacemaker (SA node). The AV node then becomes the pacemaker, discharging at an intrinsic rate of 40 to 60 beats per minute. This serves as a safety mechanism, maintaining cardiac output and preventing cardiac standstill.

Etiology. Junctional escape rhythms have several etiologies. These include increased vagal tone, pathologically slow sinus node discharge or heart block, digitalis toxicity, and acute inferior wall myocardial infarction.

ECG Characteristics/Lead II Monitoring. (Figure 3–22.)

- Rate: 40 to 60/min, but may be less
- Rhythm: Essentially regular
- Pacemaker site: Escape pacemaker in the AV junction
- P waves: Inverted; may appear before or after the QRS complex or be absent (buried within the QRS complex)
- PR interval: If the P wave precedes the QRS complex, the PR interval will be less than 0.12 sec. If the P wave follows the QRS complex, the R–P interval is less than 0.20 sec.
- QRS complex: Usually normal (0.04 to 0.12 sec), unless a preexisting intraventricular conduction disturbance is present.

Clinical Implication. Signs and symptoms and clinical significance of junctional escape rhythms are the same as those in sinus bradycardia. The slow heart rate can decrease cardiac output, thus precipitating or worsening angina and other cardiac disorders.

Prehospital Management. If the patient is asymptomatic, close observation is all that is necessary. Treatment is only required if hypotension or ventricular irritability is present. In this situation, administer atropine 0.5 to 1.0 mg every 3 to 5 minutes until a satisfactory rate has been achieved or a total of 3 mg of the drug has been given. Early application of transcutaneous cardiac pacing may also be beneficial.

Accelerated Junctional Rhythm

Description. An accelerated junctional rhythm is one that results from increased automaticity in the AV junction causing the AV junction to discharge faster than its intrinsic rate. If the rate is fast enough (> 60), the AV node can override the SA node.

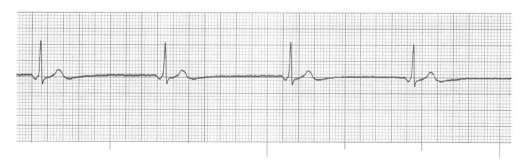

Figure 3–22.
Junctional rhythm.

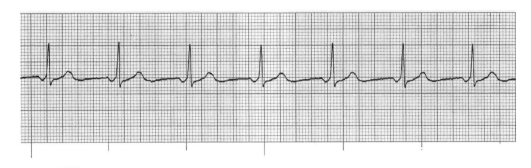

Figure 3–23.
Accelerated junctional rhythm.

Etiology. Accelerated junctional rhythms often result from ischemia of the AV junction, acute myocardial infarction (especially inferior wall infarction), and digitalis toxicity.

ECG Characteristics/Lead II Monitoring. (Figure 3–23.) All the characteristics described for junctional escape rhythm apply, except for ventricular rate. In accelerated junctional rhythm the ventricular rate is between 60 and 100 beats per minute.

Clinical Implication. Accelerated junctional rhythm is usually well tolerated. However, because ischemia or infarction are often etiologic events, the patient should be closely monitored.

Prehospital Management. Treatment is usually unnecessary. Investigation as to and correction of the underlying cause is the goal of therapy.

Paroxysmal Junctional Tachycardia

Description. Paroxysmal junctional tachycardia (PJT), a form of paroxysmal supraventricular tachycardia, develops when rapid AV junctional depolarization overrides the natural firing rate of the SA node. It may be caused by increased automaticity or a reentry circuit within the AV node of junctional tissue.

Etiology. Paroxysmal junctional tachycardia may occur at any age and may be associated with underlying heart disease. It is frequently associated with arteriosclerotic heart disease, rheumatic heart disease, myocardial infarction, heart failure, and digitalis toxicity.

ECG Characteristics/Lead II Monitoring. (Figure 3–24.)

- Rate: 100 to 180/min
- Rhythm: Essentially regular, except at its onset and termination
- Pacemaker site: Ectopic pacemaker in the AV junction
- P waves: P waves may be present or absent. When present, they either precede or follow each QRS complex and are inverted. Their absence indicates that the P wave is buried within the QRS complex.
- PR interval: If the P wave occurs before the QRS complex, the PR interval will be less than 0.12 sec. If it occurs after the QRS complex, the R–P interval is less than 0.20 seconds.
- QRS complex: Usually normal (0.04 to 0.12 sec), unless ventricular conduction is delayed

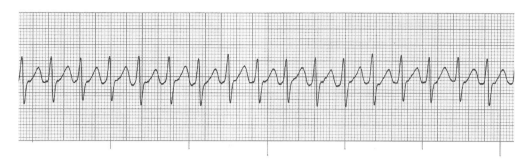

Figure 3–24.
Paroxysmal junctional tachycardia.

Clinical Implication. PJT may be well tolerated for a short period of time in healthy hearts with good cardiac reserve. Eventually, rapid rates will compromise cardiac output and coronary artery perfusion due to inadequate ventricular filling and a reduction in the length of diastole. PJT may precipitate angina, hypotension, or congestive heart failure.

Prehospital Management. Treatment for PJT is identical to that of paroxysmal supraventricular tachycardia. Therapy includes vagal stimulation, pharmacologic (Adenocard, verapamil, and diltiazem), and electrical intervention.

DYSRHYTHMIAS ORIGINATING IN THE VENTRICLES

Ventricular dysrhythmias are rhythm disturbances caused by ectopic impulses that originate below the AV node in any part of the ventricles. Many factors, including ischemia, hypoxia, increased sympathetic tone, and adverse medication effects have been identified as causes. Since the abnormal impulses originate in the ventricle, the normal route of depolarization is bypassed. This prevents the simultaneous depolarization of the right and left ventricles that normally occurs. Instead, the impulse must travel a longer circuitous route in order to stimulate the ventricles. This results in a widened, bizarrely shaped QRS complex that is greater than 0.12 seconds in duration. In addition, P waves will be absent because atrial activation does not occur. Ventricular dysrhythmias of major importance include ventricular escape complexes and rhythms, premature ventricular complexes, ventricular tachycardia, ventricular fibrillation, and asystole.

Ventricular Escape Complexes and Rhythms (Idioventricular Rhythm)

Description. A ventricular escape beat, or ventricular escape rhythm, is a dysrhythmia that results when impulses from higher pacemakers fail to reach the ventricles or the rate of discharge of the higher pacemakers becomes less than that of the ventricles (20 to 40 beats per minute). Ventricular escape rhythms serve as a safety mechanism to prevent cardiac standstill.

Etiology. Ventricular escape complexes and ventricular rhythms have several etiologies. These include slowing of supraventricular pacemaker sites or high-degree AV block, acute MI, and cardiomyopathy. Frequently, they are the first organized rhythms seen following successful defibrillation.

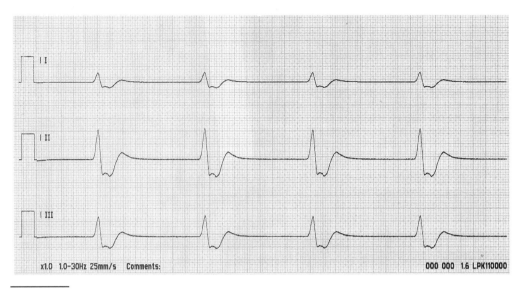

Figure 3–25.
Idioventricular rhythm.

ECG Characteristics. (Figure 3–25.)

- Rate: 20 to 40/min (occasionally less)
- Rhythm: Irregular, if a single escape complex is present. Regular, if a ventricular escape rhythm is present unless the pacemaker site originates very low in the conduction system.
- Pacemaker site: Ventricle
- P waves: None
- PR interval: None
- QRS complex: Greater than 0.12 sec and bizarre in shape

Clinical Implication. Slow heart rate can significantly decrease cardiac output. Hypotension and decreased perfusion to the brain and other vital organs may occur. The ventricular escape rhythm serves as a safety mechanism and should not be suppressed. Escape rhythms can be classified as perfusing (those with pulses) or nonperfusing (those without pulses) and treated accordingly.

Prehospital Management. If the escape rhythm is perfusing, therapy is directed at increasing the heart rate (refer to Figure 3–18). Administer 0.5 to 1.0 mg of atropine every 3 to 5 minutes until a satisfactory rate has been obtained or a total of 3 mg of the drug has been given. Early application of transcutaneous pacing must also be considered. If the rhythm is nonperfusing, follow the pulseless electrical activity (PEA) protocol.

Premature Ventricular Complexes (Contractions)

Description. A premature ventricular complex (PVC) is a single ectopic impulse, arising from an irritable focus in either ventricle, that occurs earlier than the next expected beat of the underlying rhythm. It may result from increased automaticity in the ectopic cell or a reentry mechanism. PVCs appear wide and bizarre because ventricular depolarization does not follow the normal conduction pathway. This abnormal depolarization sequence also results in an abnormality of repolarization, causing the T wave to be directed opposite the QRS complex. PVCs do not usually depolarize the SA node. Therefore, the prolonged pause following a PVC is fully compensatory. This means that the duration of two cycles, including the premature ventricular complex, is the same as the duration of two normal cycles. A compensatory pause is commonly observed because the ventricular ectopic impulse traveling retrogradely fails to reach the SA node. Sinus discharge remains undisturbed, and the basic underlying rhythm is preserved. On the ECG it is assessed by measuring the distance between the two normally conducted sinus beats that flank the PVC and comparing them with the baseline R–R interval.

Etiology. PVCs may occur in healthy persons with apparently healthy hearts and without apparent cause. Frequent PVCs may be caused by increased sympathetic tone (as in emotional stress), stimulants (e.g., alcohol, caffeine, and tobacco), excessive administration of digitalis or sympathomimetic drugs, hypoxia, ischemia, electrolyte imbalance, or congestive heart failure. PVCs often occur in the setting of acute myocardial infarction, and in this case require suppression as they can trigger more lethal ventricular dysrhythmias.

Types of PVCs.

- Infrequent PVCs: Less than five PVCs/min
- Frequent PVCs: Five or more PVCs/min
- Isolated PVCs: PVCs occurring independently
- Interpolated PVCs: PVC sandwiched between two normal sinus beats that does not disturb the underlying rhythm
- Paired PVCs (couplet): Two PVCs in succession
- Group beats (salvos): PVCs occurring in groups of two or more
- R on T phenomenon: PVC occurs on or near the peak of a previous T wave (relative refractory period). This is a vulnerable period of ventricular repolarization when PVCs may predispose a patient to ventricular tachycardia or fibrillation.
- Ventricular tachycardia: Three or more PVCs in succession
- Uniform PVCs (also known as unifocal): PVCs of identical shape that originate from a single ectopic focus
- Multiform PVCs (also known as multifocal): PVCs that vary in their site of origin and hence their appearance. Multiform PVCs are typically associated with myocardial ischemia and are therefore considered more dangerous than unifocal.

Patterns of PVCs.

- Bigeminy: PVC occurring every other beat
- Trigeminy: PVC occurring every third beat
- Quadrigeminy: PVC occurring every fourth beat

ECG Characteristics. (Figure 3–26.)

- Rate: Depends on the underlying rhythm and rate of PVCs
- Rhythm: Irregular; PVCs interrupt the regularity of the underlying rhythm
- Pacemaker site: An ectopic pacemaker in the ventricle, specifically in the bundle branches, Purkinje fibers, or ventricular myocardium
- P waves: None preceding the ectopic QRS complex
- PR interval: None
- QRS complex: Greater than 0.12 sec and bizarre in morphology as the ectopic impulse takes longer than normal to depolarize the

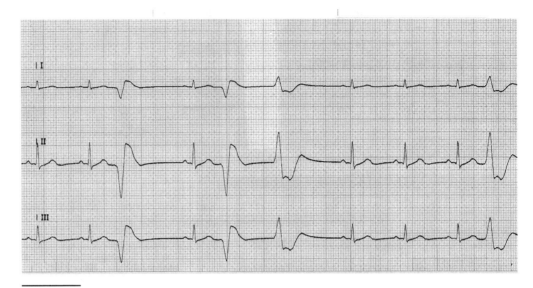

Figure 3–26.
Premature ventricular complexes.

ventricles. The ST segment and T wave slope in the opposite direction from the QRS complex.

Clinical Implication. Isolated premature ventricular complexes in patients without underlying heart disease are usually of no significance and do not require treatment. In patients with myocardial ischemia or infarction, PVCs may indicate ventricular irritability and predispose individuals to more lethal ventricular dysrhythmias. Certain situations have been identified in which PVCs pose an increased risk of triggering ventricular tachycardia or fibrillation. These are summarized below in the rules on malignancy.

- More than 6 PVCs per minute
- R on T phenomenon
- Couplets or runs of ventricular tachycardia
- Mutiform PVCs
- PVCs associated with ischemic chest pain

Prehospital Management. Treatment of PVCs should be guided by the clinical setting. If the patient has no history of cardiac disease and no symptoms, and if the PVCs are nonmalignant, no treatment is required. If the patient has a history of heart disease or symptoms, or if the PVCs are malignant, administer lidocaine at a dose of 1.0 to 1.5 mg/kg. Additional lidocaine by bolus or infusion can be given every 5 to 10 minutes if necessary, until a total of 3.0 mg/kg has been administered. If lidocaine fails to suppress the PVCs, procainamide or bretylium should be considered. (See Chapter 9)

Ventricular Tachycardia

Description. Ventricular tachycardia (VT) is a rapid rhythm created by three or more premature ventricular complexes in succession at a rate in excess of 100 beats per minute. This rhythm overrides the primary pacemaker of the heart and results in atrioventricular dissociation (atria and ventricles function independently). P waves may occasionally be seen, but have no relationship to the QRS complexes. Ventricular tachycardia is often associated with dramatic clinical signs and symptoms, and if left untreated may degenerate into fatal ventricular fibrillation.

Etiology. Ventricular tachycardia usually occurs in the presence of significant heart disease. Most commonly, it occurs in the presence of coronary artery disease, particularly in the setting of myocardial ischemia and infarction. Electrolyte disturbances, increased sympathetic tone, and digitalis toxicity are also responsible for the development of ventricular tachycardia.

ECG Characteristics. (Figure 3–27.)

* Rate: 100 to 250/min (approximately)
* Rhythm: Usually regular, but may be slightly irregular
* Pacemaker site: Ectopic pacemaker in the ventricle
* P wave: If present, they are usually of the underlying rhythm and bear no relation to the QRS complexes (P waves may be found preceding, following, or buried within the QRS).
* PR interval: None
* QRS complex: Greater than 0.12 sec and bizarre in morphology. Usually they are identical but may vary slightly. When the QRS complexes vary greatly, gradually changing back and forth from one shape and direction to another, the VT is called *torsades de pointes* (Figure 3–28).

Clinical Implication. Clinically, ventricular tachycardia can have dire consequences. The rapid ventricular rate prevents adequate filling time for the heart, so cardiac output and coronary perfusion are drastically reduced, and patients suffer from hypotension. In addition, it may degenerate into ventricular fibrillation and cardiac arrest. Ventricular tachycardia may be either perfusing or nonperfusing, and this dictates the type of intervention.

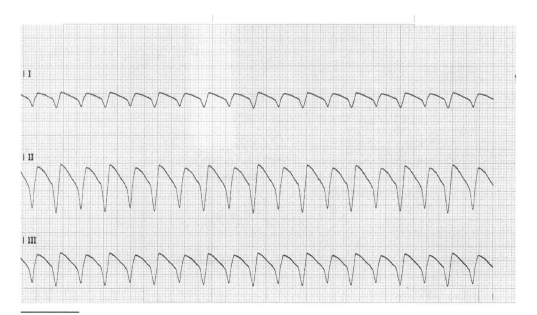

Figure 3–27.
Ventricular tachycardia.

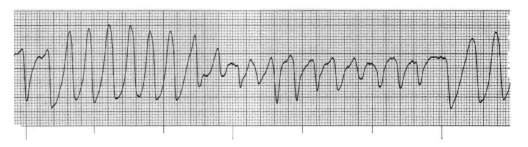

Figure 3–28.
Torsades de pointes.

Prehospital Management. Treatment of ventricular tachycardia depends on the clinical setting and the ability of the patient to tolerate the dysrhythmia. Some patients tolerate runs of ventricular tachycardia well and are able to maintain adequate cardiac output, while others experience precipitous falls in blood pressure and become pulseless. If the patient has no pulse (nonperfusing or pulseless VT), treat as for ventricular fibrillation. If the patient is stable or tolerating the rhythm (i.e., conscious, acceptable vital signs, no chest pain, etc.), proceed with intravenous lidocaine, procainamide, and/or bretylium. If VT persists or if the patient's condition becomes unstable, deliver one or more electrocardioversions at 100-200-300-360 joules. If the initial presentation of the patient is one that is unstable (e.g., unconscious, hypotension, chest pain, etc.), proceed directly to electrocardioversion at the energy setting previously described.

Ventricular Fibrillation

Description. Ventricular fibrillation (VF) is a chaotic ventricular rhythm usually resulting from the presence of many reentry circuits within the ventricles. It is a catastrophic dysrhythmia characterized by total disorganization of electrical activity in the heart. There is no ventricular depolarization or contraction and subsequently no cardiac output (pulselessness).

Etiology. A wide variety of causes have been associated with ventricular fibrillation. Most cases result from advanced coronary artery disease, myocardial ischemia, myocardial infarction, and third-degree atrioventricular block.

ECG Characteristics. (Figure 3–29.)

- Rate: None; no organized rhythm
- Rhythm: No organized rhythm
- Pacemaker site: Multiple ectopic foci throughout the ventricles
- P waves: Absent
- PR interval: Absent
- QRS complex: Absent, fibrillatory waves are present

NOTE: VF has no identifiable ECG waveforms. Instead an undulating, wavy baseline is present, composed of waveforms that vary in amplitude and morphology. Early in the course of VF, these fibrillatory waveforms are exaggerated and the rhythm is described as coarse VF. After several minutes of ventricular fibrillation, the fibrillatory waveforms become smaller and smaller, and the rhythm is

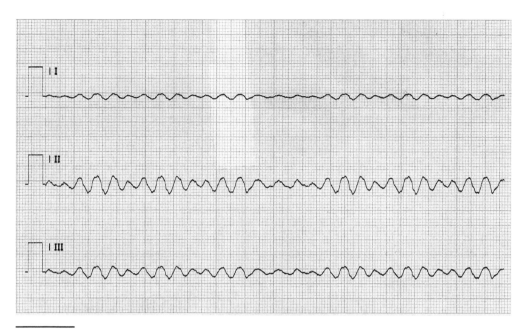

Figure 3–29.
Ventricular fibrillation.

described as fine VF. Fine ventricular fibrillation can commonly be mistaken for asystole.

Clinical Implication. Ventricular fibrillation is a lethal dysrhythmia. There is no cardiac output or organized electrical pattern, thus resulting in cardiac arrest.

Prehospital Management. Ventricular fibrillation and nonperfusing ventricular tachycardia are treated identically. Initiate CPR, and follow this with one or more immediate electrical defibrillations (countershocks) at 200-300-360 joules. Subsequently, control the airway and establish intravenous access. Epinephrine 1:10,000 is the drug of first choice and should be delivered every 3 to 5 minutes as required. If unsuccessful, consider lidocaine, bretylium, magnesium, or possibly sodium bicarbonate.

Asystole (Cardiac Standstill)

Description. Ventricular asystole is characterized by the complete absence of all cardiac electrical activity.

Etiology. Asystole may be the primary event in cardiac arrest when the dominant pacemaker (SA node) and/or escape pacemaker in the AV junction fail to generate electrical impulses or when the electrical impulses are blocked from entering the ventricle. It is usually associated with massive myocardial ischemia, injury, and necrosis.

ECG Characteristics. (Figure 3–30.)

- Rate: None; no electrical activity
- Rhythm: None; no electrical activity
- Pacemaker site: None
- P waves: Absent

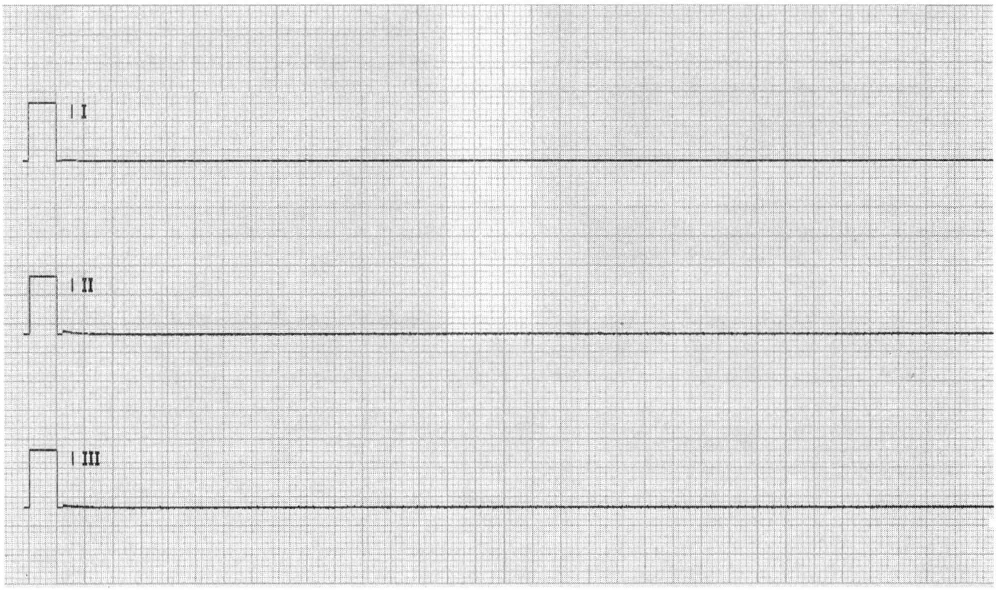

Figure 3–30.
Asystole.

- PR interval: Absent
- QRS complex: Absent

Clinical Implication. Asystole results in cardiac arrest. The prognosis for resuscitation is poor.

Prehospital Management. Asystole is treated with CPR, airway management, oxygenation, and medications. If there is any doubt as to whether the rhythm is asystole or fine ventricular fibrillation, attempt defibrillation. Pharmacological therapy includes epinephrine, atropine, and in certain situations, sodium bicarbonate. Transcutaneous pacing may also be beneficial for asystole.

ARTIFICIAL PACEMAKER RHYTHMS

Description. An artificial pacemaker rhythm is a rhythm created by an electronic device that generates and transmits an electrical signal to the heart through an electrode implanted in the atria, ventricle, or both. The pacemaker lead may be implanted in any of several locations in the heart, although it is most often placed in the right ventricle or in both chambers (dual-chambered pacemakers). Most pacemakers function as an electrical backup system, keeping the heart rate fast enough to prevent rate-related clinical symptoms.

Pacemakers may be implanted on a temporary or permanent basis, depending on the clinical condition. Temporary pacing is appropriate in emergency situations (i.e., ventricular asystole) or if there is risk of symptomatic bradycardia, as in patients with transient atrioventricular block (especially associated with myocardial ischemia). Permanent pacing does not automatically follow temporary pacing and is used in acquired third-degree block, AV block associated with myocardial infarction, and sick sinus syndrome with episodes of severe bradycardia. Both temporary and permanent pacemakers are easily recognized by the presence of vertical spikes, which are the electrical impulses released by the pacemaker generator and conducted to the heart.

Types of Pacemakers. There are two basic models of pacemakers: fixed rate and demand. Fixed rate pacemakers are designed to fire constantly at a preset rate without regard to the patient's own inherent beats. Demand pacemakers contain a sensing device that will only discharge when the natural rate of the heart falls below the preset value established for the pacemaker.

Single Versus Dual Chamber Pacing. Pacemakers can be single chamber pacemakers that pace either the ventricles or atria or, dual chamber pacemakers (AV sequential pacemakers) that pace both the atria and ventricles. Dual chamber pacemakers stimulate the atria first and then the ventricles. These are beneficial for patients with marginal cardiac output who require the extra atrial stimulation (atrial kick), thus ensuring adequate ventricular filling.

ECG Characteristics. (Figure 3–31.)

* Rate: Varies with the present rate of the pacemaker; usually between 60 to 70/min

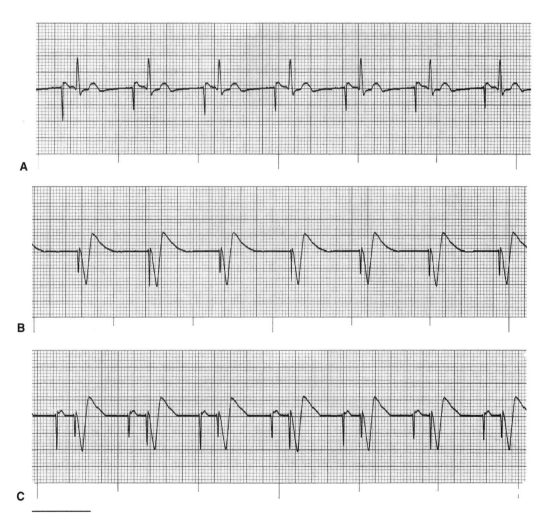

A

B

C

Figure 3–31.
Artificial pacemaker rhythms.
(A) Atrial pacemaker. (B) Ventricular pacemaker. (C) Dual–chambered pacemaker.

- Rhythm: Regular if pacing constantly; irregular if pacing on demand
- Pacemaker site: Depends on electrode placement of the pacemaker. Ventricular pacing is commonly positioned in the apex of the right ventricular cavity, while atrial pacing is positioned in the right atrium.
- Pacemaker spikes: Electrical discharge from an artificial pacemaker produces a narrow upward or downward deflection (biphasic) from the isoelectric line. This deflection, known as a pacemaker spike, is an artifact created each time the pacemaker discharges. A pacemaker lead positioned in the atria produces a spike followed by a P wave. In contrast, a pacemaker lead positioned in the ventricles produces a spike followed by a wide (0.12 sec and greater) and bizarre QRS complex. A P wave or QRS complex following a pacemaker spike indicates electrical capture. A pacemaker spike not followed by a P wave or QRS complex indicates that the pacemaker is discharging, but not capturing. Mechanical capture (myocardial contraction) is evidenced by the presence of a palpable pulse.
- P waves: No P waves are produced by ventricular pacemakers. Sinus P waves may be seen, but are unrelated to the paced QRS complexes. Dual-chambered pacemakers produce a P wave behind each atrial spike.
- PR interval: If present, may be normal (0.12 to 0.20 sec) or abnormal depending on the rhythm
- QRS complex: QRS complexes associated with pacemaker rhythms are 0.12 sec or greater and bizarre in morphology. Each ventricular pacemaker spike should be followed by a QRS complex.

Problems with Pacemakers. The majority of pacemaker malfunctions result from abnormalities in sensing, firing, or capturing. Sensing is the ability of the pacemaker to process (or see) intrinsic electrical signals. Failure to sense is the inability of the pacemaker to properly identify ECG waveforms (P waves and/or QRS complexes), resulting in paced beats appearing too early, too late, or not at all. Pacemaker firing indicates that the pacemaker generator has delivered a stimulus to the myocardium and a spike is produced. Therefore, failure to fire means that a pacing spike fails to appear when it should and both electrical and mechanical activity do not occur. Failure to capture implies that the expected waveform fails to appear after the pacing spike and depolarization of the heart does not occur. This is common with temporary pacemakers. Additionally, although rare, battery failure and a runaway pacemaker may occur, resulting in no pacing or a rapid rate of electrical discharge.

Considerations for Management. Treatment of bradydysrhythmis, asystole, and ventricular fibrillation resulting from pacemaker failure are treated with standard intervention. Caution should be exercised, however, when defibrillating patients with implanted pacemakers. Never discharge the defibrillatory paddles directly over the battery pack. Position the paddles (or pads) a few inches away from the battery pack and deliver the shock as usual. Patients with pacemaker failure should be promptly transported without prolonged field intervention, as definitive care consists of battery replacement or temporary pacemaker insertion.

DYSRHYTHMIAS RESULTING FROM DISORDERS OF CONDUCTION (AV BLOCKS)

Atrioventricular (AV) blocks represent prolonged, intermittent, or absent conduction between the atria and ventricles. These dysrhythmias are caused by pathology of the AV junctional tissue or less often a physiological block, such as occurs with atrial fibrillation or flutter. Specific etiologies include AV junctional ischemia or necrosis, degenerative disease of the conduction system, and drug toxicity (especially digitalis). AV block is classified into three types: (1) first-degree atrioventricular block, which is only a prolongation in the time for each atrial impulse to reach the ventricles; (2) second-degree atrioventricular block, in which some of the atrial impulses are not conducted to the ventricles; (3) third-degree atrioventricular block or complete block, in which none of the atrial impulses are conducted to the ventricles. All three varieties are diagnosed by carefully examining the relationship of the P wave to the QRS complexes.

First-Degree Atrioventricular Block

Description. A first-degree AV block is not an actual block, but rather a delay in conduction at the level of the AV node. The wave of depolarization spreads normally through the atria, but upon reaching the AV node is held up for longer than the usual one-tenth of a second. As a result, the PR intervals are prolonged (> 0.20 sec), but every atrial impulse eventually makes its way through to activate the ventricles (P wave precedes each QRS). First-degree AV block is not a rhythm in itself, but a condition superimposed upon another rhythm. Therefore, when diagnosing first-degree block, the underlying rhythm must also be identified (for example, sinus bradycardia with first-degree AV block).

Etiology. AV block can occur in healthy hearts. However, ischemia at the AV junction is the most common cause. Other causes include drug toxicity, hyperkalemia, and myocardial infarction (especially inferior wall MI).

ECG Characteristics. (Figure 3–32.)

- Rate: Depends on the underlying rhythm. Atrial and ventricular rates are typically the same.
- Rhythm: Usually regular. However, it can be slightly irregular.
- Pacemaker site: SA node or the atria
- P waves: Normal
- PR interval: Greater than 0.20 sec (diagnostic)
- QRS complex: Usually normal (< 0.12 sec), unless a preexisting intraventricular conduction disturbance is present.

Clinical Implication. First-degree block does not by itself produce symptoms and is usually of no danger. However, a newly developed first-degree block may be a forerunner of a more advanced block.

Prehospital Management. Generally, no treatment is required except observation and continuous ECG monitoring.

Second-Degree Atrioventricular Block (Mobitz Type I or Wenckebach)

Description. A second-degree AV block (Mobitz I) is an intermittent block most often occurring at the level of the AV node. It is the result of progressive impairment of conduction through the AV node. Mobitz I produces a characteristics cyclic pattern in

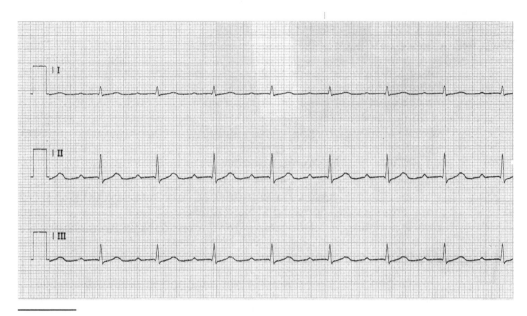

Figure 3–32.
First-degree atrioventricular block.

which each successive atrial impulse encounters a longer and longer delay in the AV node until one impulse (usually every third or fourth) fails to make it through (not conducted). What you see on the ECG is a progressive lengthening of the PR interval with each beat, until a QRS complex fails to appear after a P wave (dropped beat). Following the dropped beat, during which no QRS appears, the sequence repeats itself over and over, often with impressive regularity. The ratio of conduction (P waves to QRS complexes) is commonly 5:4, 4:3, 3:2, or 2:1. This pattern may be constant or variable depending on the ability of the AV node to recover following the interruption of transmission.

Etiology. AV blocks most commonly represent defective conduction of the electrical impulse through the AV node. Typically, ischemia at the level of the AV junction is the most common cause, but increased parasympathetic tone and drug effects (e.g., digitalis, propranolol, and diltiazem or verapamil) are also common etiologies.

ECG Characteristics. (Figure 3–33.)

- Rate: Atrial rate is that of the underlying rhythm. Ventricular rate will be less than the atrial rate because of the nonconducted impulses.
- Rhythm: Atrial rhythm is essentially regular. Ventricular rhythm is irregular (R–R interval) owing to the dropped beats, causing the QRS complexes to appear clustered together (pairs or groups of beats).
- Pacemaker site: SA node or atria
- P waves: Normal; some P waves are not followed by QRS complexes
- PR interval: Gradual progression until a QRS complex is dropped. The first PR interval in a group of beats may be normal or prolonged. Subsequent PR intervals lengthen in smaller and smaller increments. The cycle is then repeated.

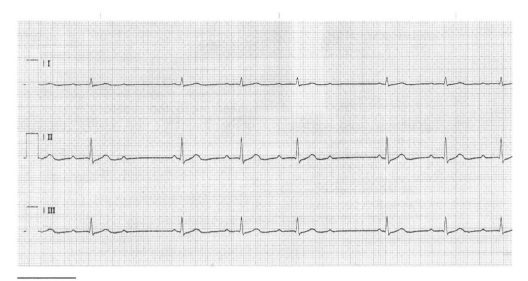

Figure 3–33.
Second-degree atrioventricular block Mobitz Type I.

- QRS complex: Usually less than 0.12 sec. It may be bizarre in shape if a preexisting intraventricular conduction disturbance is present.

NOTE: The diagnosis of Mobitz I requires the progressive lengthening of each successive PR interval until one P wave fails to penetrate the AV node and is therefore not followed by a QRS complex.

Clinical Implication. If impulse transmission is frequently blocked, second-degree block can compromise cardiac output and produce associated symptoms (e.g., syncope, angina, etc.). Often, Mobitz I is a transient and reversible phenomenon that occurs immediately following an inferior wall infarction.

Prehospital Management. Because most patients remain clinically asymptomatic, definitive therapy is usually unnecessary. In the majority of patients, observation and continuous ECG monitoring is all that is required. If extreme or symptomatic bradycardia does develop, the administration of 0.5 to 1.0 mg of atropine every 3 to 5 minutes is warranted. If atropine fails to accelerate the dysrhythmia or a total of 3 mg has been administered, transcutaneous pacing should be immediately employed.

Second-Degree Atrioventricular Block (Mobitz Type II)

Description. Second-degree AV block (Mobitz II), like Mobitz I, describes a situation in which not every atrial impulse is conducted to the ventricles. However, progressive lengthening of the PR interval does not occur. Instead, conduction is an all-or-none phenomenon. The ECG displays two or more normal beats with normal PR intervals and then a P wave that is not followed by a QRS complex (dropped beat). The cycle is then repeated. The ratio of conduction (P waves to QRS complexes) is commonly 4:1, 3:1, or 2:1 and may be constant or variable. In addition, the location of the Mobitz II block is found most often below the bundle of His (within the bundle branch system). Because the block is further down the conduction system, the ventricles do not depolarize simultaneously; hence, the QRS complex may be prolonged or widened.

Etiology. Second-degree AV block (Mobitz II) is usually associated with acute anterior wall myocardial infarction and septal necrosis. Unlike Mobitz I, it rarely results from increased parasympathetic tone.

ECG Characteristics. (Figure 3–34.)

- Rate: Atrial rate is that of the underlying rhythm. Ventricular rate is typically less than that of the atrial rate and is usually bradycardic.
- Rhythm: Atrial rhythm is regular. Ventricular rhythm is regular or irregular depending upon whether the conduction ratio is constant or variable.
- Pacemaker site: SA node or atria
- P waves: Normal; some P waves are not followed by QRS complexes.
- PR interval: Constant or fixed for the conducted beats; may be greater than 0.20 sec.
- QRS complex: May be normal (< 0.12 sec), but is often greater because of the abnormal ventricular depolarization sequence (bundle branch block).

NOTE: The diagnosis of Mobitz II requires the presence of a dropped beat without progressive lengthening of the PR interval.

Clinical Implication. Clinically, Mobitz II block reflects progressive disease of the conduction system. Cardiac output is often compromised, causing problems such as syncope, angina, and decreased coronary perfusion. Because this block is often associated with myocardial infarction, it is considered much more dangerous than Mobitz I. Many Mobitz II blocks progress to full blocks (third-degree) or asystole.

Prehospital Management. Definitive treatment of Mobitz II block requires the insertion of an electronic pacemaker. In the field, 0.5 to 3.0 mg total of atropine may be adminis-

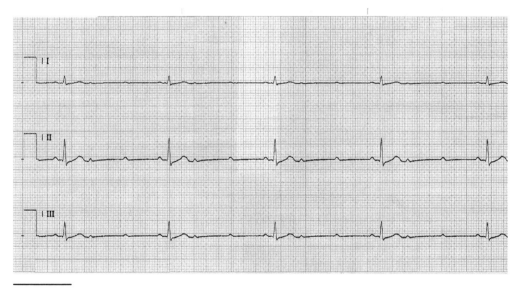

Figure 3–34.
Second-degree atrioventricular block Mobitz Type II.

tered, along with the immediate application of transcutaneous pacing. Never delay the use of transcutaneous pacing while awaiting IV access or for atropine to take effect. Atropine should be used cautiously in patients with high-grade blocks (Mobitz II and third-degree), as it may accelerate atrial rate, but worsen the AV nodal block. If the patient continues to remain clinically unstable, an infusion of dopamine or epinephrine may be considered.

Third-Degree Atrioventricular Block

Description. A third-degree AV block, also called complete heart block (CHB), is the absence of conduction between the atria and the ventricles resulting from complete electrical obstruction at or below the AV node. The atria and ventricles subsequently pace the heart independent of each other. In other words, P waves appear at one rate, whereas QRS complexes, unrelated to the P waves, appear at a slower rate. Because the block is complete (i.e., no atrial impulses are conducted to the ventricles), a secondary pacemaker will arise in the automatic cells of the atrioventricular junction or Purkinje system. The rate at which these ectopic pacemakers will fire is dependent upon their inherent automaticities. For example, a junctional pacemaker will discharge at 40 to 60 beats per minute, while a Purkinje pacemaker will fire approximately 30 times per minute. Thus, the ventricular rhythm in third-degree block usually produces severe bradycardia. In addition, the location of the pacemaker will determine the morphology of the QRS complex.

Etiology. The causes of third-degree block are immense and include all the conditions that produce first- and second-degree blocks, but in more advanced forms. In elderly individuals it most commonly results from chronic degeneration of the conduction system.

ECG Characteristics. (Figure 3–35.)

- Rate: Atrial rate is that of the underlying rhythm. Ventricular rate is 40 to 60/min if the escape pacemaker is junctional. It is less than 40/min if the escape pacemaker is from the ventricles.
- Rhythm: Both atrial and ventricular rhythms are usually regular.

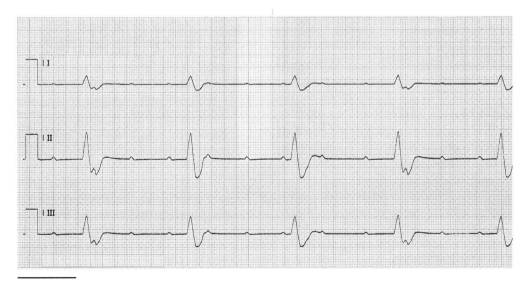

Figure 3–35.
Third-degree atrioventricular block (complete heart block).

- Pacemaker sites: SA node and AV junction or ventricle
- P waves: Normal in morphology, but atrioventricular dissociation is present (no relationship between P waves and QRS complexes).
- PR interval: No relationship between P waves and R waves
- QRS complex: Greater than 0.12 sec if the pacemaker is ventricular; less than 0.12 sec if the pacemaker is junctional.

NOTE: The diagnosis of third-degree block requires the presence of AV dissociation in which the ventricular rate is slower than the sinus or atrial rate.

Clinical Implication. Third-degree AV block is a serious conduction abnormality because it leads to the formation of secondary pacemakers that produce severe bradycardia. Cardiac output is dangerously compromised and blood flow to vital organs may be inadequate.

Prehospital Management. Because third-degree block is often accompanied by rate-related symptoms, therapy is designed either to accelerate conduction through the AV node or to support the ventricular rate. In patients with a transient block who are symptomatic, a temporary electronic pacemaker is employed, whereas patients with chronic third-degree block require permanent artificial pacing. In the field, immediate transcutaneous pacing is necessary for the treatment of symptomatic third-degree block with wide QRS complexes (regardless of the cause) and for asymptomatic third-degree block with wide QRS complexes in the setting of acute anterior wall myocardial infarction. Additionally, the intravenous administration of atropine in therapeutic doses (0.5 mg) may be given.

KEY POINTS SUMMARY

The Electrocardiogram

1. The electrocardiogram (ECG) is a graphic display of the electrical forces generated by the heart. Evidence of these forces is detected by electrodes placed on the surface of the body. Electrical forces may be seen as either a positive (upright) deflection or a negative (downward) deflection on the ECG.

ECG Leads

2. ECG leads are of two types, bipolar and unipolar. Bipolar leads measure electrical forces between a negative and positive electrode. Unipolar leads use a single positive electrode and an indifferent reference point created electronically.
3. Bipolar leads are leads I, II, and III. Lead II is the most common monitoring lead used in out-of-hospital cardiac care.
4. Unipolar leads consist of three augmented voltage leads and six precordial (chest) leads. These leads are used primarily for diagnostic (12-lead) electrocardiography.

ECG Graph Paper

5. ECG graph paper is specialized paper used to record the sequence of electrical events as they occur through the conduction system. The paper is standardized to allow for comparative analysis of ECG waveforms and intervals. Horizontal lines measure time in seconds and distance in millimeters. Vertical lines measure voltage in millimeters. Each small square represents 0.04 sec of time or 1 mm. Each large box represents 0.20 sec of time or 5 mm. Standard calibration of the ECG is 10 mm or 1 mV.

Sequence of Electrical Conduction

6. The flow of current in the heart's electrical field normally originates in the atria with right atrial activation preceding the left. Following stimulation of the atria, the impulse activates the AV node and travels down the bundle of His. Ventricular activation follows, beginning with the septum. Once the septum has been activated, the impulse spreads to both the right and left ventricular walls. All of these events are represented on the ECG as a series of complexes and intervals.

Electrocardiographic Waveforms

7. The electrocardiogram consists of five waveforms or deflections arbitrarily labeled the P, QRS, and T waves.
8. The P wave represents depolarization of the atria. The normal P wave is small and round and less than 3 mm in amplitude and width.
9. The QRS complex represents depolarization of the ventricles. Its normal duration (width) is 0.04 sec to 0.12 sec.
10. The QRS complex is a collective term that consists of three distinct waveforms, a Q wave, R wave, and S wave.
    - The Q wave is the first negative deflection following the P wave. It represents depolarization of the intraventricular septum. When present, Q waves are narrow and small (< 25% of the succeeding R wave).
    - The R wave is the first positive deflection following the P wave. R waves represent the majority of ventricular depolarization.
    - The S wave is the first negative deflection following the R wave. S waves represent the final stages of ventricular depolarization.
11. The T wave represents repolarization of the ventricles. Its shape is normally round and asymmetrical.
12. An additional wave, the U wave, is a small rounded wave of low voltage occasionally seen following the T wave. Its origin remains unclear, but it is suggested to represent repolarization of the Purkinje fibers.

Segments and Intervals

13. Segments and intervals are the different straight lines on the ECG connecting the various waves on the ECG. These include the PR interval, ST segment, and QT interval.
14. The PR interval represents atrial depolarization and a delay at the AV junction. Its duration is between 0.12 and 0.20 sec and is measured from the beginning of the P wave to the beginning of the QRS complex.

15. The ST segment represents the period of time between ventricular depolarization and repolarization. It is the straight line connecting the end of the QRS complex with the beginning of the T wave. The ST segment is normally isoelectric (flat) and gradually blends into the upslope of the T wave. Elevation of the ST segment is the hallmark of myocardial injury, while ST segment depression is highly suggestive of ischemia.

16. The QT interval represents the depolarization and repolarization sequence of the ventricles. It is measured from the beginning of the QRS complex to the end of the T wave. Normal QT intervals vary with heart rate, sex, and age.

17. The R–R interval represents the time between two ventricular depolarizations. It is measured from the beginning of the R wave in one complete cycle to the onset of the R wave in the next cycle. The R–R interval is used to calculate ventricular rate and regularity.

Rhythm Strip Analysis and Interpretation

18. ECG analysis and interpretation requires a systematic approach to ensure the proper evaluation of all complexes and intervals. The following steps provide the necessary information needed to analyze rhythm strips and interpret dysrhythmias.
    - Obtain a 6-second rhythm strip and ensure proper calibration (1 mV)
    - Determine the cardiac rate
    - Determine the regularity of the rhythm
    - Analyze the P waves to ensure their presence and regularity
    - Measure the PR interval
    - Examine the QRS complex for its presence, regularity, and duration
    - Measure the QT interval

Dysrhythmogenesis (Origin of Dysrhythmias)

19. A dysrhythmia is defined as a disturbance in the heart's normal rate and rhythm.

20. Factors that influence the development of dysrhythmias include ischemia, electrolyte disturbances, autonomic nervous system imbalances, hypothermia, drug effects or toxicity, electrical shock, and many other causes. All of these potentiate the formation of dysrhythmias by altering automaticity, conductivity, or a combination of the two.

Classification of Dysrhythmias

21. Dysrhythmias are commonly classified according to their anatomical site of origin. These include dysrhythmias that originate in the sinoatrial node, atrioventricular node, atrioventricular junction, and ventricles. Two other classes of dysrhythmias include artificial pacemaker rhythms and dysrhythmias resulting from disorders of conduction.

BIBLIOGRAPHY

Atwood S, Stanton C, Storey J. *Introduction to Basic Cardiac Dysrhythmias*. St. Louis, MO: Mosby; 1990.

Blesdsoe BE, Porter RS, Shade BR. *Paramedic Emergency Care*. Englewood Cliffs, NJ: Prentice-Hall Inc.; 1994.

Caroline NL. *Emergency Care in the Streets*. Boston, MA: Little, Brown, and Company; 1995.

Conover MB. *Understanding Electrocardiography: Arrhythmias and the 12-Lead ECG*. St. Louis, MO: Mosby; 1992.

Foster DB. *Twelve Lead-Electrocardiography for ACLS Providers*. Philadelphia, PA: WB Saunders; 1996.

Huszar RJ. *Basic Dysrhythmias: Interpretation and Management*. St. Louis, MO: Mosby; 1994.

Johnson R, Swartz MH. *A Simplified Approach to Electrocardiography*. Philadelphia, PA: WB Saunders; 1986.

Lipman BC, Casio T. *ECG: Assessment and Interpretation*. Philadelphia, PA: FA Davis Company; 1994.

Marriot HJ. *Practical Electrocardiography*. Baltimore, MD: Williams and Wilkins; 1988.

Sanders MJ. *Mosby's Paramedic Textbook*. St. Louis, MO: Mosby; 1994.

Thaler MS. *The Only EKG Book You'll Ever Need*. Philadelphia, PA: JB Lippincott; 1988.

Walraven G. *Basic Arrhythmias*. Englewood Cliffs, NJ: Prentice-Hall Inc.; 1995.

4

The 12-Lead ECG and Electrical Axis

1. Describe the normal sequence of current flow in the heart.
2. Discuss two types of emergency electrocardiography and describe their roles.
3. Describe the 12-lead electrocardiogram and discuss the benefits associated with its use.
4. Describe the bipolar (frontal plane) leads and identify their anatomical placement.
5. Describe the unipolar (frontal plane) limb leads and identify their anatomical placement.
6. Differentiate a unipolar lead from a bipolar lead.
7. Describe the precordial (horizontal plane) leads and identify their anatomical placement.
8. Discuss the common ECG characteristics of limb and precordial leads.
9. Describe R wave progression and relate its importance to the electrocardiogram.
10. Describe modified chest leads and explain their monitoring and diagnostic significance.
11. Discuss special monitoring and diagnostic leads and identify those leads investigating the right ventricle.
12. Describe and discuss the use of 3-, 5-, and 10-wire portable monitoring systems.
13. Describe the four anatomical quadrants of the left ventricle as reflected in the 12-lead electrocardiogram.
14. Describe the acquisition of a 12-lead ECG utilizing a 12-lead ECG machine and a 3-lead ECG machine with a 12-lead ECG selection box.
15. Name the clinical uses of axis determination.
16. Describe the hexaxial reference system.
17. State the normal axis (in degrees) of the ventricular depolarization current.
18. Define left axis deviation, right axis deviation, and extreme axis deviation.
19. Discuss the different methods of calculating QRS axis.

INTRODUCTION

Your advanced life-support rescue unit is dispatched to a patient complaining of chest pain and difficulty breathing. Upon arrival, you and your crew find a 48-year-old male who is pale, diaphoretic, and clutching his chest. The patient states that he is suffering from a sudden onset of retrosternal chest discomfort with radiation into the left shoulder and arm. He describes the discomfort as crushing, occurring without exertion, and approximating two hours in duration. The patient rates the pain at seven on a scale of one to ten and reports that it has been up to ten. The patient also advises you that he has a family history of cardiovascular disease and is currently medicated for hypertension. Blood pressure is 142/88; pulse 86, regular and strong; respirations 24 and chest equal and clear bilaterally. The patient has palpable pulses in all extremities and the abdomen is soft and nontender.

Treatment of your patient begins with the application of oxygen via a nasal cannula. Pulse oximetry is applied, identifying an oxygen saturation of 96%. The patient is then placed on the cardiac monitor to ascertain a baseline tracing. An IV of lactated ringers is established at a keep open rate and two children's aspirin are administered by mouth (PO). Nitroglycerin is administered sublingually for pain, but the patient denies any relief. The acquisition of a 12-lead ECG is obtained and you verify the presence of a probable acute anterior wall myocardial infarction (MI). Immediately following, you contact the receiving medical center and initiate a cardiac alert. The attending emergency physician advises to continue with the implementation of acute myocardial infarction (AMI) protocol and administer morphine 1 to 3 mg IV, as required (PRN) for chest pain. En route to the hospital you complete a thrombolytic prescreening checklist of the patient and submit it along with your assessment findings to the physician and nursing team upon arrival. The patient's condition is rapidly reevaluated and he is successfully thrombolized within minutes.

The preceding scenario represents a typical event in the delivery of emergency medical care. Out-of-hospital recognition and treatment of acute myocardial infarction is an important paramedic skill. Proficiency not only requires the ability to adequately assess and perform a physical examination, but also the ability to interpret electrocardiographic data. For years prehospital health care practitioners have successfully employed the use of cardiac monitoring devices for interpreting the electrocardiogram (ECG) rhythm and identifying dysrhythmias. Today, however, with thrombolytic reperfusion the established therapy for acute myocardial infarction, the field use of diagnostic-quality 12-lead ECGs has become an integral part of the paramedic's arsenal for the early detection of infarction.

THE PHYSIOLOGICAL BASIS OF ELECTROCARDIOGRAPHY

As outlined in Chapters 2 and 3, the currents in the heart's electrical field flow in repetitive patterns with each cardiac cycle. Electrical flow normally originates in the atria, with right atrial activation preceding the left. Following stimulation of the atria, the impulse (electrical wave of depolarization) activates the atrioventricular (AV) node and travels down the bundle of His, which provides the electrical connection between the atria and ventricles. Ventricular activation follows, beginning with the septum (see Chapter 2). Septal activation proceeds in a left-to-right direction. Once the septum has been activated the impulse spreads to both the right and left ventricular walls. The right ventricle is activated first (a fraction of a second before the left) because it is a thinner muscle. Left ventricular activation then follows. Because of its large muscle mass, the left ventricle requires the greatest amount of electricity.

The electrical current produced during the cardiac cycle can be recorded on the surface of the body by an electrocardiograph. The electrocardiograph utilizes electrodes placed at various sites on the body to complete an electrical circuit and produce an ECG. These various electrode sites each produces a different view of the heart's electrical impulse with each referred to individually as a lead.

TYPES OF EMERGENCY ELECTROCARDIOGRAPHY

Emergency electrocardiography consists of two distinct and separate functions: (1) single-lead monitoring for dysrhythmia interpretation and (2) diagnostic 12-lead electrocardiography for identification of infarct and other cardiac disorders.

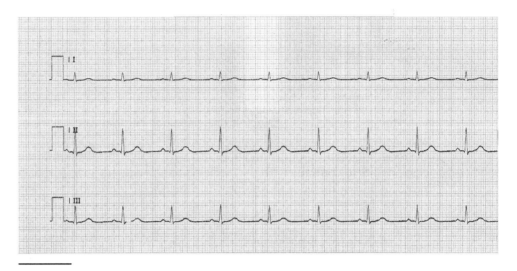

Figure 4–1.
Rhythm strip generated utilizing a monitor-quality device.
Note that all complexes and intervals are within normal limits and the ST segment is isoelectric. Monitor-quality devices are set at a narrow frequency window and are used only for dysrhythmia recognition.

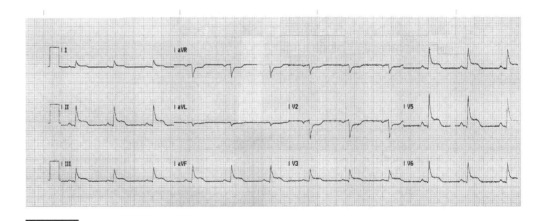

Figure 4–2.
Diagnostic electrocardiogram of the rhythm in 4–1.
Note that the ST segment is elevated throughout the tracing. Diagnostic devices are set at a wider frequency band in comparison to monitor devices and are thus able to provide accurate ST segment analysis.

MONITORING FOR DYSRHYTHMIAS

Identification of dysrhythmias is an essential prehospital skill outlined in Chapter 3. This mode of emergency electrocardiography generates tracings that show mainly the rhythm of cardiac events. Traditionally, dysrhythmia monitoring has been accomplished using monitor-quality devices that allow for evaluation of the relationship and intervals of the P, QRS, and T waves. In order to eliminate unwanted artifacts (60 cycle interference, muscle tremor, etc.), these devices are set at a narrow frequency window (Figure 4–1). That is, monitor-quality devices have less bandwidth and thus provide less information, making them useful only for rhythm monitoring. Accurate ST segment evaluations *cannot* be accomplished in monitor-quality ranges, therefore ST segment analysis should not be attempted with standard monitors. The advanced circuitry (greater bandwidth) of diagnostic monitors enables the acquisition of more information, thus allowing for accurate ST segment evaluation and the ability to anatomically locate pathology (Figure 4–2).

DIAGNOSTIC ELECTROCARDIOGRAPHY

Beyond dysrhythmia interpretation, a subset of emergency patients may benefit from a diagnostic surface electrocardiogram. These include those with chest pain (or any anginal equivalent), syncope, severe weakness and/or collapse, certain dysrhythmias, dyspnea, and a variety of other factors. The wide frequency band of the diagnostic ECG, when combined with the standard twelve leads and occasionally additional specific leads, is capable of providing the examiner with a plethora of diagnostic evidence. In addition to a host of cardiac disorders, the diagnostic ECG can provide evidence to support or establish the diagnosis of certain pulmonary disorders, electrolyte disturbances, hypothermia, etc. (see Chapter 7). Medical directors should provide clear guidelines within each system's protocol to establish the appropriate use of the diagnostic ECG. Some of the newer portable monitors have the ability to select either monitor or diagnostic modes of operation. The diagnostic frequency range allows for ST segment analysis and pacer spike identification.

THE 12-LEAD ELECTROCARDIOGRAM

The 12-lead ECG is a noninvasive diagnostic surface electrocardiogram composed of twelve leads that record the electrical activity in the heart from twelve different views. Each lead provides a unique picture of the electrical impulses transmitted from different regions within the heart to the surface of the body. The diagnosis of myocardial ischemia and infarction, as well as other cardiac disorders, requires the use of a multilead ECG. When cardiac monitoring is limited to a single lead, such as lead II, the eleven other views of myocardial electrical activity that can be recorded with a 12-lead electrocardiogram are omitted.

A 12-lead ECG consists of three bipolar leads and nine unipolar leads. Each lead is used to record atrial depolarization (P wave), ventricular depolarization (QRS complex), and ventricular repolarization (T wave). Of the twelve leads, six are frontal plane leads that utilize the patient's limbs as electrode sites and six are horizontal plane leads placed across the precordium. As with any cardiac monitoring device, 12-lead ECGs will record or demonstrate only the electrical activity of the heart. Mechanical activity must be evaluated through other means, such as pulse and blood pressure measurements.

TABLE 4–1 • **Major Prehospital Benefits of 12-Lead Electrocardiography**

1. Early recognition of myocardial injury patterns
2. Identification of the area of the heart involved in myocardial infarction
3. Identifying ischemic changes within myocardial tissues
4. Detection of prehospital ischemia that resolves prior to hospital arrival
5. Differentiation of high-risk cardiac patients vs. low-risk
6. Identification of those patients who are at risk for developing complete heart block
7. Differentiating wide-complex tachycardias
8. Electrical axis identification
9. Early delivery of thrombolytic therapy

BENEFITS OF 12-LEAD ELECTROCARDIOGRAPHY

The benefits associated with the use of 12-lead electrocardiography are immense (Table 4–1). Many studies have demonstrated the importance, accuracy, and effectiveness of utilizing multilead diagnostic electrocardiography in the field. The benefits of 12-lead ECGs include, but are not limited to, early recognition of myocardial injury patterns; identification of the area involved in infarction; differentiation of high-risk cardiac patients versus low-risk; identification of those patients who are at risk for developing complete heart block; differentiation of wide complex tachycardias; identification of ischemic changes within the myocardial tissues; and the detection of patients with prehospital ischemia that resolves prior to hospital arrival. The most significant prehospital benefit of 12-lead electrocardiography is a reduction in the amount of time elapsed between a patient's entry into the EMS system and the point at which an MI can be identified and thrombolytic therapy initiated. Furthermore, once infarction has been recognized and localized, certain specific complications may be anticipated. This allows for the design of improved treatment plans regarding pain relief, AV block, and hypotension.

FRONTAL PLANE LEADS

Three of the frontal plane leads utilize a negative electrode and a positive electrode in order to measure the difference in potential of the connected limbs. These leads are called bipolar limb leads and are referred to as lead I, lead II, and lead III. As previously described in Chapter 3, a bipolar lead consists of two electrodes of opposite polarity; one is a positive electrode and the other a negative electrode. When these electrodes are placed on the skin they measure the amount and direction of electrical forces (vector) generated between the two.

The bipolar limb leads constitute what is known as Einthoven's triangle (see Figure 3–2B). In lead I, the negative electrode is placed on the right arm and the positive electrode is placed on the left arm. Thus the measurement of electrical activity in lead I is from the right shoulder to the left shoulder so the axis of lead I runs from shoulder to shoulder (Figure 4–3). In lead II, the negative electrode is placed on the right arm and the positive electrode is placed on the left leg, so that the measurement of electrical activity in lead II is from the right shoulder to the left leg (Figure 4–4). In lead III, the negative electrode is placed on the left arm and the positive is placed on the left leg. Thus the measurement of electrical activity in lead III is from the left shoulder to the left leg (Figure 4–5). All three bipolar leads are placed an equal distance from the heart and visualize the heart as the central source of electricity. Therefore, the triangle they form is equilateral.

Traditionally, the electrodes for the bipolar limb leads are placed on the limb itself. However, placing the electrode in the torso near the root of the limb is also acceptable, particularly in the prehospital setting where movement artifact presents a constant challenge (Figure 4–6). The arm electrodes are best placed in the soft area just below the clavicle near the limb. The left leg electrode, if not attached to the leg, should be placed *be-*

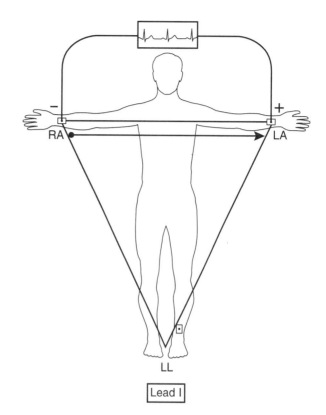

Figure 4–3.

Einthoven's triangle showing the measurement of electrical current from right arm to left arm: Recording positive ECG complexes.

Modified from R. Huszar, *Basic Dysrhythmias Interpretation and Management*, 2nd ed. St. Louis: Mosby, 1994.

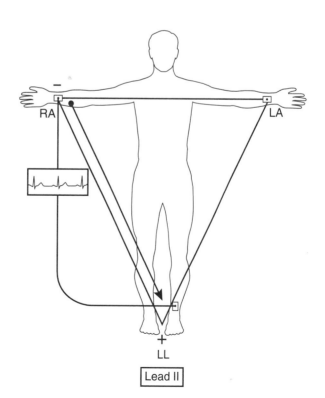

Figure 4–4.

Einthoven's triangle showing the measurement of electrical activity from right arm to left leg: Recording positive ECG complexes.

Modified from R. Huszar, *Basic Dysrhythmias Interpretation and Management*, 2nd ed. St. Louis: Mosby, 1994.

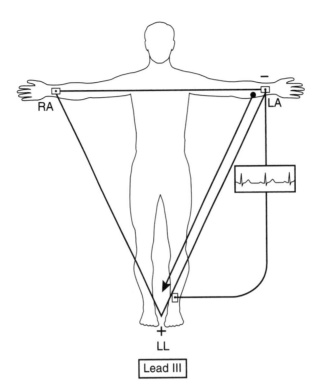

Figure 4–5.

Einthoven's triangle showing the measurement of electrical current from left arm to left leg: Recording positive ECG complexes.

Modified from R. Huszar, *Basic Dysrhythmias Interpretation and Management*, 2nd ed. St. Louis: Mosby, 1994.

low the rib cage near the anterior axillary line. Care should be taken not to place this electrode too high, as it begins to resemble V_4 or V_5 when placed on the thorax. Common ECG characteristics that exist among the bipolar leads include (Table 4–2):

1. All recorded deflections should be positive. The normal electrical axis of each lead is directed toward the positive electrode.
2. Lead II will have the greatest voltage (amplitude) and lead I will have the least voltage.
3. The voltage of lead I added to the voltage of lead III equals the voltage of lead II.
4. Lead I may present with physiological (normal) Q waves and all three leads visualize the heart in the frontal plane (Figure 4–7).

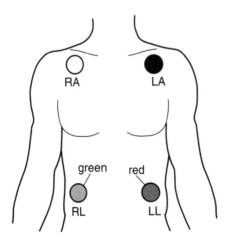

Figure 4–6.

Prehospital limb lead electrode placement and standard color-coded designations.

Right arm (RA)—white; left arm (LA)—black; right leg (RL)—green; left leg (LL)—red.

TABLE 4–2 • **Common Characteristics of Standard Bipolar Limb Leads**

• All recorded deflections should be positive
• Lead II has the greatest voltage (amplitude)
• Lead I has the least voltage
• Lead III may have physiological Q waves

```
PR    176   (NSR  ). Normal sinus rhythm, rate 58 - - - - - -   Normal P axis, PR, rate & rhythm
QRSD   63                                - NORMAL ECG -
QT    422
QTc   414

--AXES--
P      81
QRS    64
T      55
```

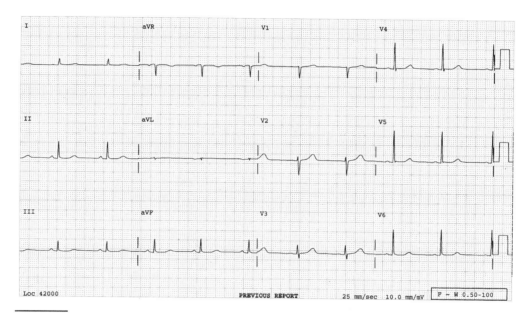

Figure 4–7.
12-lead ECG recording demonstrating the characteristics of the bipolar leads.
Note that lead II has the greatest voltage, lead I has the least voltage, and all three leads are positive (upright) in deflection.

UNIPOLAR LIMB LEADS (FRONTAL PLANE)

Unipolar limb leads are produced by utilizing all of the limb electrodes as a common negative. This leaves the positive electrode as the sole influence on the recording. These leads are designated as V (unipolar) leads. They are called unipolar because each lead uses only one electrode at a time to record the electrical forces generated from the heart. For each unipolar limb lead, the specific limb electrode is the positive (+) electrode, which records the electrical forces in relation to a negative central reference point (center of the heart) created electronically. By placing the positive electrode on one limb, the ECG records the potential at the root of that limb exclusively (as opposed to the difference in potential of the connected limbs with bipolar leads). Unipolar limb leads are identified by the placement of their positive pole. When the positive is on the left leg, VF (F for foot) is used. When the positive is on the left arm, VL (L for left arm) is used, and when the positive electrode is on the right arm, VR (R for right arm) is used. Since the multiple negative currents used reduce the QRS size, these leads must be augmented

TABLE 4–3 •	**Common Characteristics of Augmented Voltage Leads**
• All leads have low voltage • aVF has the greatest voltage • aVL has the least voltage • aVR has a negative deflection • aVR is not used for infarct recognition	

(amplified) and are therefore designated aVR, aVL, and aVF (see Figure 3–3). Common ECG characteristics that exist among the augmented voltage leads include (Table 4–3):

1. All leads have low voltage.
2. aVF has the greatest voltage because the net electrical forces are moving toward this lead; aVL has the least voltage. Both leads are mostly positive (upright) in deflection.
3. aVR will have a negative deflection because the net electrical forces are moving away from the positive electrode of this lead.
4. aVR is not used for infarct recognition.
5. Augmented voltage leads record electrical activity of the heart in the frontal plane (refer to Figure 4–7).

HORIZONTAL PLANE LEADS

The horizontal plane leads (also known as chest leads, precordial leads), like the unipolar limb leads, are V leads. That is, they utilize all of the limb electrodes as a common negative and allow the positive as the sole influence on the recording. Each chest electrode records electrical forces in relation to a negative central reference point, the center of the heart (Figure 4–8). The chest electrodes are placed on the anterior, left lateral chest wall (see Figure 3–4). Their proper placement is essential for accurate recording of the chest leads, especially when acquiring serial (repeated) tracings. Six specific precordial points have been identified for placement of the chest leads:

V_1: Fourth intercostal space to the right of the sternum
V_2: Fourth intercostal space to the left of the sternum
V_3: Directly between leads V_2 and V_4
V_4: Fifth intercostal space at the midclavicular line
V_5: Horizontally level to V_4 at the left anterior axillary line
V_6: Horizontally level to V_4 at the left midaxillary line

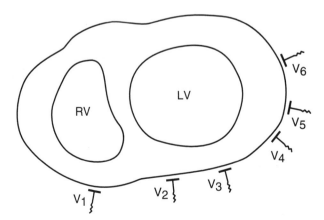

Figure 4–8.
Unipolar chest leads V_1 through V_6 record electrical forces between a positive precordial electrode and a negative central reference point (center of the heart) created electronically.

Modified from B. Lipman and T. Cascio, *ECG Assessment and Interpretation.* Philadelphia: F.A. Davis Company, 1994.

Leads V_1 through V_6 provide an excellent view of the septal, anterior, posterior, and lateral surface of the left ventricle. The right ventricle is underrepresented on the standard 12-lead ECG.

R WAVE PROGRESSION THROUGH THE PRECORDIAL LEADS

R wave progression is the gradual increase in the height of the R wave (QRS complex) as the chest electrodes (V_1 through V_6) move across the precordium toward the left ventricular muscle (Figure 4–9). The initial portion of QRS deflection in chest leads V_1 through V_6 represents depolarization of the septum. The remaining balance of the QRS complex represents depolarization of both ventricular walls. Because the left ventricle contains two to three times the mass of the right ventricle, it has the most electrical force or potential with which to influence the ECG pattern. Thus, depolarization of the left ventricle contributes to the majority of QRS deflection.

Leads V_1 and V_2 view the heart from the right side. They see depolarization of the septum (activation from the left side to the right side) as current flowing toward them. The initial part of the QRS complex in leads V_1 and V_2 is recorded as a small positive R wave. The remainder of depolarization in the ventricles is produced by activation of the left ventricle as current flows away from electrodes V_1 and V_2. Thus, the remainder of

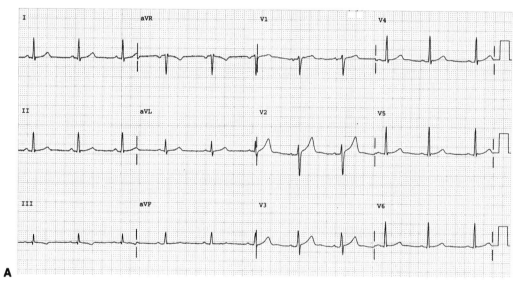

A

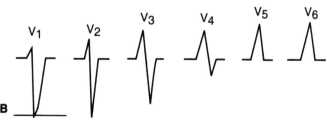

B

Figure 4–9.

(A) 12-lead ECG recording demonstrating normal R wave progression through the precordial leads (V_1 through V_6).
Note the gradual increase in the height of the R wave through these leads. This phenomenon represents the spread of electrical forces toward the left ventricle.
(B) Graphic representation of R wave progression.
Note the small r waves and deep S waves in V_1 and V_2, followed by an equiphasic (equally positive and negative) complex in V_3 and positive R waves in V_4 through V_6.

the QRS complex is negative, creating a large S wave as the forces are seen moving away from these electrodes. Common characteristics of V_1 and V_2 include:

- Focus is on the septum
- Placement is over the right atrial tissue
- They will have small R waves and deep S waves (predominant negative deflection)
- The R wave in V_2 will be slightly taller than the R wave in V_1
- Referred to as right-sided chest leads

Leads V_3 and V_4 are referred to as transitional leads. Transitional refers to placement in between the right-sided chest leads and the left-sided chest leads. V_3 is equiphasic (equally positive and negative) and V_4 is biphasic in deflection. Common characteristics of V_3 and V_4 include:

- Placement is over the interventricular septum
- The R wave is taller in these leads than in V_1 and V_2, with equally deep S waves

Leads V_5 and V_6 are left-sided chest leads that look at the ventricles from the left side. They view depolarization of the septum as current flowing away from them. The initial deflection of the QRS complex in these leads is recorded as a small negative deflection (septal Q wave). The remainder of ventricular depolarization is seen moving toward the recording electrode. Leads V_5 and V_6 record the large amount of current directed toward them as a large positive deflection (R wave). Common characteristics of V_5 and V_6 include:

- Placement is over the left ventricular tissue
- They show physiological Q waves that reflect septal depolarization
- Demonstrate large R waves and minimal S waves
- Referred to as left-sided chest leads

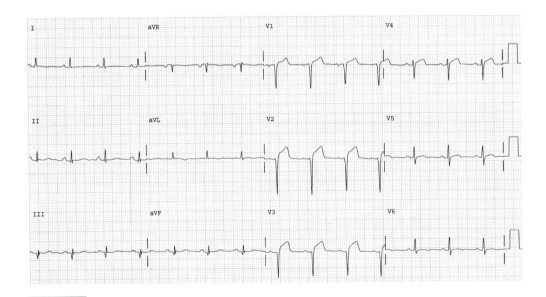

Figure 4–10.
12-lead ECG recording demonstrating the absence of R wave progression in the presence of an acute infarction to the anterior wall of the left ventricle.
Note the ST segment elevation in the leads overlying the anterior wall (V_1 through V_4). The tissue in this area is electrically silent due to infarction.

Poor R wave progression or its absence occurs when the QRS complex does not become predominately positive by lead V_4. This may indicate the loss of electrical activity in an area of the myocardium and subsequent altered hemodynamic function. The lost R wave is often replaced by a pathological (disease causing) Q wave indicating myocardial necrosis. Abnormal R wave progression results from infarction, ventricular hypertrophy (dilation of the ventricles), and other cardiac disorders (Figure 4–10).

MODIFIED CHEST LEADS

When only a basic monitoring system is available, obtaining true V leads is impossible. This is because the V leads require three of the four limb electrodes to be negative, thus producing a common central terminal, which has little to no influence on the ECG, leaving the positive electrode as the sole contributor to the tracing. However, modified precordial V leads can be produced using the negative and positive wires of a bipolar system. When the positive electrode is placed near the heart and the negative electrode is placed on a limb, it is obvious that the positive electrode will contribute more to the tracing. This will closely duplicate the precordial V leads. The letter C is used to designate the use of the bipolar system in the precordial or *chest* lead positions (C = chest).

In C leads the positive electrode is called the exploring electrode. It is placed in any of the precordial positions previously described. The negative electrode can be placed on any limb, but experience and tradition leads us to place it on the left arm, or more specifically, on the root of the left arm, often just below the distal clavicle (Figure 4–11). The designation L is used to indicate that the negative electrode is on the left arm. M is used to indicate that we have modified the position slightly and brought the negative to the root of the limb. The designation MCL means that we have *m*odified a *c*hest lead by placing the negative on the *l*eft shoulder. The final designator is the position of the positive electrode. Numbers 1 through 6 are used to indicate the corresponding V lead position and an R designates leads placed in the right precordial positions. MCL_1 and MCL_6 are two monitoring and diagnostic leads of prehospital relevance. Their description is as follows:

- MCL_1 is negative on the left shoulder, positive in the V_1 position. This is a popular and effective monitoring lead.
- MCL_6 is negative on the left shoulder, positive in the V_6 position. This is an excellent lead for the differential diagnosis of certain dysrhythmias.

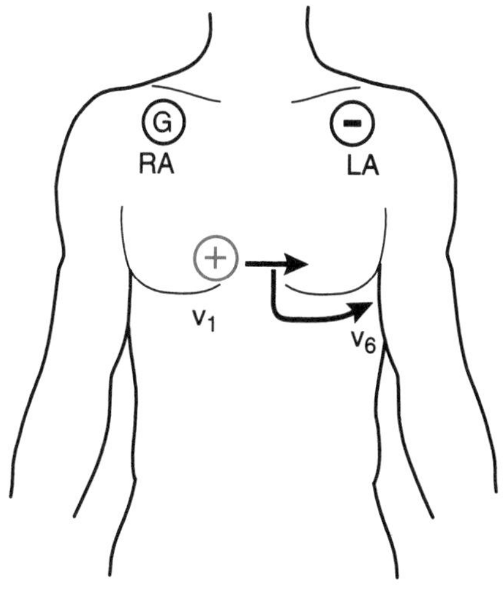

Figure 4–11.
Modified chest leads identifying the placement of the negative and positive electrodes.
Note the positive electrode is placed in the V_1 through V_6 position and the negative is placed on the left arm or shoulder.

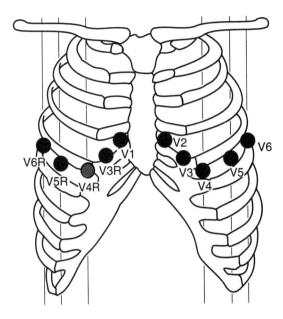

Figure 4–12.
Placement of the right-sided chest leads for viewing the right ventricle.
Note that these leads are placed in the identical position as the left-sided chest leads, but on the right side of the chest.

MCL leads are essentially equivalent to the precordial leads and can be used along with leads I, II, and III to identify infarct if the monitor has a diagnostic frequency range option. This 9-lead ECG is usually sufficient for identification of infarct since aVR is not used for infarct recognition, aVF is flanked by the other inferior wall leads (II and III), and aVL is only one of the four leads investigating the lateral wall.

MCL_1 or MCL_5 or MCL_6 are useful for identifying left and right bundle branch block, and therefore can be used to separate supraventricular complexes with aberration from complexes of ventricular origin (see Chapter 7). This explains why they are used extensively in CCUs and MICUs. Monitor-quality frequency ranges are usually adequate for dysrhythmia interpretation.

SPECIAL MONITORING AND DIAGNOSTIC LEADS

For the purposes of infarct recognition, the standard twelve leads provide an adequate view of the left ventricle and can detect a majority of myocardial infarctions. However, the right ventricle can infarct as well, and does so in a small percentage of all infarcts. Recognition of right ventricular infarction accompanying infarction to the inferior wall of the left ventricle is an important diagnostic skill. Knowledge of this enables the clinician to modify treatments in regard to fluid administration, pain control, and atrioventricular block (see Chapter 6). In order to "see" the right ventricle, electrodes must be placed over the right precordium. These leads, designated V_3R through V_6R, are placed in the V_3 through V_6 positions on the right side of the chest (Figure 4–12). V_4R is by far the most sensitive indicator of right ventricular infarction and its use as the sole right-sided chest lead is all that is necessary in the prehospital setting. Additionally, left precordial leads can be extended to the posterior thorax via V_7, V_8, and V_9. These are placed at the same horizontal plane as V_4, utilizing the posterior axillary line for V_7, the angle of the scapula for V_8, and the spine for V_9. It is interesting to note that these leads exist. However, at the present time, these have little practical use in the field.

MODERN PORTABLE MONITORING SYSTEMS

Contemporary portable monitoring systems are combination units capable of defibrillation, synchronized cardioversion and, in some cases, pacing, diagnostic frequency range capability, multichannel 12-lead recording, and cellular phone communication. Many systems also include computers capable of ECG interpretation. These computerized programs have proven to be very accurate and reliable. Their use should help decrease the concern over paramedics or other allied health care professionals making "diagnostic decisions" in the absence of a cardiologist. All systems consist of basic components including an oscilloscope, printer, amplifier, cable system, and control panel. Care providers should become familiar with all equipment they are subject to work with. Manufacturer operating manuals are beneficial in this regard and can usually be readily obtained from the distributor or manufacturer. Most monitors use one or more of three basic cabling systems: 3-wire, 5-wire, and 10-wire, each providing a different range of functions.

3-Wire Cabling

The 3-wire cable is the standard basic cable for the past generation of portable monitors. Most monitors using this system require the user to attach the cable wires to electrodes in the lead II position (RA−, LAG, LL+). An internal switch is then employed to change the cable polarity internally. Leads I, II, and III can then be obtained. Since this system is purely bipolar, it is not capable of duplicating leads aVR, aVL, and aVF or pure precordial leads. However, modified chest left (MCL) leads (Figure 4–13) can be obtained with this system. With the lead wires in the lead II position and the switch on lead III, the electrode on the left shoulder is negative. This is the proper position of the negative

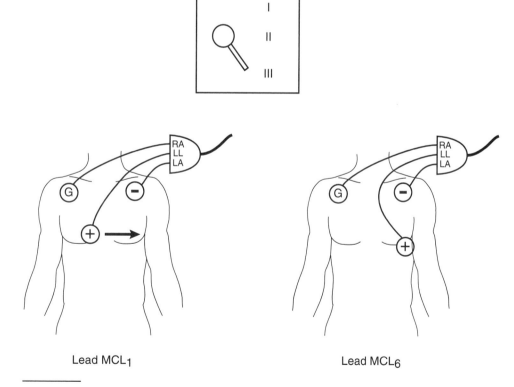

Lead MCL₁   Lead MCL₆

Figure 4–13.

When using a 3-wire cable system, modified chest leads MCL₁ through MCL₆ are created by placing the positive electrode (LL) in the desired precordial position. The negative electrode (LA) is placed under the left clavicle and the ground electrode (G) is placed under the right clavicle.
Note: This modified configuration requires the selection of lead III on the monitoring device.

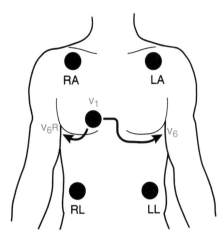

Figure 4–14.
**The 5-wire cable system uses the four limb elec-
trodes (RA, LA, RL, LL) in the conventional locations,
with the fifth electrode being placed in the desired
V_1 through V_6 or V_3R to V_6R position.**

electrode for the MCL leads. All that remains for the user to do is pull the positive (left leg) lead wire from its electrode, attach it to a suction cup adapter, and probe the V leads by placing the suction cup in the proper position. MCL_1 through MCL_6 and MCL_3R through MCL_6R can be obtained in this manner.

5-Wire Cabling

The 5-wire cable is an excellent setup for dysrhythmia monitoring and provides an easier and more complete 12-lead ECG than the 3-wire system. With this cable system, one electrode is placed on each limb (LA, RA, LL, RL) and a fifth chest (C) electrode is placed in the V_1 position (Figure 4–14). The chest wire can be moved across the precordium to obtain a full set (V_1 through V_6, V_3R through V_6R) of true precordial leads. The four limb electrodes provide access to the frontal plane leads (I, II, III, and aVR, aVL, and aVF). As with the 3-wire system, monitor quality is usually sufficient for dysrhythmia interpretation. The diagnostic-quality frequency range is required for infarct detection and most other diagnostic evidence.

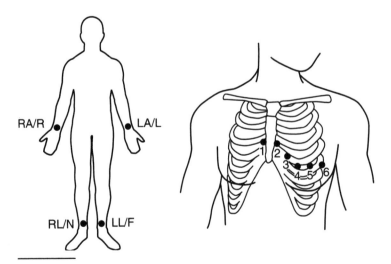

Figure 4–15.
Standard limb and precordial electrode placement for the 12-lead ECG using the 10-wire cable.

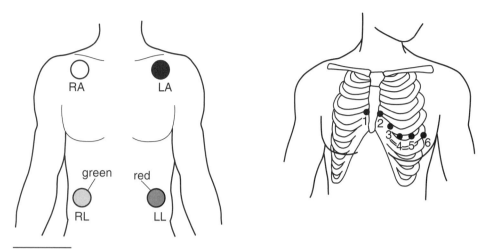

Figure 4–16.
The prehospital limb and precordial electrode placement.
The limb electrodes are moved toward the root of the limb to reduce arti-
fact from extremity movement.

10-Wire Cabling

The 10-wire cable is the standard set used for 12-lead acquisition. Four limb electrodes and six precordial electrodes are attached in the traditional format (Figure 4–15). When used in the emergency or prehospital setting, the limb leads are often moved toward the root of the limb to provide a more stable tracing (Figure 4–16). Right precordial leads are obtained by moving the V_3 through V_6 electrodes to their respective positions on the right side of the chest and recording an additional tracing. Right precordial leads should be marked (V_3R, V_4R, V_5R, V_6R) by the technician to avoid confusion. Ten-wire units may be an integral part of the monitoring device or be attached via a switchbox. The switchbox provides a rapid 12-lead selection system for monitors without integral 10-wire cabling.

LEAD REFLECTION AND IDENTIFICATION

Identification of electrocardiographic disorders requires knowledge of the heart's surface reflection (epicardial or exterior wall of the left ventricle) in the twelve different leads. This is especially true for the recognition of infarction. Both the prognosis and therapy of an infarction are largely determined by which area of the heart has died. Since myocardial infarctions usually involve the left ventricle (not surprising, since the left ventricle performs the hardest work), the following section discusses the four anatomical quadrants of the left ventricle as reflected in the twelve leads (Table 4–4).

TABLE 4–4 • **ECG Lead Reflection (Left Ventricle)**	
Anterior surface:	V_1, V_2, V_3, V_4
Lateral surface:	I, aVL, V_5, V_6
Inferior surface:	II, III, aVF
Posterior surface:	RECIPROCAL V_1-V_2

Inferior Wall

The leg or foot electrode faces directly toward the inferior surface of the left ventricle. The leads that use the leg or foot as the positive electrode are leads II, III, and aVF. Therefore, leads II, III, and aVF can be said to reflect the electrical activity of the inferior surface of the left ventricle. Primary changes in an inferior wall MI will be seen in these leads.

Lateral Wall

When the left arm is used as the positive electrode, the lateral portion of the left ventricle is displayed. The leads that use the left arm as the positive electrode are leads I and aVL. Additionally, the positive precordial leads V_5 and V_6 look at the lateral surface of the left ventricle. These leads are located on the anterior left lateral chest wall. Therefore, leads I, aVL, V_5, and V_6 will show primary changes associated with lateral wall MIs.

Anterior Wall

Damage to the anterior wall of the left ventricle is observed in the precordial leads V_1 through V_4. This lead group lies directly on the anterior surface of the chest, observing the anterior wall of the left ventricle.

Posterior Wall

Because there are no electrodes employed with a 12-lead ECG that overlie the posterior surface of the myocardium, no primary changes will be displayed. Diagnosis of posterior injury is made by looking for reciprocal (mirror image) changes in the anterior leads (V_1 and V_2). More on this and all of the lead groups will follow in Chapter 6.

ACQUIRING A 12-LEAD ECG

Any monitor is capable of producing a 12-lead ECG. The following represents two diagnostic units commonly employed in the prehospital setting.

Using a 12-Lead ECG Machine

1. Turn the power on and adjust the contrast as needed.
2. Identify the appropriate electrode sites on the patient.
   - Limb lead electrodes are typically placed on the wrists and ankles. It is acceptable to place the limb electrodes at the root of the limbs.
   - Chest leads are placed on specific locations previously described. Proper placement is important for accurate diagnosis.
3. Tips for precordial lead placement
   - Locate the V_1 position:
   - V_1 (fourth intercostal space) is the reference point for the placement of the remaining V leads.
   - Place your finger at the notch in the top of the sternum.
   - Move your finger downward about 1.5 inches until you feel a slight horizontal ridge or elevation. This is the angle of Louis, where the manubrium joins the body of the sternum (Figure 4–17).
   - Locate the second intercostal space on the right side, lateral to and just below the angle of Louis.

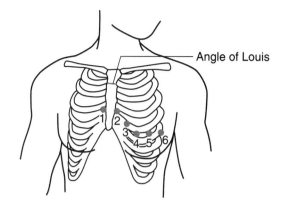

Angle of Louis

Figure 4–17.
Precordial lead electrode placement identifying the angle of Louis.

- Move your finger down two more intercostal spaces to the fourth intercostal space which is the V_1 position.
4. Other important chest lead considerations:
   - When placing electrodes on female patients, always place leads V_3 through V_6 under the breast rather than on the breast.
   - Never use the nipples as reference points for locating the electrodes for men or women patients because nipple locations may vary widely.
5. Prepare the patient's skin for electrode application.
   - Shave excessive hair at the electrode site
   - Avoid locating electrodes over tendons and major muscle masses
   - For oily skin, clean the skin with an alcohol pad
   - Prepare the site with a brisk rub
6. Apply the ECG electrodes.
   - Inspect the electrode package for its expiration
   - Attach an electrode to each of the ten lead wires
   - Inspect the electrode gel to ensure that it is intact
   - Hold the electrode taut with both hands and apply the electrode flat to the skin
7. Encourage the patient to remain as still as possible, and provide support as needed.
8. Press the mechanism to acquire and print the 12-lead ECG report.

Using a 3-Lead Machine with a 12-Lead ECG Selection Box

The selection box is an accessory for some monitors which allows users to obtain a true 12-lead ECG. It replaces the 3-lead patient cable set and provides bipolar and unipolar recordings. Its use is described below.

1. Turn the machine on and calibrate a 1-mV signal for accurate ECG analysis.
2. Switch to the diagnostic quality mode.
3. Identify the appropriate electrode sites as previously described.
4. Prepare the patient's skin for electrode application.
5. Attach the electrodes to the ten lead wires.
6. Attach the limb and chest lead electrodes.
7. Encourage the patient to remain as still as possible.
8. Select lead II on the monitor.

9. With the monitor set at lead II, push record and dial through each of the 12-lead settings. Record only 2 to 2.5 seconds of each lead.
10. Mark the selected leads on the ECG paper.

NOTE: V₄R may be obtained with both systems by removing lead V_4 (left-sided chest lead) and reattaching it to the desired location (fifth intercostal space right midclavicular line).

DETERMINING AXIS

The QRS axis is the sum total of all electrical currents generated by the ventricular myocardium during depolarization. The direction of this current can be plotted and assigned a value.

QRS axis determination plays a relatively minor role in emergency electrocardiography. Clinical uses of QRS axis determination in the emergency setting include the diagnosis hemiblock, differentiation of wide-complex tachycardia, and the recognition of acute pulmonary emboli (Chapter 7).

We know as the wave of depolarization moves toward a positive electrode, the oscilloscope displays a positive deflection, and conversely, when the wave of depolarization moves away from the positive electrode, a negative deflection is displayed. Perpendicular movement across a positive electrode creates an equiphasic complex. Using this basic principle, we can examine the frontal plane leads and plot the direction of depolarization.

THE HEXAXIAL REFERENCE SYSTEM

The six frontal leads create six poles intersecting at the center of the heart. Each pole has a positive and negative axis. This forms what is known as a hexaxial reference (Figure 4–18). The positive and negative end of each pole is assigned a value expressed in degrees.

The hexaxial reference can be divided into quadrants (Figure 4–19). The area between 0 degrees and +90 degrees is traditionally considered the normal axis quadrant.

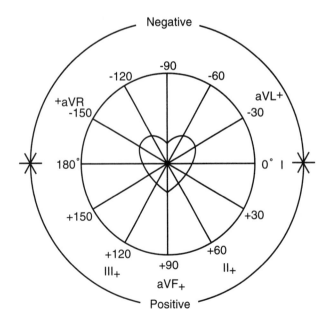

Figure 4–18.
The hexaxial reference system intersects the lead axis of the six-limb leads at a common center point.
Note that the positive and negative ends of each lead axis are assigned specific degrees.
Modified from B. Lipman and T. Cascio, *ECG Assessment and Interpretation*. Philadelphia: F.A. Davis Company, 1994.

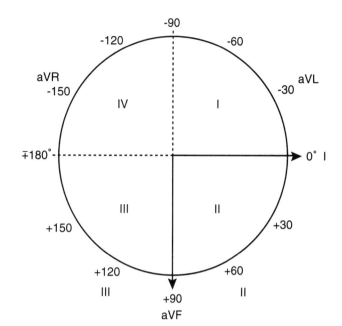

Figure 4–19.
The four quadrants of the hexaxial reference figure.

The area from 0 degrees to −90 degrees is said to be the left axis quadrant, +90 degrees to 180 degrees is the right axis quadrant, and −90 degrees to 180 degrees is the right shoulder axis quadrant. (This quadrant is also referred to as no man's land, extreme right axis, extreme left axis, northwest axis, and intermediate axis). These values are convenient for teaching and understanding basic axis calculation methods. However, most experts regard the normal axis to be between −30 degrees and +120 degrees, slight left axis deviation (0 to −30 degrees), and slight right axis deviation (+90 to +120 degrees) are usually considered physiological (Figure 4–20). The reader should consider these differences when examining the various methods of axis calculation.

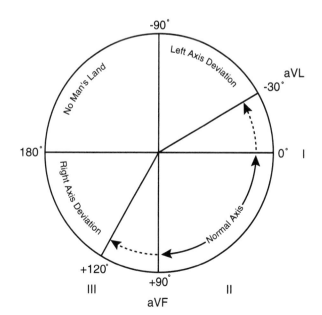

Figure 4–20.

Normal and abnormal QRS axis.
(A) Normal QRS axis: −30 degrees to +120 degrees; (B) Left axis deviation: −30 degrees to −90 degrees; (C) Right axis deviation: +120 degrees to +180 degrees; (D) "No man's land": −90 degrees to +180 degrees.

METHODS OF CALCULATING QRS AXIS

Methods of axis calculation are divided into sections based on the different monitoring systems presently available and in use in the emergency setting.

Diagnostic Monitoring Systems

The latest generation of portable diagnostic monitoring systems utilize ten cable setups and interpretive programs that print the QRS axis in the data margin. This is by far the most accurate method of determining QRS axis. Users will note that the axis values are printed in a 360 degree format (Figure 4–21) in lieu of the "minus and plus" system of the traditional hexaxial reference. This simplifies computer programming. Conversion to this format is simple and self-explanatory.

5-Wire System (No Interpretive Program)

The 5-wire system described earlier has four limb wires (RA, LA, LL, RL) and a single chest lead wire. These systems typically lack the interpretive program of the newer diagnostic monitoring systems.

By providing the user with access to leads aVF and I, the traditional quadrant method of axis determination can be utilized. Although this method lacks the accuracy required to separate slight left and slight right physiological deviation from pathological deviation, it remains the best method of gaining an understanding of how QRS axis is determined. The reader is encouraged to examine this section carefully.

aVF and I, the Quadrant Method

Consider the hexaxial reference a sphere divided in half from left to right by the pole of aVF (−90 degrees to +90 degrees) and top to bottom by I (0 degrees to 180 degrees) (Figure 4–22). If the QRS complex in I is positive or mostly positive (sum total), then the axis is moving toward I of the left side (patient's left) of the sphere (Figure 4–23). If aVF is positive or mostly positive the axis is moving toward the bottom half of the sphere. This indicates that the axis points down and to the patient's left, or in the normal range. If the

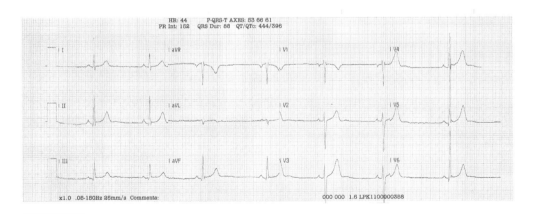

Figure 4–21.
Interpretive program of electrical axis providing P, QRS, and T wave axes.
Note the axis data provided at the top of the tracing. This form of axis determination is the most accurate. Focus on the axis data in the 12-lead tracing, especially the QRS data of "66." Also note P wave and T wave axes.

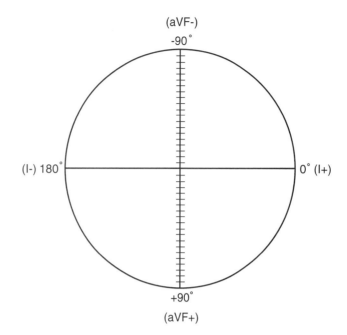

Figure 4–22.
Hexaxial reference is a sphere divided in half from left to right by the poles of aVF and top to bottom by the pole of lead I.

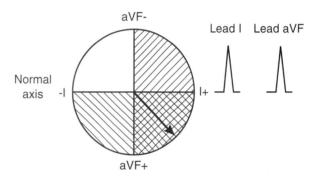

Figure 4–23.
Normal QRS axis using the quadrant method.
The axis is moving toward I and aVF. Note the positive QRS deflection in both leads.
Modified from B. Lipman and T. Cascio, *ECG Assessment and Interpretation.* Philadelphia: F.A. Davis Company, 1994.

QRS complex in lead I is mostly negative, then the axis must be toward the right side (patient's right) of the sphere. If aVF is negative, the axis must be toward the top of the sphere, and so the axis would be in the right shoulder axis quadrant (Figure 4–24). If the QRS is positive in I and negative in aVF, that places the axis in the left axis quadrant (Figure 4–25). And lastly, if the QRS is negative in I and positive in aVF, the axis is in the right axis quadrant (Figure 4–26).

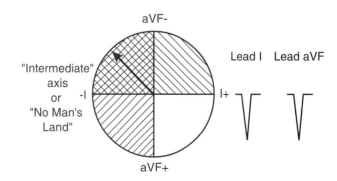

Figure 4–24.
Abnormal right shoulder axis as identified by the negative QRS deflection in I and aVF.
Modified from B. Lipman and T. Cascio, *ECG Assessment and Interpretation.* Philadelphia: F.A. Davis Company, 1994.

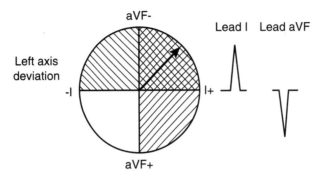

Figure 4–25.
Left axis deviation identified by the positive QRS deflection in lead I and negative deflection in aVF.
Modified from B. Lipman and T. Cascio, *ECG Assessment and Interpretation.* Philadelphia: F.A. Davis Company, 1994.

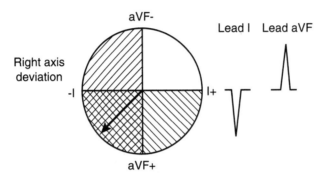

Figure 4–26.
Right axis deviation identified by the negative QRS deflection in lead I and positive deflection in aVF.
Modified from B. Lipman and T. Cascio, *ECG Assessment and Interpretation.* Philadelphia: F.A. Davis Company, 1994.

Equiphasic Complex Method

An equiphasic (equally positive and negative in deflection) complex indicates an axis that is moving perpendicular (90 degrees) to the lead in which the equiphasic complex is found. Perpendicular leads are I and aVF, II and aVL, and III and aVR. Examine all of the frontal plane leads (I, II, III, aVR, aVL, aVF) and locate the most equiphasic complex. Find the lead perpendicular to the equiphasic lead. Examine the QRS of the perpendic-

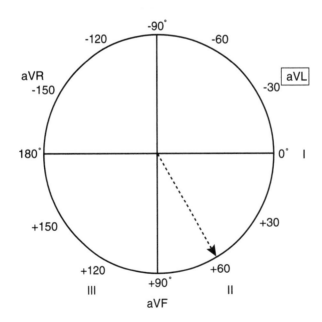

Figure 4–27.
Equiphasic complex method.
Using the limb leads, aVL is the most equiphasic. Compare aVL to its perpendicular lead (II) and examine the QRS deflection of this lead. Lead II is upright, therefore the axis is moving toward the positive pole of lead II. The QRS axis is approximately 60°. Note the interpretative axis of 64° in the data margin of Figure 4–7.

TABLE 4–5 • **"Quickie" Axis**

LEAD 1		LEAD 2		AXIS
↑	+	↑	=	Normal
↑	+	↓	=	LAD
↓	+	↑	=	RAD
↓	+	↓	=	No man's

ular lead. If the QRS of the perpendicular lead is positive, then the axis is moving toward the positive pole of that lead. If the QRS of the perpendicular lead is negative, then the axis is moving away from the positive pole of the perpendicular lead; see, for example Figure 4–27 and Figure 4–7. Lead aVL is equiphasic (sum total 0), and lead II is the perpendicular lead to aVL, so examine lead II. Lead II is upright, so the axis must be moving toward the positive pole of lead II, the QRS axis is therefore +60 degrees. Practice on the examples provided.

3-Wire Cable System

Leads I and II can be used in combination with the quick reference chart (Table 4–5) to quickly identify pathological axis changes in the emergency setting. When I and II are upright the axis is normal. Abnormal left axis deviation (greater than 30 degrees) displays a positive QRS in lead I and a negative QRS in lead II. Abnormal right axis deviation displays a negative lead I and a positive lead II. Right shoulder axis (no man's land) usually presents with I and II as negative, however this combination can also represent a right axis between 150 and 180 degrees. This system is usually adequate for hemiblock identification, but may lack the precision required when differentiating wide complex supraventricular tachycardias from ventricular tachycardia by axis (Chapter 7).

KEY POINTS SUMMARY

Types of Emergency Electrocardiography

1. Emergency electrocardiography consists of single-lead monitoring and diagnostic 12-lead electrocardiography. Single-lead monitoring is used for the recognition of dysrhythmias, whereas diagnostic electrocardiography is used for the identification of infarct and other cardiac disorders.

Monitor Versus Diagnostic Quality Devices

2. Monitoring for dysrhythmias is accomplished with the use of monitor-quality devices. These devices are set at a narrow frequency range that provides less information in comparison to the wide frequency band of diagnostic-quality devices. Accurate ST segment analysis can only be accomplished with the use of diagnostic-quality (12-lead ECG) devices.

The 12-Lead Electrocardiogram

3. A 12-lead ECG is a noninvasive diagnostic surface electrocardiogram composed of twelve leads that record the heart's electrical activity from twelve different viewpoints. Each lead records atrial depolarization, ventricular depolarization, and ventricular repolarization.
4. Of the twelve leads, six are frontal plane limb leads and six are horizontal plane chest leads.

Benefits of Out-of-Hospital 12-Lead Electrocardiography

5. Early recognition of myocardial ischemia, injury, and infarction.
6. Localization of the area of ischemic heart muscle.
7. Detection of prehospital ischemia that resolves prior to hospital arrival.
8. Identification of patients who are at risk for developing complex heart block.
9. Differentiation of wide-complex tachycardias.
10. Reduction in the time from admission to thrombolytic therapy.

Frontal Plane Leads (Bipolar and Augmented Voltage Leads)

11. Frontal plane leads include the three bipolar limb leads and the three unipolar augmented voltage leads.

Bipolar Leads

12. Bipolar leads are leads I, II, and III. Each lead utilizes a negative and positive electrode in order to measure the difference in electrical potential between connected limb sites. Lead I measures electrical activity from the negative right shoulder to the positive left shoulder. Lead II measures electrical activity from the negative right shoulder to the positive left leg, while lead III measures electrical activity from the negative left shoulder to the positive left leg.
13. Because the net electrical flow is toward the positive pole of each bipolar lead, all recorded deflections should be positive (upright).

Augmented Voltage Leads

14. Unipolar augmented voltage leads are produced by utilizing all of the limb electrodes as a common negative. This leaves the positive electrode as the sole influence on the recording. Augmented leads are identified by the placement of their positive pole. aVR is placed on the right arm, aVL the left arm, and aVF on the foot.

Horizontal Plane Leads

15. Unipolar horizontal chest leads record electrical forces in relation to a negative central reference point (center of the heart) created electronically. Six electrodes are placed across the anterior and left lateral chest wall in the following anatomical positions:
    - V_1: Fourth intercostal space to the right of the sternum
    - V_2: Fourth intercostal space to the left of the sternum
    - V_3: Between V_2 and V_4
    - V_4: Fifth intercostal space midclavicular line
    - V_5: Fifth intercostal space anterior axillary line
    - V_6: Fifth intercostal space midaxillary line

R Wave Progression Through the Precordial Leads

16. R wave progression is the gradual increase in the height of the R wave (QRS complex) as the chest electrodes (V_1 through V_6) move across the precordium toward the left ventricle.
17. Normal R wave progression is as follows:
    - V_1 and V_2 are predominately negative
    - V_3 is equiphasic
    - V_4, V_5, and V_6 are positive

Modified Chest Leads (MCL Leads)

18. Modified chest leads are produced by using the negative and positive wires of a bipolar system. The positive electrode is placed on the chest near the heart in the same anatomical position as the precordial V leads, while the negative electrode

is placed on the limb. The descriptions MCL$_1$ through MCL$_6$ are used to identify the anatomical placement of the positive electrode.

Special Monitoring and Diagnostic Leads

19. Leads V$_3$R through V$_6$R (R designating the right side of the chest) are specialized leads used to investigate the right ventricle. These leads are placed in the same anatomical position as their left-sided counterparts, but on the right precordium. Lead V$_4$R is the most sensitive and specific indicator of right ventricular infarction.

Portable Monitoring Systems

20. Portable monitors utilize either a 3-wire, 5-wire, or 10-wire cabling system. The 3-wire cable is the standard basic cable used with most portable monitors. Its use requires the examiner to attach the cable wires in the lead II position.
21. The 5-wire cable system is good for dysrhythmia monitoring and provides an easier and more complete 12-lead ECG than the 3-wire system. Four of the five electrodes are placed on the limbs, while the fifth electrode is placed in the V$_1$ through V$_6$ positions.
22. The 10-wire system is the standard arrangement used for 12-lead ECG acquisition. Four limb electrodes and six chest electrodes are attached in the traditional format.

Lead Reflection

23. Recognition of infarction requires knowledge of those leads that view the four anatomical quadrants of the left ventricle. Quadrants of the left ventricle include the anterior, inferior, lateral, and posterior aspects, with the following leads observing their respective surfaces:
    • Anterior wall: Leads V$_1$ through V$_4$
    • Inferior wall: Leads II, III, and aVF
    • Lateral wall: Leads I, aVL, V$_5$, and V$_6$
    • Posterior wall: Reciprocal (mirror image) changes in V$_1$ and V$_2$

Electrical Axis

24. QRS axis is the sum total of all electrical currents generated by the ventricular myocardium during depolarization. Determination of electrical axis plays a relatively minor role in emergency electrocardiography, but does assist in the diagnosis of hemiblock, the differentiation of wide-complex tachycardia, and the recognition of acute pulmonary disorders. A number of methods exist for determining axis whether utilizing a 3-wire, 5-wire, or 10-wire cabling system.

BIBLIOGRAPHY

Aufderheide TP, Hendley GE, Thakur RK, et al. The diagnostic impact of prehospital 12-lead electrocardiography. *Annals of Emergency Medicine*. 1990;19:1280–1287.

Canan S, Taigman M. Recognition of acute myocardial infarction: Advanced EKG interpretation. *Journal of Emergency Medical Services*. 1987;12(10):49–53.

Canan S, Taigman M. The only constant is change: The push for 12-lead ECGs. *Journal of Emergency Medical Services*. 1992;17(4):65–69.

Conover MB. *Understanding Electrocardiography: Arrhythmias and the 12-Lead ECG*. St. Louis, MO: Mosby; 1992.

Cummins RO, Eisenberg MS. From pain to reperfusion: What role for the prehospital 12-lead ECG? *Annals of Emergency Medicine*. 1990;19:1343–1346.

Gibler WB, Kereiakes DJ, Dean EN, et al. Prehospital diagnosis and treatment of acute myocardial infarction: A north south perspective. *American Heart Journal*. 1991;121(1):1–11.

Huszar RJ. *Basic Dysrhythmias: Interpretation and Management*. St. Louis, MO: Mosby; 1994.

Johnson R, Swartz MH. *A Simplified Approach To Electrocardiography*. Philadelphia, PA: WB Saunders; 1986.

Jones SE. Prehospital 12-lead ECGs. *Annals of Emergency Medicine*. 1991;20:942–943.

Kowalenko T, Kereiakes DJ, Gibler WB. Prehospital diagnosis and treatment of acute myocardial infarction: A critical review. *American Heart Journal*. 1992;123(1):181–190.

Kudenchuck PJ, Ho MT, Litwin PE, Martin JS, Weaver WD. Accuracy of cardiologist vs computerized ECG analysis in selecting patients for out-of-hospital thrombolytic therapy. *Circulation*. 1988;78(suppl. II):II–110.

Langer F. *12-Lead Electrocardiography: Advanced Dysrhythmias*. Orlando, FL: Florida Hospital Medical Center; 1992.

Lipman BC, Cascio T. *ECG: Assessment and interpretation*. Philadelphia, PA: FA Davis Company; 1994.

Marriot HJ. *Practical Electrocardiography*. Baltimore, MD: Williams and Wilkins; 1988.

Mercer S. 12-lead ECGs: Ready to hit the streets? *Emergency*. 1993;(11):46–49.

Setaro JF, Cabin HS. Right ventricular infarction. *Cardiology Clinics*. 1992;10(1):69–90.

Thaler MS. *The Only EKG Book You'll Ever Need*. Philadelphia, PA: JB Lippincott; 1988.

White RD. Prehospital 12-lead ECG. *Annals of Emergency Medicine*. 1992;21:586.

Willems J, et al. The diagnostic performance of computer programs for the interpretation of electrocardiograms. *New England Journal of Medicine*. 1991;325:1767–1773.

Practice Exercises
In Axis Determination

1. Find the limb lead with the equiphasic (or smallest) QRS.

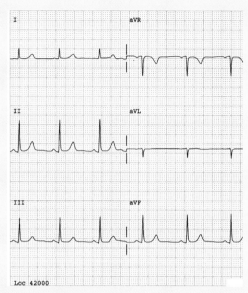
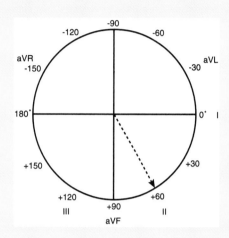

Problem 4-1.

2. Look at the lead perpendicular to this lead and note its QRS deflection.
   a. I–aVF
   b. II–aVL
   c. III–aVR

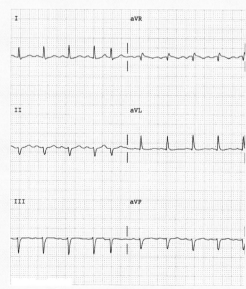
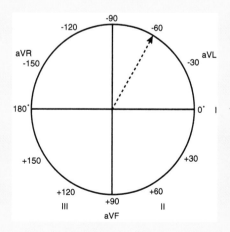

Problem 4-2.

3. Read the degrees in this lead (based on QRS polarity).

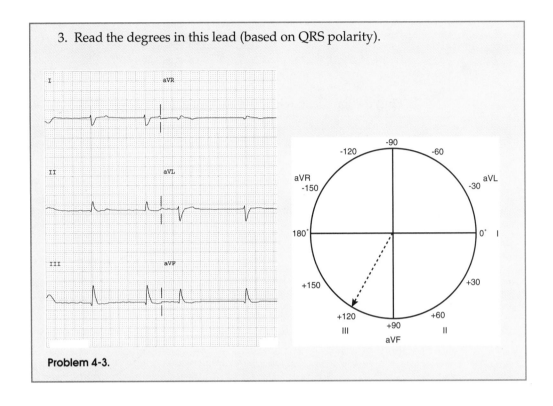

Problem 4-3.

Chapter 4 Practice Exercises/Axis Determination

1. **4-1:**   Lead aVL has the smallest QRS.
   Lead II is perpendicular to lead aVL.
   Lead II is positive (upright) in deflection equaling
     a normal electrical axis of +60 degrees.

2. **4-2:**   Lead aVR has the smallest and most equiphasic
     QRS.
   Lead III is perpendicular to lead aVR.
   Lead III is negative (downward) in deflection
     equaling an abnormal electrical axis of −60
     degrees (left axis deviation).

3. **4-3:**   Lead aVR has the smallest and most equiphasic
     QRS.
   Lead III is perpendicular to lead aVR.
   Lead III is positive (upright) in deflection
     equaling an abnormal electrical axis of +120
     degrees (right axis deviation).

5

Electrocardiographic Diagnosis of Myocardial Ischemia, Injury, and Infarction

LEARNING OBJECTIVES

1. Describe the pathophysiology of myocardial infarction.

2. List and describe the electrocardiographic evolution of myocardial ischemia, injury, and infarction.

3. Define myocardial ischemia, myocardial injury, and myocardial infarction.

4. List and identify the abnormal ECG findings of myocardial ischemia, myocardial injury, and myocardial infarction.

5. Explain the significance of ST segment depression, ST segment elevation, T wave inversion, and hyperacute T waves.

6. Explain anatomically contiguous ST segment elevation and relate its significance to infarct detection.

7. Discuss and identify reciprocal ECG changes.

8. List and describe the ischemic ST segment elevation pattern.

9. List and identify the different forms of ST segment elevation.

10. Discuss the following nonischemic causes of ST segment elevation: technical malfunctions, benign early repolarization, acute pericarditis, and left bundle branch block.

11. Define transmural and nontransmural myocardial infarction and differentiate the two types.

12. Define the terms physiological and pathological Q waves.

13. Explain the difference between Q wave and non-Q wave infarctions.

14. Discuss the significance of a loss of R wave progression and identify its ECG characteristics.

15. Discuss dating an infarct and identify its three stages.

INTRODUCTION

Myocardial ischemia, injury, and infarction represent a continuum of electrical changes that occur as the heart is progressively deprived of an adequate blood supply. Ischemia and injury are reversible conditions, infarction is not. Therefore, myocardial infarction delineates an end point in a dynamic cellular response to oxygen deprivation. It is incumbent on the prehospital care provider to understand the nature of the myocardial response to oxygen deprivation and the resulting alterations in the physiological function of myocardial cells under hypoxic conditions. When these physiological changes are coupled with an understanding of basic electrocardiography, a rational and systematic approach for interpreting ECGs in the face of myocardial ischemic injury or infarction can be utilized. Prehospital interventions can then be individualized, based on clinical findings and supporting electrocardiographic information, to institute appropriate and effective therapy to cardiac patients in all phases of the spectrum of ischemic heart disease. This chapter will introduce the pathophysiological evolution of infarction, followed by a detailed discussion of the electrocardiographic manifestations associated with this illness.

PATHOPHYSIOLOGY OF INFARCTION

The process of myocardial infarction occurs when a coronary artery is unable to sufficiently supply a segment of myocardial tissue with oxygen and other metabolic substrates. Typically, this process begins as a result of atherosclerosis (fatty deposition along with plaque formation in the coronary arteries), followed by the development of a blood clot in the immediate area of an incomplete fixed obstructive lesion. The cause of the clot is multifactorial, but it often occurs from the rupture of an atherosclerotic plaque followed by secondary platelet aggregation. Once obstruction by a clot occurs, myocardial cells instantly undergo a hypoxic evolution of ischemia (oxygen deprivation), followed by injury (worsened ischemia), and then infarction (tissue death). Patterns of these events are recorded on the electrocardiogram as a series of electrical changes. Knowledge of these changes will help to establish the presence, location, and extent of myocardial ischemia and/or infarction, as well as prepare the paramedic for certain complications.

ELECTROCARDIOGRAPHIC EVOLUTION OF INFARCTION

The evolution of electrocardiographic changes following coronary artery occlusion is well known. Recognition of these abnormalities involves the detection of morphological (configuration) changes of the QRS complex, ST segment, and T wave. Changes in the size, shape, or displacement of these waveforms occur in relation to certain pathological events during infarction. They often occur in a predictable pattern and are easily recognized on the ECG with continued practice. However, the period of time during which these changes are seen is often highly variable. In fact, one, all, or none of the findings may be recorded during an evolving infarction.

The earliest change that one is likely to observe (especially in the prehospital setting) is an increase in the amplitude and symmetry of the T wave (Figure 5–1). The T wave assumes a tall and sharply peaked appearance, which has been described as the hyperacute phase of infarction. T wave changes occur during the first few hours of infarction and may last for hours. As time and ischemia progress, the peaked T wave is replaced by ST segment elevation, signifying the acute phase of myocardial infarction. ST segment elevation typically occurs within the first hour to few hours of infarction and may be accompanied by T wave inversion. Several hours later, the appearance of significant (large) Q waves begins, providing evidence of myocardial tissue death. In time,

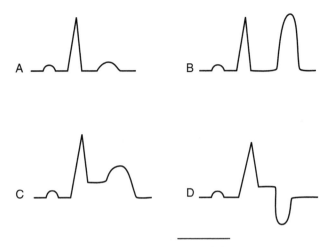

Figure 5–1.
The ECG evolution of infarction.
(A) Normal ECG. (B) Hyperacute phase, identified by the presence of abnormally large peaked T waves. (C) Acute phase, identified by the presence of ST segment elevation without T wave inversion. (D) Acute phase, with the presence of ST segment elevation accompanied by T wave inversion. (E) Old phase, with presence of large Q waves and the return of the ST-T waves to the baseline.

as well as through intervention, the ST segment returns to the baseline and the T wave gradually regains its normal contour. The Q waves, however, remain as permanent features of the ECG.

Evolving ECG Pattern of Infarction

- Sharp peaked T waves lasting minutes to hours (hyperacute phase)
- ST segment elevation occurs within an hour to a few hours (acute phase)
- Q wave formation within several hours (tissue death)

It should be noted again, however, that the evolving ECG changes described above are by no means absolute. Not every infarction will follow this pattern, and in fact, some infarctions do not produce appreciable changes on the ECG. Therefore, *a normal ECG does not exclude the diagnosis of infarction.* The emergency care provider should never rely on sole use of the electrocardiogram for evidence of infarction. The ECG is employed only as a tool to support historical and physical examination findings. Nevertheless, once the ECG changes of infarction are understood, they can be applied to individual patient conditions and used as a reference point.

MYOCARDIAL ISCHEMIA

Definition and Description

Myocardial ischemia represents the first phase in the degeneration of electrical function under hypoxic stress. It denotes a temporary, reversible reduction of blood supply to the heart muscle and is the earliest manifestation of reduced coronary perfusion.

As the oxygen requirements of the myocardium may vary, ischemia should be considered in relation to the myocardium's oxygen requirement under a given set of circumstances. For example, during periods of inactivity, diminished blood flow through atherosclerotic coronary arteries may still be sufficient to meet the metabolic needs of the myocardium. However, during periods of physical or emotional exertion, the needs of the myocardium will temporarily exceed the available blood supply. Cardiac ischemia, therefore, represents an imbalance between myocardial oxygen supply and demand.

Electrocardiography of Myocardial Ischemia

As blood supply diminishes, ischemic electrocardiographic changes will occur. Blood flow diminishes first and foremost in the subendocardium (innermost portion of the heart), while epicardial (outer wall) blood flow remains preserved. The reason for this is that the innermost portion of the heart is farthest away from the coronary arteries. The coronary arteries first supply the epicardium and then divide into small penetrating branches coursing deep into the endocardium. As a result, the subendocardium is the first area to experience early myocardial ischemic events when blood flow is compromised.

The electrophysiological basis of ST segment changes in myocardial ischemia has not been completely clarified. When oxygen delivery to the myocardial cells is deficient it is believed that the oxygen-dependent, sodium-potassium pump on the cell membrane becomes incapacitated. Sodium, chloride, and water accumulate inside the cell and potassium, normally in higher concentration inside the cell, moves extracellularly. The net result of these movements is a swelling of the myocardial cells, as well as a decrease in the potassium mediated resting action potential from approximately -90 mV to approximately -65 mV (see Chapter 2).

Electrical Alterations in Myocardial Ischemia

The net effect of the ion movements described above is a delay in repolarization. The ischemic zone (subendocardium) is electrically more negative than the unaffected area during the recovery phase. This creates a difference in electrical potential between ischemic and nonischemic (unaffected) tissue. As a result, current flows away from normal cells in the epicardium toward ischemic cells in the endocardium. An electrode that overlies such an ischemic area will record ST segment depression as the current now flows away from its positive pole (Figure 5–2).

Ischemia is also represented by T wave abnormalities on the ECG. Remember that the T wave represents repolarization of the ventricular myocardium and ischemia produces a delay in repolarization. The ischemic area is electrically more negative than the unaffected area during the repolarization phase and the electrical forces, therefore, point away from it. An exploring electrode overlying the ischemic area records a negative (inverted) T wave (refer to Figure 5–2).

Abnormal ECG Findings in Myocardial Tissue Ischemia

While the ECG is often normal in patients complaining of chest pain, certain ECG patterns of acute ischemia are characteristic. As noted previously, a delay in repolarization of ischemic myocardial tissue produces ST segment depression and T wave inversion, respectively.

ST Depression

The earliest change one is likely to see is ST segment depression. It is important to remember that ST segment depression may be reflective of ischemia over the recorded area or may be the result of reciprocal injury (i.e., the mirror image of ST elevation in an-

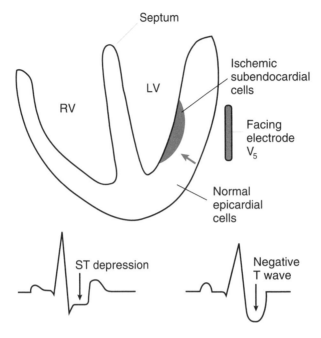

Figure 5–2.
Schematic view of the left ventricle showing the flow of current during stimulation (systole) from healthy cells in the epicardium toward ischemic cells in the subendocardium.
Note the current flow (arrow) is away from the facing (V_5) electrode. This results in ST segment depression and a negative (inverted) T wave in relation to the QRS.
Modified from D.B. Foster. *Twelve Lead Electrocardiography for ACLS Providers.* Philadelphia: W.B. Saunders, 1996.

other area). Reciprocal changes are very important in determining the significance of many ECG findings. They apply not only to ST segments, but also to T waves and Q waves. The concept and identification of reciprocal changes will be discussed later in this chapter.

To truly call the ST segment depressed the ECG should be of good quality with little artifact and smooth baselines. The ST segment should be compared with the overall level of the TP segment and the former should be depressed visibly in relation to the latter (Figure 5–3). The segments should be compared in the same lead and, as will be discussed, the ST depression should ideally be seen in contiguous lead groups, II, III, and aVF for inferior ischemia; I, aVL, V_5, and V_6 for lateral ischemia; and V_1 through V_4 for anterior ischemia.

As a general rule, the deeper the ST depression, the more severe the ischemia. The American Heart Association criterion for significant ST segment depression is > 1 mm at 0.08 seconds (two small squares) after the end of the QRS. Furthermore, ST segment depression associated with nontransmural (subendocardial) ischemia is either horizontal (flat) or downsloping, and the segment is altogether straight. Finally, the ST segment in ischemia typically intersects with the T wave at a sharp angle, which is in contrast to other causes of ST depression (Table 5–1).

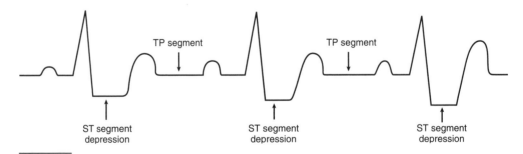

Figure 5–3.
ST segment depression reflective of myocardial ischemia.
Evaluation of the ST segment involves comparison to the level of the TP segment.

TABLE 5-1 • **Primary Causes of ST Depression**

- Myocardial ischemia
- Left ventricular hypertrophy (enlargement of the left ventricle)
- Intraventricular conduction defects
- Medications (e.g., digitalis)

The T Wave

The T wave represents the recovery period of the ventricles and should be examined with regard to its shape, symmetry, and height in relation to its corresponding QRS complex throughout the twelve leads of the ECG. Normal T wave polarity can be summarized as follows:

- Normally upright in leads I, II, and V_3 through V_6
- Normally inverted in lead aVR
- Variable in all other leads

In general, it is helpful to think of a common agreement in axis (deflection) between the net QRS axis and the net T wave axis. On initial overview, the T waves should, with minor variation, be *concordant* (same deflection) with the respective QRS in the limb leads and have the same general trend as those QRS complexes in the chest leads (Figure 5–4). This is true, however, only in the setting of a narrow (< 0.12 sec) QRS without ventricular hypertrophy (enlargement of the ventricle) (see Chapter 7). The T wave should appear rounded and usually have an asymmetrical curve. The height of the T wave is also important in reading the ECG. T waves are normally not greater than 5 mm (one large box) in any standard limb lead and not above 10 mm (two large boxes) in the precordial leads.

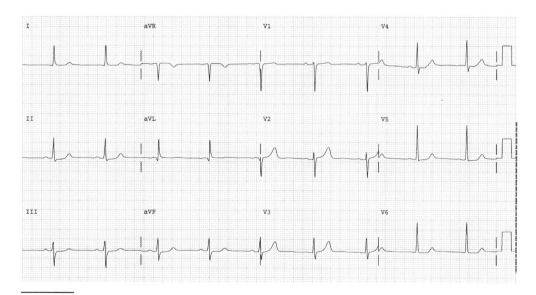

Figure 5–4.
12-lead ECG recording of normal sinus rhythm.
Note the characteristic rounded asymmetrical T wave of less than 5 mm in the limb leads (I, II, III, aVR, aVL, aVF) and less than 10 mm in the precordial leads (V_1 through V_6). Furthermore, note the concordant deflection of the T wave with the respective QRS.

Abnormal T Waves

As mentioned, T waves should normally be rounded and usually less than 5 mm in the limb leads and 10 mm in the chest leads. While a range of normal exists, certain generalizations can be made about abnormalities in T wave polarity and morphology. These include T waves which are extremely tall (i.e., as large as or larger than the corresponding QRS) and those which are more pointed than they are round.

Hyperacute T Waves

One class of T waves deserving of special attention are those referred to as hyperacute (enlarged) T waves (Figure 5–5A). These are seen in the earliest stages of myocardial infarction, often before changes are seen in the QRS or ST segments. Hyperacute T waves are typically symmetrical and peaked. ST segment elevation (indicating myocardial injury) may or may not coexist. Other signs of acute myocardial infarction (e.g., Q wave formation) usually follow within a short time, however.

The combination of large hyperacute T waves with an elevated ST segment give the T wave a large tombstone appearance (Figure 5–5B). Special note should be made of these changes by the paramedic, as their sudden appearance is usually indicative of ongoing acute injury to acute infarction.

T Wave Inversion

Although seen less frequently than ST segment depression, T wave inversion is another potential indicator of myocardial ischemia. T waves become inverted because ischemia reverses the sequence of repolarization, causing it to occur in the endocardial to epicar-

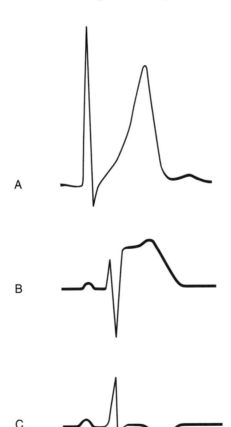

A

B

C

Figure 5–5.
(A) Hyperacute T wave present in the early stage of infarction. The normal rounded asymmetrical T wave becomes symmetrical and peaked. (B) Tombstone T wave characterized by the combination of ST segment elevation and hyperacute T waves. Their presence is of great significance, reflecting ongoing myocardial injury. (C) Symmetrical T wave inversion often seen in myocardial ischemia.

TABLE 5–2 • **Primary Causes of T Wave Inversion**

- Myocardial ischemia
- Left ventricular hypertrophy
- Myocarditis
- Pericarditis
- Electrolyte imbalances
- Intraventricular conduction defects
- Normal variant in certain leads (e.g., aVR)

dial direction rather than the normal epicardial to endocardial pattern. The normally upright asymmetrical T wave becomes deeply inverted and symmetrical, reflecting the underlying ischemic process (Figure 5–5C). However, it is important to remember that T wave inversion may represent a normal variant or occur from other causes such as ventricular hypertrophy, myocarditis, pericarditis, and electrolyte imbalances (Table 5–2). T wave inversion is usually seen during episodes of acute transmural wall ischemia, but may not appear for hours or even days following the initial event. It typically follows the stage of ST segment elevation, occurring independently or in conjunction with ST depression.

In summary, ST and T wave changes may be early warning signs of impending infarction. It is imperative that these changes be considered with regard to the overall condition of the patient. Beginning inappropriate treatment based on inaccurate or overzealous reading of ST-T waves should be avoided. It is only with repeated review and practice that true ischemic versus other nonischemic changes can be confidently diagnosed.

MYOCARDIAL INJURY

Definition and Description

As the imbalance between oxygen supply and demand continues, myocardial tissue evolves from being ischemic to being injured. Injury reflects a degree of cellular damage beyond that of mere ischemia, but it too is potentially reversible if blood flow to areas of jeopardized myocardium is restored before tissue death ensues. Furthermore, myocardial injury, unlike ischemia, is not exclusively due to increased demand. It is often the result of a diminishing supply of oxygen.

Electrical Alterations in Myocardial Injury

In myocardial injury, the myocardium is depolarized incompletely. Injured myocardium is electrically more positive than surrounding uninjured myocardium at the end of depolarization. An electrode overlying the injured area will record this as a positive charge, resulting in ST segment elevation (Figure 5–6). ST segment elevation is the result of subepicardial injury (injury confined to the outer ventricular wall), often appearing within minutes following the acute event. Additionally, an ECG lead placed opposite the injured area over normal myocardium will record ST depression, since the net depolarization force is now away from that electrode.

Abnormal ECG Findings in Myocardial Tissue Injury

At the point in the evolution of ischemia to injury, quick and appropriate understanding and intervention by EMS personnel is of critical importance. The injured myocardium is still viable if adequate oxygenation and perfusion can be restored. How-

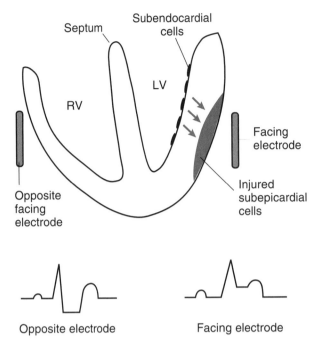

Figure 5–6
Schematic view of the left ventricle demonstrating the flow of electrical current from uninjured subendocardial cells toward injured subepicardial cells (arrows). The injured subepicardial cells are electrically more positive than the surrounding uninjured areas. This is recorded as ST segment elevation in those leads overlying injured areas and ST segment depression in those leads opposite the injured area.

ever, if blood flow and/or oxygen delivery to the area remains inadequate, within hours the cell membrane will lose its integrity, lose its ability to maintain its resting action potential, and the heart's ability to produce normal pumping action will be lost. At this point a vicious cycle of decreased cardiac output leading to decreases in perfusion of other marginally at-risk areas ensues. Therefore, it is crucial to recognize ST elevation and intervene quickly to prevent progression to larger and more hemodynamically significant ischemia and/or infarction.

ST Segment Elevation

As we have stated earlier, injured myocardium incompletely depolarizes. Therefore, it remains electrically more positive than surrounding uninjured myocardium at the end of depolarization. The ECG will record this injury as ST segment elevation when the lead is placed over the injured (epicardial) area, and ST segment depression when it is placed opposite, or reciprocally, to the area of injury. Thus, it may be said that the classic and earliest ECG finding in acute injury is characterized by contiguous ST segment elevation of those leads directly over the injured area with reciprocal ST depression in contiguous leads opposite the injury site. Furthermore, because ST segment elevation is reasonably specific to infarction, its presence provides the strongest ECG evidence of the acute event.

Anatomically Contiguous ST Segment Elevation

When ST segment elevation or other indicative changes of ischemia or infarction are present on the electrocardiogram, they are diagnostic only when present in anatomically contiguous leads. Anatomically contiguous leads are those leads which "view" the same region of the heart (Table 5–3). For example, leads II, III, and aVF all look at adjoining tissue of the inferior wall of the left ventricle. If ST elevation is present in at least two of the three leads, enough evidence exists to suspect injury to the inferior wall (Figure 5–7). However, when ST segment elevation is seen in two or more leads that are not anatomically contiguous (i.e., do not view the same region of the heart), injury or infarction is

TABLE 5–3 • **Anatomically Contiguous Leads**
• II, III, and aVF: View the inferior wall of the left ventricle • I, aVL, V_5, and V_6: View the lateral wall of the left ventricle • V_1 and V_2: View the anterior septum • V_4 and V_5: View the anterior wall of the left ventricle

Note: V_1 through V_4 are all considered anterior leads.

not present. For example, if ST elevation is present in leads II and V_4, infarction would not necessarily be suspected. This is because leads II and V_4 are not anatomically contiguous. Lead II looks at the inferior wall of the left ventricle, while V_4 looks at the anterior wall. Therefore, knowledge of the different anatomical lead groups is mandatory for infarct recognition.

Reciprocal Changes

The concept of reciprocal changes is quite simple. Essentially, reciprocal changes are sometimes recorded on the ECG from leads positioned opposite the area of ischemia or infarction. In other words, ST segment elevation in one lead will be recorded by an opposite lead as ST depression, since each lead is observing electrical forces from different viewpoints (Figure 5–8). For example, acute anterior wall infarction with associated ST segment elevation in the anterior leads (V_1 through V_4) may be accompanied by ST segment depression in the opposing inferior leads (II, III, and aVF) (Figure 5–9). Likewise, inferior infarction with ST elevation in the inferior leads may be associated with simultaneous ST depression in the opposing lateral leads (I and aVL). The presence of reciprocal changes greatly enhances the diagnosis of acute myocardial injury and/or infarction (Table 5–4).

ECG Evaluation of ST Segment Elevation

ST segment elevation is the hallmark of acute cardiac injury; however, numerous other nonischemic conditions may produce ST segment elevation. Therefore, it is critical for the EMS provider to become familiar with the characteristics of what we will call the ischemic ST elevation pattern. In order to help differentiate ischemia from nonischemic

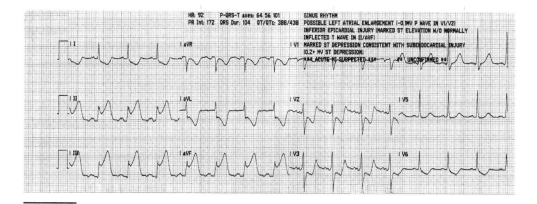

Figure 5–7.
12-lead ECG recording of an acute inferior wall infarction.
Note the presence of contiguous ST segment elevation in the inferior leads (II, III, and aVF). Contiguous ST elevation is the classic ECG marker of injury/infarction.

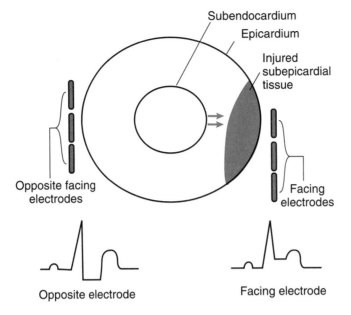

Figure 5–8.
Schematic view of the left ventricle demonstrating the concept of reciprocal ST segment depression.
Note the flow of electrical current toward the injured subepicardium (arrows). This is recorded as ST segment elevation in those leads facing the injured area and ST segment depression in those leads opposite the injured area.

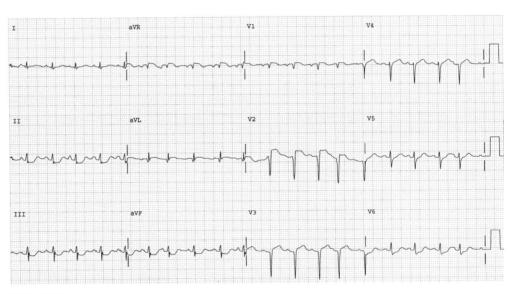

Figure 5–9.
12-lead ECG recording of an acute anterior wall infarction.
Note the presence of ST segment elevation in the anterior leads (V_1 through V_4) with reciprocal ST segment depression in the opposing inferior leads (II, III, and aVF). The simultaneous presence of reciprocal changes enhances the ECG diagnosis of infarction.

TABLE 5–4 • **Reciprocal Leads**

ECG LEADS	RECIPROCAL CHANGES
I, aVL, V_5, and V_6 (lateral leads)	II, III, and aVF
II, III, aVF (inferior leads)	I and aVL
V_1 through V_4 (anterior leads)	II, III, aVF

TABLE 5–5   •   **Ischemic ST Segment Elevation Pattern**

- 1 mm or more ST segment elevation in two or more anatomically contiguous leads
- 2 mm or more ST segment elevation in the precordial leads
- ST segment elevation with the simultaneous presence or reciprocal changes

patterns, certain general rules regarding ST segment elevation apply. They are as follows (Table 5–5).

The Ischemic ST Segment Elevation Pattern

- 1 mm or more of ST segment elevation in two or more anatomically contiguous limb leads
- 2 mm or more of ST segment elevation in the precordial lead
- ST elevation with the simultaneous presence of reciprocal changes

It is still unclear whether reciprocal ST depression is simply the result of a loss of the net positive forces over injured myocardium. It may also represent ischemia of other areas of muscle at points distant from the area of injury. However, the presence of reciprocal ST depression makes the likelihood of contiguous ST segment elevation being due to injury more likely. It should also be noted again that if there is subendocardial injury hiding under an area of well perfused epicardial muscle, ST segment elevation may be hidden as well.

The ST segment is also a quantitative representation of the amount of muscle undergoing injury. It is often assumed that the amplitude of the ST segment approximates the amount of muscle at risk. This means that the greater the ST segment displacement, the more ischemic and injured cells are present (Figure 5–10). Typically, this is true; however, there are limitations to this kind of quantitative interpretation. For example, the ST segment must be looked at in relation to the height of the respective QRS complex. In left ventricular hypertrophy, leads V_1 and V_2 may have large, associated ST segment elevation (see Chapter 7).

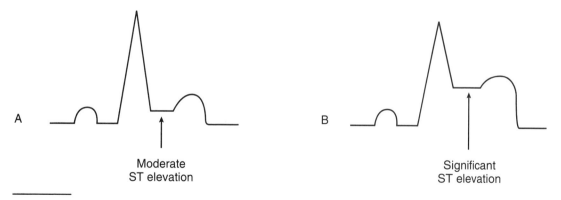

A   Moderate
ST elevation

B   Significant
ST elevation

Figure 5–10.
ST segment elevation.
Note the difference in amplitude between the ST segment in A versus that
of B. Generally, the greater the ST elevation, the more significant the injury.

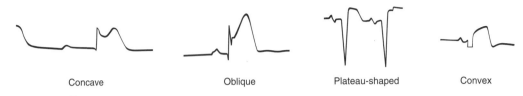

Figure 5–11.
Different forms of ST segment elevation.

Types of ST Segment Elevation

Characteristic changes in the shape and polarity of the ST segment herald the evolution from injury to infarction. While many of these changes are subtle, this recognition by the EMS provider may be helpful in assessing the patient's response to intervention.

The earliest or acute stage of myocardial injury is seen as a concave elevation of the ST segment (Figure 5–11). Its presence in the patient with a characteristic clinical picture of ischemic heart disease (e.g., chest pain, diaphoresis, difficulty breathing, etc.) is highly suggestive of early injury. As injury progresses with time, the ST segment will take on a more oblique shape. It is at this point that the T wave may appear either upright, flattened, or inverted. It is also at this point that the interpreter should look closely at the QRS complex for the appearance of new Q waves or deepening and widening Q waves in the injury leads. Following this stage, the ST segment usually appears more plateau-shaped, but with faster heart rates may take on more of a convex domed appearance. A distinct J-point (see Chapter 3) may or may not be present, so the correct assessment of what constitutes the beginning and end of the ST segment may be difficult.

NONISCHEMIC CAUSES OF ST SEGMENT ELEVATION

ST segment elevation, as we have discussed, is the hallmark of the acute injury pattern. However, ST elevation itself is not limited exclusively to myocardial infarction. It is vitally important therefore, for EMS personnel to not overread or misinterpret ST segment elevation as acute injury when it occurs as the result of benign or nonischemic conditions. It cannot be overemphasized that making clinical decisions in the out-of-hospital setting based solely on ECG interpretation of presumed acute myocardial injury is unacceptable and potentially life-threatening. Among the numerous other conditions producing ST segment elevation a few merit special attention and will be introduced. These include technical malfunctions, benign early repolarization, acute pericarditis, and left bundle branch block.

Technical Malfunctions

Because of the nature and environment in which prehospital ECGs are performed, especially in the emergency setting, numerous technical and operator-dependent factors may produce artificial elevations of the ST segment; among them, poor lead and electrode contacts producing a wandering baseline, poor skin-electrode contact, and the presence of a ventricular pacemaker or pacer wires interfering with the normal tracing. The possibility of a technical error should be considered if the ST segment is elevated on a poor quality tracing or if the patient is moving, hyperventilating, or otherwise uncooperative.

Benign Early Repolarization

Benign early repolarization is a distracting electrocardiographic finding that may confuse the diagnosis of acute infarction. It is characterized by ST segment elevation of up to 2 mm in the precordial leads, and occasionally up to 4 mm in the left precordial leads (V_4 and V_5) because of elevation of the J-point. The ST elevation seen often has a downward saddleback or caved shape, rather than an upward convex shape, which lowers but does not eliminate suspicion of myocardial ischemia. Furthermore, benign early repolarization shows no reciprocal ST depression and is most prevalent in young black males who are clinically asymptomatic (see Chapter 7, Figure 7–4).

Acute Pericarditis

The normal pericardial space is formed by the visceral pericardium, which envelopes the epicardium, and the outer parietal pericardium. Normally, this space contains less than 50 cc of pericardial fluid. With acute inflammation, however, fluid accumulates within this space, producing acute pericarditis. Acute pericarditis often causes chest pain that is retrosternal and left precordial, referred to the back and shoulders. Often the pain is pleuritic (sharp), aggravated by inspiration, coughing, and changes in body position. Therefore, confusion with myocardial infarction is common as the clinical symptoms indicate.

Distinguishing between acute myocardial injury and acute pericarditis is also complicated by the fact that on the ECG, acute pericarditis often presents with diffuse ST elevation (Figure 5–12). The important point to emphasize about ST segment elevation in acute pericarditis is that it is diffuse. In other words, ST elevation is not isolated to one anatomically contiguous lead group (i.e., II, III, and aVF for inferior injury), but is

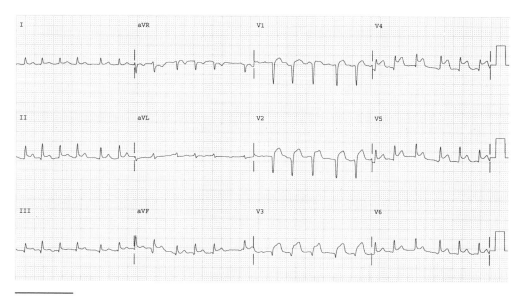

Figure 5–12.
12-lead ECG recording of acute pericarditis.
Note the widespread ST segment elevation throughout the tracing. Diffuse ST elevation scattered about the limb and precordial leads is the primary finding of acute pericarditis. The ECG recognition of acute pericarditis is often extremely difficult to distinguish from acute myocardial infarction. Historical and physical examination findings, in combination with the ECG, are paramount to proper diagnosis.

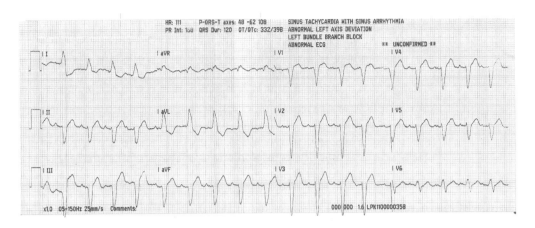

Figure 5–13.
12-lead ECG recording of left bundle branch block.
Note the enlarged QRS (. 0.12 sec) complexes and the difference in deflection between QRSs and T waves. Furthermore, note the elevated ST segment primarily in the chest leads (V_1 through V_5), making the diagnosis of infarction in the presence of LBBB very difficult.

widespread and usually present in all leads except aVR. In myocardial infarction, the ST segment is more localized and is accompanied by reciprocal ST depression in the opposite leads.

Left Bundle Branch Block

Left bundle branch block (LBBB) is the complete blockage of electrical conduction down the left bundle branch. It often is the result of ischemic heart disease, long-standing hypertension, or cardiomyopathy. When any of these or other conditions cause complete blockage of conduction down the left bundle branch, the net result is prolongation of the QRS because the right and left sides of the conduction system are now conducting slightly out of sequence. The QRS complex will be longer than 0.12 seconds (three small squares) and the net depolarization vector will shift toward the blocked side (e.g., to the left in LBBB) (Figure 5–13).

Because left bundle branch block alters the normal sequence of depolarization, changes in repolarization also occur. The net result is a discordance between the normal QRS axis and the T wave axis. Simply put, in LBBB, in any lead which has a positive QRS complex, the associated T wave will be predominantly negative and vice versa (refer to Figure 5–13). The abnormal relationship between repolarization and depolarization may produce secondary ST elevation, seen primarily in the chest leads. The appearance of this elevation, in association with a small or negative QRS in those leads makes them appear more ominous, but it should be realized that they are the result of a conduction rather than a primary ischemic pattern. A further discussion of these and other causes of nonischemic ST segment elevation will follow in Chapter 7.

MYOCARDIAL INFARCTION

Definition and Description

As oxygen deprivation to the myocardium continues, eventually the cellular damage becomes irreversible. At this point, infarction or necrosis (death) of myocardial tissue occurs and the affected cells are without function, both electrically and mechanically.

Electrical Alterations in Myocardial Infarction

From the standpoint of ECG manifestation of myocardial infarction, the key point to remember is that infarcted tissue is electrically silent (i.e., it is no longer able to conduct electricity). The net electrical forces, therefore, are directed away from the infarcted area. An electrode facing the infarcted tissue will record an abnormal negative deflection during depolarization, a Q wave. This is because the electrode "looks through" the infarcted tissue and records only those electrical forces moving through undamaged muscle in the endocardial surface of the opposite wall. Since depolarization proceeds from endocardium to epicardium, this electrode now records the electrical current as going away in the opposite wall (Figure 5–14).

Transmural Versus Nontransmural Infarction

Myocardial infarction may involve either the complete thickness or only a partial thickness segment of the ventricular wall (Figure 5–15). While ultimately the process which produces myocardial necrosis is similar in transmural and subendocardial infarction, an important point needs to be made about their electrically different manifestations. Since transmural infarction by definition involves the full thickness myocardium, a surface electrode overlying the infarcted area will record the net vector as being negative, or away. This may not be the case in subendocardial infarction where a layer of intact muscle may overlie the necrotic area. As we will discuss, the ECG manifestation of those two entities will often vary. It should never be assumed that the absence of a typical ECG pattern of myocardial infarction precludes the possibility of either subendocardial or even early transmural necrosis.

Abnormal ECG Findings in Myocardial Infarction

Myocardial infarction (MI) is defined as the point at which irreversible necrosis or cell death occurs. From a physiological perspective, it is the end result of the evolution of the myocardial cell's response to hypoxic stress. However, in a practical sense, it is critical to remember that the ECG significance in infarction is in itself a dynamic one. The ECG

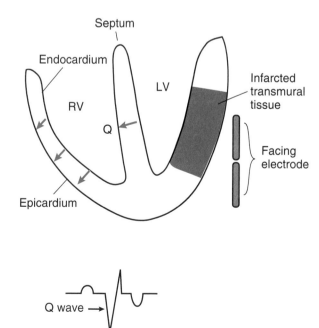

Figure 5–14.
Mechanism of Q wave formation. Schematic of the ventricular myocardium representing a transmural (full thickness) infarction. Infarcted (dead) tissue is electrically silent, unable to conduct an electrical current. As a result, electrodes facing the infarcted area "look through" the dead tissue and record impulses on the opposite wall. Normal forces in the opposite wall are going away from the electrodes, traveling from endocardium to epicardium, inscribing a large negative Q wave (arrows).

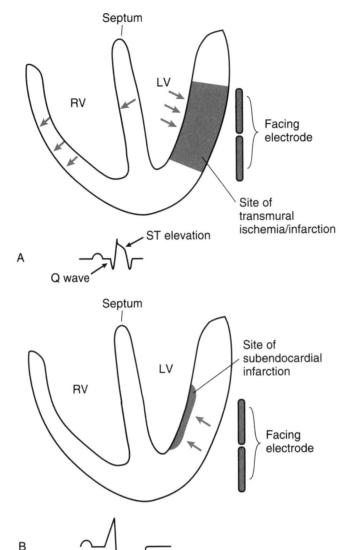

Figure 5-15.
(A) Schematic view of the left ventricle identifying a transmural (full thickness) infarction. Electrodes facing the injured/infarcted tissue will record ST segment elevation as the current flows (arrows) toward the damaged area.
(B) Schematic of the left ventricle identifying a subendocardial (partial thickness) infarction. Electrodes facing the injured/infarcted tissue will record this as ST segment depression as the current flows away from the electrodes toward the damaged area (arrows).

should be viewed, by the emergency care worker, as a road map of the evolution of an MI rather than as a simple positive or negative type test.

The ECG hallmarks of evolving MI

- ST segment elevation (with or without hyperacute T waves)
- Inverted T waves
- Development of Q waves

As you recall, the first indication of an acute infarction is injury. This is represented by ST segment elevation in the area overlying the injury, followed variably by T wave inversion and the presence of reciprocal changes in opposing leads. As injury progresses, some of the cells begin to infarct (die) from anoxia. This results in the appearance of new pathologic (deep and wide) Q waves, indicating that irreversible myocardial cell death has occurred.

TABLE 5–6   •   **Q Waves**

DURATION	HEIGHT
Physiological (normal): < 0.04 sec	< 25% of the succeeding R wave
Pathological (abnormal): > 0.04 sec	> 25% of the succeeding R wave

Normal (Physiological) Versus Abnormal (Pathological) Q Waves

Although Q waves are often thought of as the hallmark of infarction, it is important to remember that Q waves are present as part of the normal ECG. Septal Q waves describe the left-to-right rapid, early depolarization of the septum. They are seen in the lateral leads I, aVL, V_6 (and occasionally V_5). They are typically narrow and small, less than 0.04 seconds in duration and less than 25% of the corresponding R wave amplitude (Table 5–6).

Pathological Q waves are generally greater than 0.04 seconds in duration and have an amplitude greater than 25% of the associated R wave (Figure 5–16). They represent areas of myocardium that have become electrically silent, with a resultant shift in the initial depolarization force away from the infarcted area. Pathological Q waves may develop in any lead, and the more extensive the infarction, the more leads in which they will be displayed. Furthermore, because significant Q waves represent tissue death, they will remain as part of a patient's ECG for a lifetime. In the patient with a history of previous MI, comparison with a prior ECG to determine whether the Q waves represent new acute changes is often very helpful. In the absence of a prior tracing, however, Q waves in the prehospital setting should be presumed to be acute.

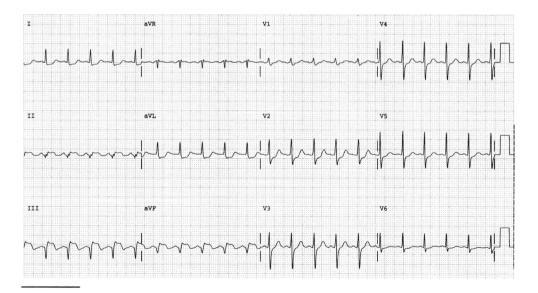

Figure 5–16.
12-lead ECG recording of an acute inferior wall myocardial infarction.
Note the presence to large (pathological) Q waves accompanied by ST elevation in the inferior leads (II, III, aVF). Pathological Q waves denote dead myocardial tissue.

Q Wave Versus Non-Q Wave Infarction

Because an ECG essentially records surface forces only, it was believed that if the myocardium overlying an infarct remained normal (i.e., a nontransmural or subendocardial infarct), that the ECG would be nondiagnostic. However, ischemic changes can effect the net electrical forces manifested on an ECG even when the outermost layers of the heart remain intact. While it is often taught that myocardial infarction can be divided into transmural versus nontransmural (subendocardial) infarction, it is more useful to think in terms of Q wave versus non-Q wave infarction, keeping in mind that other ECG derangements of evolving MI, hyperacute T waves, ST elevation, and T wave inversion may be present either with or without associated Q waves.

If infarction involves the entire thickness of the ventricular wall (i.e., from subendocardium to epicardium) an abnormal (pathological) Q wave will usually develop on the ECG. This type of infarction, termed Q wave infarction, is usually associated with extensive myocardial death. On the other hand, if infarction involves only the innermost or subendocardial layer, a pathological Q wave will not develop on the ECG. This type of infarction, termed non-Q wave infarction, usually implies less myocardial tissue death than a Q wave infarction, and is accompanied by fewer complications.

Loss of R Wave Progression

Another diagnostic ECG feature of myocardial infarction is the loss of R wave progression. Recall from the previous chapter that the normal pattern for R waves is to increase in height in the leads V_1 through V_4. This is representative of the dominance of the anteroseptal wall of the left ventricle in the production of the main depolarization force. It has been classically taught that poor R wave progression through these leads is indicative of anterior wall injury/infarction. While in theory this may be true, as a practical matter, poor R wave progression probably has more to do with variations in the placement of the precordial leads than with ischemia. However, the loss of R wave progression on serial (repeated) tracings (especially with identical lead placement) is more likely to represent pathology, especially if clinical and other ECG findings (ST elevation) are also suggestive of acute ischemia/infarction (Figure 5–17).

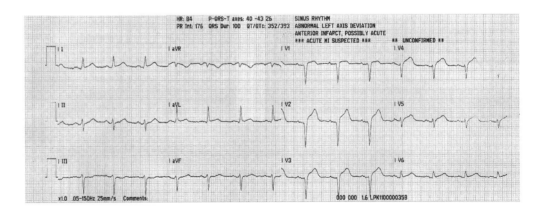

Figure 5–17.
12-lead ECG recording of an acute anterior wall myocardial infarction.
Note the loss of R wave progression through the anterior leads (V_1 through V_4), coupled with the presence of ST segment elevation. This combination greatly enhances the diagnosis of myocardial injury/infarction.

TABLE 5–7 • **Dating an Infarct**

- Acute infarction: Contiguous ST segment elevation with or without T wave inversion
- Resolving infarction: ST segment returns to the baseline and the T wave regains its normal contour
- Old infarction: Presence of pathological Q waves

Dating an Infarct

As we have emphasized throughout this chapter, myocardial infarction is the end point of the dynamic process of ischemia. However, electrocardiographic changes continue and the complete ECG picture of an infarct may not be manifested until weeks or even months later. This has often been described as dating an infarct and it may be summarized as follows (Table 5–7):

- Acute infarction: Contiguous ST segment elevation with without T wave inversion.
- Resolving infarction: ST segment returns to the baseline and the T wave regains its normal contour.
- Old infarction: Presence of pathological Q waves.

It is essential to remember that ST segment elevation is the earliest ECG indicator of infarction. Because it occurs so early in the course of infarction, ST elevation is well suited for prehospital detection. Other signs of infarction, T wave inversion, and/or the appearance of Q waves may not be present in the stage of infarction when patients are encouraged to seek treatment.

SUMMARY

As the role of the prehospital provider expands, he or she will be called upon to make rapid diagnostic and treatment decisions on patients presenting with the entire spectrum of ischemic heart disease. A basic understanding of the physiology of acute ischemia, injury, and infarction are prerequisite to proper ECG interpretation. When used properly and appropriately, the ECG offers an essential and often lifesaving addition to the didactic and practical skills EMS providers can employ on behalf of their patients.

KEY POINTS SUMMARY

Pathophysiology of Infarction

1. Myocardial infarction occurs when a coronary artery is unable to sufficiently supply a segment of myocardial tissue with oxygenated blood. Usually this process begins as the result of atherosclerosis followed by the formation of a blood clot in the immediate area of an incomplete fixed obstruction lesion. Once obstruction occurs, the myocardial cells instantly undergo a hypoxic evolution of ischemia, followed by injury, and then infarction.

Electrocardiographic Evolution of Infarction

2. ECG evolution of infarction begins with an increase in the amplitude and symmetry of the T wave (hyperacute T waves). This is followed by ST segment elevation (acute phase) and T wave inversion. Finally, the development of large (pathological) Q waves occurs, providing evidence of myocardial tissue death.
3. The paramedic should note that the evolving ECG changes of infarction are by no means absolute. One, all, or none of the findings may be recorded during infarction.

Myocardial Ischemia

4. Myocardial ischemia is the first phase of tissue hypoxia. It is usually the result of diminished subendocardial blood flow and is often reversible with little or no permanent cell damage if prompt intervention is initiated.

5. The electrical alterations of myocardial ischemia are due to a delay in repolarization. ECG evidence of myocardial ischemia is thus represented by ST segment depression and T wave inversion.

Myocardial Injury

6. Myocardial injury is the result of unresolved myocardial ischemia, but it too is potentially reversible with prompt intervention (i.e., thrombolytic therapy).

7. The electrical alterations of myocardial injury are due to incomplete depolarization of the myocardium. ECG evidence of myocardial injury is represented by anatomically contiguous ST segment elevation in those leads overlying the injured heart muscle.

Myocardial Infarction

8. Myocardial infarction (tissue necrosis) is the culminating lethal response to unresolved myocardial ischemia. The myocardial cells are both electrically and mechanically dead.

9. The electrical alterations of myocardial infarction are due to the electrically inactive muscle. ECG evidence of myocardial infarction is represented by the development of pathological (abnormally enlarged) Q waves.

Transmural Versus Nontransmural Infarction

10. A transmural infarction (Q wave infarct) is a full thickness infarction of the myocardium. A nontransmural (subendocardial or non-Q wave) infarction involves only a segment of the myocardium (partial thickness).

Reciprocal ECG Changes

11. Reciprocal (mirror image) changes are sometimes recorded on the ECG from leads positioned opposite the area of injury/infarction. ST segment elevation in one lead is recorded as ST segment depression in an opposite lead. The presence of reciprocal changes (ST depression) enhances the diagnosis of myocardial infarction.

Loss of R Wave Progression

12. The loss of R wave progression through the anterior and left lateral chest leads is another diagnostic feature of infarction. This loss, coupled with the simultaneous presence of ST segment elevation, is highly suggestive of anterior, lateral, or anterolateral myocardial infarction.

Nonischemic Causes of ST Segment Elevation

13. ST segment elevation is not limited exclusively to myocardial infarction. Other nonischemic causes of ST segment elevation include technical malfunctions, benign early repolarization, acute pericarditis, and left bundle branch block.

BIBLIOGRAPHY

Braunwald E. *Heart Disease: A Textbook of Cardiovascular Medicine.* Philadelphia, PA: WB Saunders; 1980.

Chou TC. *Electrocardiography in Clinical Practice.* Philadelphia, PA: WB Saunders; 1991.

Conover MB. *Understanding Electrocardiography: Arrhythmias and the 12-Lead ECG.* St. Louis, MO: Mosby; 1992.

Foster DB. *Twelve-Lead Electrocardiography for ACLS Providers.* Philadelphia, PA: WB Saunders; 1996.

Goldberger AL. *Myocardial Infarction, Electro-*

cardiographic Differential Diagnosis. 4th ed. St Louis, MO: Mosby; 1991.

Goldman MJ. *Principles of Clinical Electrocardiography.* 11th ed. Los Altos, CA: Lange Medical Publications; 1982.

Huszar RJ. *Basic Dysrhythmias: Interpretation and Management.* 2nd ed. St. Louis, MO: Mosby; 1994.

Johnson R, Swartz MH. *A Simplified Approach To Electrocardiography.* Philadelphia, PA: WB Saunders; 1986.

Langer F. *12-Lead Electrocardiography: Advanced Dysrhythmias.* Orlando, FL: Florida Hospital Medical Center; 1992.

Lipman BC, Cascio T. *ECG: Assessment and Interpretation.* Philadelphia, PA: FA Davis Company; 1994.

Marriot HJ. *Practical Electrocardiography.* 8th ed. Baltimore, MD: Williams and Wilkins; 1988.

Otto LA, Aufderheide TP. Evaluation of ST segment elevation criteria for the prehospital electrocardiographic diagnosis of acute myocardial infarction. *Annals of Emergency Medicine.* 1994;23:1, 17–24.

Thaler MS. *The Only EKG Book You'll Ever Need.* Philadelphia, PA: JB Lippincott; 1988.

Infarct Localization and Systematic Analysis

1. Describe the anatomy of the coronary circulation and list the structures supplied by the right and left coronary arteries.

2. Discuss the pathophysiology of coronary artery disease.

3. Describe the precipitating events of myocardial infarction.

4. List and identify the ECG changes associated with myocardial ischemia/infarction.

5. Discuss the classifications of myocardial infarction.

6. Define Q wave and non-Q wave infarctions and identify their ECG characteristics.

7. Describe the pathology of anterior, inferior, lateral, and posterior infarction.

8. Predict the site of coronary artery obstruction for anterior, inferior, lateral, and posterior infarction.

9. List those leads that reflect the anterior, inferior, lateral, and posterior myocardial surfaces of the left ventricle.

10. Identify anterior, inferior, lateral, and posterior myocardial infarction on the electrocardiogram.

11. Discuss the common complications associated with anterior and inferior myocardial infarction.

12. Discuss the pathophysiology of right ventricular infarction and list those leads that reflect the right ventricular surface.

13. List and describe the clinical symptoms of right ventricular infarction.

14. Discuss the treatment strategy for right ventricular infarction.

15. Describe reciprocal ECG changes and relate their significance to infarct detection.

16. List and describe the steps for the systematic 12-lead ECG analysis.

INTRODUCTION

Previous chapters have introduced both the basic concepts of 12-lead electrocardiography and the evolutionary patterns of infarction. In this chapter, the reader will learn how to localize the area of the heart muscle (myocardium) which is ischemic. Localization allows anticipation of complications and will influence therapeutic choices for the treatment of acute myocardial infarction. By anticipating the specific complications associated with infarction in each region of the heart, morbidity and mortality may be reduced as appropriate interventions are accomplished in a timely manner. The reader will also be provided with a systematic approach to the interpretation of 12-lead electrocardiographs.

Myocardial ischemia may be isolated to the anterior wall, inferior wall, lateral wall, posterior wall, and septum of the left ventricle. Infarction or ischemia in a particular area of the myocardium will produce ischemic or infarction changes (ST elevation, ST depression, Q waves, or T wave inversion) in the lead associated with that particular anatomic location of the myocardium. Both the limb leads (I, II, III, aVL, aVF) and the chest leads (V_1 through V_6) are used to localize the area of injury.

CORONARY ANATOMY

In most patients, the left anterior descending coronary artery supplies the anterior and apical regions of the left ventricle (see Chapter 2, Figure 2–6). It may also supply portions of the intraventricular septum, anterolateral wall, papillary muscles, and the inferoapical wall of the left ventricle. The left circumflex coronary artery usually supplies the lateral and inferoposterior wall of the left ventricle. Myocardium supplied by the right coronary artery includes the inferoposterior wall of the left ventricle, inferior part of the intraventricular septum, posteromedial papillary muscles, and most of the right ventricle. The right coronary artery also supplies the SA node in 60% of patients and the AV node in 90% of patients. The posterior descending coronary artery supplies the posterior left ventricular wall. A dominant right coronary artery or a dominant left circumflex coronary artery usually supplies the posterior descending coronary artery.

Collateral anastomosis (communication between vessels) of the coronary arteries are present in the normal human heart. There is great variation in the size and distribution of the collateral blood supply. In patients with normal coronary arteries, there is little clinical significance to the anastomosis. Those patients with significant coronary artery disease may have well-developed anastomotic networks. Further, a long history of angina pectoris (chest pain due to an imbalance between myocardial oxygen supply and demand) may also be associated with a significant collateral blood supply. Clinical evidence exists to support the theory that collateral circulation improves outcome by limiting necrosis.

CORONARY ARTERY PATHOLOGY

Atherosclerosis (thickening and a loss of elasticity of the arterial walls) has long been associated with ischemic coronary artery disease and myocardial infarction. Only recently has the event causing acute myocardial infarction been characterized. It is now known that thrombotic occlusion of a coronary artery is responsible for 80 to 90% of acute myocardial infarctions.

Acute myocardial infarction occurs when blood flow to the myocardium is abruptly decreased, resulting in insufficient delivery of oxygen and other metabolic substrates to the myocardium. The interaction between fixed obstructions (plaques), vasospasm, and platelet aggregation producing coronary obstruction results in acute myocardial infarction (Figure 6–1). Coronary artery disease causes luminal narrowing in the main coro-

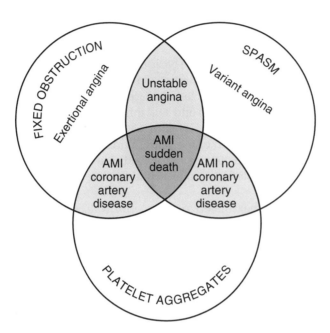

Figure 6–1.
Interaction of fixed obstruction, vasospasm, and platelet aggregates to produce acute myocardial events.

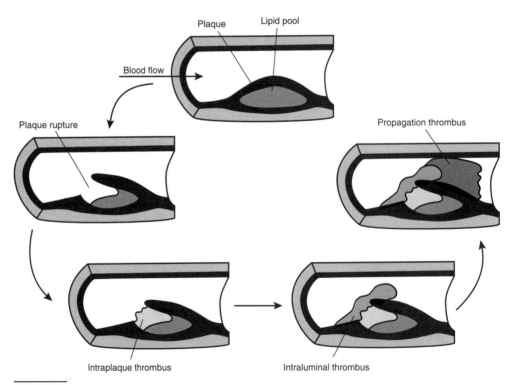

Figure 6–2.
Pathophysiology of coronary artery thrombosis.

nary arteries and their branches. The location and size of myocardial infarctions are determined by multiple factors, including location and size of atherosclerotic plaques in coronary arteries, amount of myocardium supplied by the affected artery, oxygen demand of the affected myocardium, extent of collateral blood supply, coronary artery spasm, tissue factors which modify the ischemic process, and endogenous release of both thrombotic and thrombolytic agents.

Development of an acute cardiac event begins with formation of atherosclerotic plaques within the coronary arteries. At some point in time a rupture of the plaque occurs, resulting in intraplaque hemorrhage. This causes enlargement of the plaque, thinning of the plaque's fibrous cap, and rupture. The disrupted endothelium and blood in the plaque are powerful stimulators of platelet aggregation. With platelet aggregation comes intraluminal thrombus formation. The thrombus then propagates and completely occludes the lumen of the artery (Figure 6–2). Once the blood flow is disrupted, myocardial infarction results.

REVIEW OF ECG CHANGES ASSOCIATED WITH INFARCTION

The most time-honored test to evaluate acute myocardial ischemia is the electrocardiogram. Patients with symptoms or complaints consistent with myocardial ischemia should have an immediate 12-lead ECG. It is important to note that the initial ECG is diagnostic for infarction only 25 to 50% of the time. One study found that 13% of initial ECGs were normal and 26% demonstrated only nonspecific (not clearly defined) changes in patients suffering acute myocardial infarction. The ability of the ECG to detect myocardial ischemia may be enhanced by obtaining serial (repeat) ECGs. Recurrent chest pain and sudden improvement or deterioration in the patient's clinical condition are indications for repeat ECGs. Recent experience with continuous 12-lead ECG monitoring has demonstrated that ST and T wave changes may be extremely transient at the onset of acute infarction. An expanded role for this technology is anticipated in the near future. When chest pain resolves prior to obtaining an ECG, the ischemic changes of the electrocardiogram may also have resolved. The electrocardiogram is therefore useful when diagnostic. A normal ECG does not exclude acute myocardial ischemia.

As the myocardium becomes ischemic (the blood supply, and therefore the oxygen supply, is less than adequate) T waves become flattened, then inverted. These changes are best observed in the chest leads (V_1 through V_6) because they are the closest to the myocardium. If ischemia persists, injury of the myocardium will result. Injury is characterized by ST segment elevation. Injury, if untreated, will result in infarction (death) of the myocardium producing Q waves on the ECG. Only Q waves that are 1 mm wide or at least one-third the amplitude of the QRS complex are considered significant, indicating infarction. Small, nonsignificant Q waves are often present in leads I, II, V_5 and V_6, which may be normal. Isolated Q waves in lead III only are of no consequence and do not indicate infarction ("Qs in III are free"). Additionally, ST segment depression may indicate ischemia or infarction.

CLASSIFICATION OF MYOCARDIAL INFARCTION

Traditionally, myocardial infarctions have been termed either transmural or subendocardial. Transmural myocardial infarction involves the entire thickness of the myocardium in the distribution of a coronary vessel. In contrast, subendocardial infarction is limited to the inner wall of the ventricle. It may also involve the distribution of more than one major coronary artery. Clinical differentiation between these two types of infarction has been based on their electrocardiographic appearance. Patients demonstrating new pathologic Q waves on 12-lead ECGs were thought to have transmural infarction. In the absence of new pathologic Q waves, the infarction was classified as subendocardial. Autopsy studies of patients suffering from myocardial infarction have not confirmed the association of Q waves with transmural infarction. Accordingly, current terminology classifies infarctions as either Q wave or non-Q wave, based on the evolution of the 12-lead ECG.

Q wave infarctions are often associated with complete occlusion of a major coronary artery. From 80 to 90% of Q wave infarctions had complete obstruction of at least one major coronary artery demonstrated by angiography in one study. Angiographic studies (Hillis, Braunwald, 1977; Pasternak et al., 1992) of patients with non-Q wave infarctions demonstrate coronary artery stenosis without complete occlusion. Q wave infarctions tend to be larger and carry a higher short-term mortality than non-Q wave infarctions. Patients with non-Q wave infarction have viable muscle at risk in the distribution of a diseased vessel. This results in a higher reinfarction rate and increase in long-term mortality in patients with non-Q wave infarcts.

Q Wave Infarction

Q wave infarction is defined as new Q waves of greater than 0.04 second duration and at least 25% as deep as the R wave (see Chapter 5, Figures 5–14 and 5–16). Initially the ST segment of the leads nearest the injury will be elevated. Next the T waves become tall and peaked, followed by T wave inversion. Development of the Q wave indicates myocardial necrosis. Infarction may cause bundle branch blocks if the conduction system is involved in the area of ischemia. New onset of a bundle branch block may occur with acute ischemia. In the presence of an old left bundle branch block, interpretation of ST segment changes is difficult if not impossible.

Several studies (Hillis, Braunwald, 1977; Pasternak et al., 1992) evaluating the ability of the ECG to detect acute myocardial infarction found the sensitivity to be from 43 to 65%. One study group used three ECG criteria in an attempt to detect myocardial ischemia and achieved a 79% sensitivity with only 44% specificity. These criteria assumed that the changes were new or that no old ECG was available for comparison. Probable transmural infarction was based on a greater than or equal to 1 mm ST elevation in two or more leads or pathological Q waves in two or more leads. Strain or ischemia was defined as ST segment depression greater than or equal to 1 mm in two or more leads. Also, strain or ischemia was defined as ST depression less than 1 mm with T wave inversion.

Localization of the area of ischemia is possible, based on the 12-lead ECG pattern (Table 6–1). Infarction patterns in leads V_1 through V_4 indicate anterior myocardial involvement. The lateral infarction pattern involves leads I, aVL, V_5, and V_6. Changes in leads II, III, and aVF indicate inferior myocardial injury. Remember, Q waves in lead III alone may be normal and does not indicate infarction. Often patients suffering inferior infarction will display ST depression in the anterior leads. These are called reciprocal changes and usually represent posterolateral injury in the distribution of the same coronary artery causing the inferior infarction. Reciprocal changes probably do not represent anterior ischemia. Tall R waves in V_1 or V_2 with ST depression and peaked T waves sug-

TABLE 6–1 • **Anatomical Leads and Supplying Arteries**

ANATOMICAL LEADS	SUPPLYING ARTERY
Anterior wall: V_1, V_2, V_3, V_4	Left anterior descending coronary artery
Inferior wall: II, III, aVF	Right coronary artery
Lateral wall: I, aVL, V_5, V_6	Circumflex artery
Posterior wall: V_1, V_2 (mirror images)	Right coronary or circumflex artery

gest posterior infarction. These so called mirror-image changes are analogous to Q waves, ST elevation, and inverted T waves in the other infarction patterns.

Non-Q Wave Infarction

Non-Q wave infarction is simply infarction without development of pathological Q waves. QRS morphology typically does not change; occasionally however, shortening of the R wave is observed. The classic change associated with non-Q wave infarction is precordial and lateral ST depression with or without T wave inversion (Figure 6–3).

Etiologies other than acute myocardial ischemia may produce ECG changes. ST segment and T wave changes may be produced by myocarditis (inflammation of the myocardium). Pericarditis will often cause ST elevation, usually in all or most leads. T wave inversion has been associated with hemorrhagic stroke. Ventricular aneurysm has been known to demonstrate ST segment elevation.

ANTERIOR MYOCARDIAL INFARCTION

The precordial leads V_1 through V_4 reflect the anterior surface of the myocardium, allowing localization of the ischemia/infarction to the anterior myocardium (Figure 6–4). Lead V_1 reflects the anterior right ventricular surface, V_2, and V_3 represent the intraventricular septum, and V_3, and V_4 the anterior surface of the left ventricle. Often, changes in leads V_1 and V_2 are termed septal and V_3 and V_4 anterior infarction.

The anterior wall of the left ventricle is supplied by the left anterior descending artery, which also supplies parts of the lateral wall of the left ventricle. Because the left anterior descending artery supplies such a large part of the myocardium, anterior infarctions tend to be large, often resulting in cardiogenic shock. When anterior infarction is present, anticipate cardiogenic shock and the need for pressor agents to augment blood pressure and cardiac output.

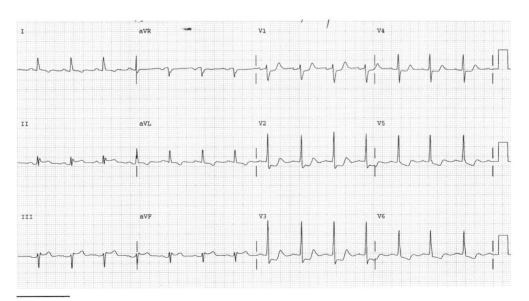

Figure 6–3.
12-lead ECG recording of a non-Q wave infarction representative of subendocardial injury.
Note the characteristic presence of ST depression and T wave inversion throughout the anterior (V_1 through V_4) and lateral (I, aVL, V_5, V_6) leads.

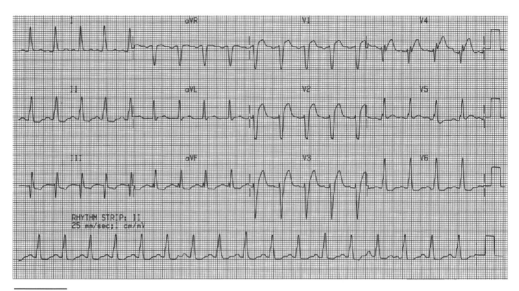

Figure 6–4.
12-lead ECG recording of an acute anterior wall myocardial infarction.
Note the presence of ST segment elevation in the anterior leads (V_1, V_2, V_3, V_4) with the simultaneous presence of reciprocal ST depression in the inferior leads (II, III, aVF). Furthermore, note the loss of R wave progression through leads V_1 through V_4.

Because the left anterior descending artery supplies large parts of the intraventricular septum, patients with anterior infarction are at risk for developing conduction abnormalities. These conduction abnormalities include second-degree AV block, left anterior hemiblock, and right bundle branch block. Some form of external pacing is often required when these conduction abnormalities develop as bradycardia may result.

INFERIOR MYOCARDIAL INFARCTION

Ischemic changes (ST elevation, Q waves, ST depression, T wave inversion) in leads II, III, and aVF represent ischemia in the inferior wall of the left ventricle (Figure 6–5). Again, knowledge of the arterial supply of the inferior wall allows the paramedic to predict the complications associated with inferior myocardial infarction. The inferior left ventricle is usually supplied by the right coronary artery, which usually supplies the AV node and the right ventricle in addition to the inferior left ventricle in most people. Inferior ischemia is therefore often associated with right ventricular infarction.

Right ventricular infarction produces hypotension not as a result of cardiogenic shock but because preload is reduced, resulting in less blood for the left ventricle to pump. Reduced preload is analogous to an inadequate water supply for a fire engine pump. The inadequate water supply results in pump cavitation and therefore low output from the fire pump. Just as pump cavitation is corrected by insuring an adequate water supply, reduced preload may be compensated for by increasing the preload with fluids (normal saline or lactated ringers). Drugs that reduce preload must also be avoided or used with great caution in the setting of inferior myocardial infarction. These drugs include morphine and nitroglycerin, agents commonly employed to treat myocardial infarction.

Conduction abnormalities are often associated with inferior myocardial infarction also. Most patients' AV node is supplied by the right coronary artery. If the AV node infarcts, a complete heart block may result. In the situation of AV nodal infarction, at-

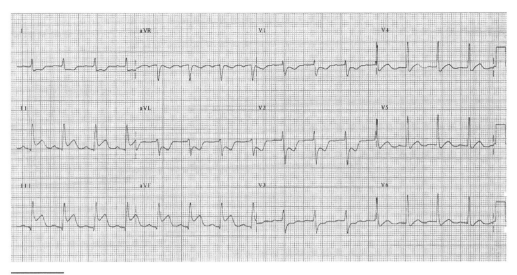

Figure 6–5.
12-lead ECG recording of an acute inferior wall myocardial infarction.
Note the presence of ST segment elevation in the inferior leads (II, III, aVF)
with reciprocal ST depression in leads I and aVL.

ropine and epinephrine are ineffective for increasing the heart rate. These patients require some form of pacing to maintain an adequate heart rate.

LATERAL MYOCARDIAL INFARCTION

Lateral myocardial infarction is characterized by changes in leads I, aVL, V_5, and V_6 (Figure 6–6). The circumflex artery most often supplies the lateral wall of the left ventricle. Proximal occlusion of the left coronary artery that divides into the left anterior descending and the circumflex artery will often produce an anterolateral myocardial infarction involving both the anterior and lateral walls of the myocardium (Figure 6–7). An easy method to remember the leads which reflect lateral infarction is to abbreviate lateral infarction "L. I." The L stands for aVL and the I for lead I. Additionally, leads V_5 and V_6, which overlay the lateral left ventricle, are involved in lateral wall infarction.

POSTERIOR MYOCARDIAL INFARCTION

Posterior myocardial infarction does not produce the usual ST elevation and Q waves in any leads of the standard 12-lead ECG. Rather, ST depression may be observed in V_1, V_2 and sometimes V_3 along with a large R wave (Figure 6–8). These changes are analogous to the ST elevation and Q waves observed in other leads with anterior, septal, lateral, and inferior infarction. In fact, if the 12-lead ECG is turned upside down and observed in a mirror, the ECG will appear to have ST elevations and Q waves in V_1 and V_2 in the presence of posterior myocardial infarction. ST depression and large R waves are produced because the depolarization wave of the posterior myocardium proceeds opposite the direction of depolarization of the anterior myocardium.

While isolated posterior myocardial infarction does occur, most often posterior infarction is associated with either inferior or lateral wall infarction. The posterior myo-

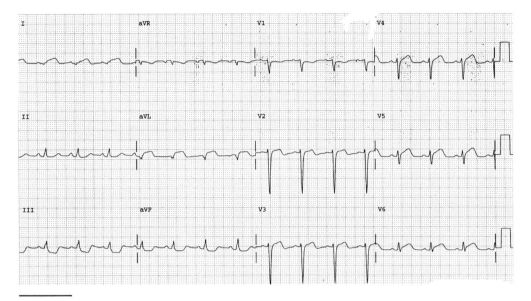

Figure 6–6.
12-lead ECG recording of an acute lateral wall myocardial infarction.
Note the presence of ST elevation throughout the lateral leads (I, aVL, V$_5$, V$_6$) with reciprocal ST depression in the inferior leads (II, III, aVF).

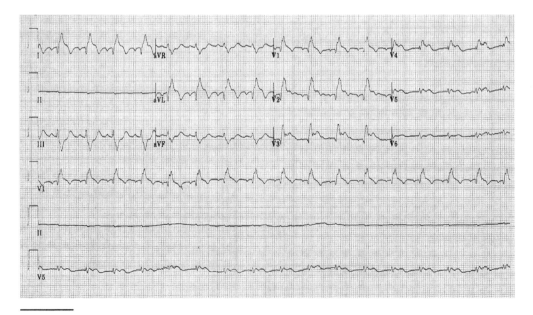

Figure 6–7.
12-lead ECG recording of an acute anterolateral myocardial infarction.
Note the presence of ST segment elevation in three contiguous anterior leads (V$_1$, V$_2$, V$_3$, V$_4$) and three contiguous lateral leads (I, aVL, V$_5$). ST segment elevation in two anatomically contiguous leads is diagnostic of ischemia/infarction.

A   B

V1

V2

V3

V4

V5

V6

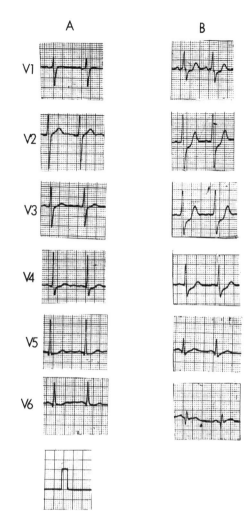

Figure 6–8.
12-lead ECG recording of an acute posterior wall myocardial infarction.
Note the presence of a large R wave and deep S wave in leads V_1 through V_4. These changes are considered mirror images of pathological Q waves and ST elevation. Reproduced with permission from Johns JA, Gold HK, Leinbash RC. "Acute Myocardial Infarction." In Eagle et al. (eds.), *The Practice of Cardiology*. 2nd ed. Boston: Little, Brown and Co., 1989. p. 412.

cardium is most often supplied by the right coronary artery as it moves posteriorly, forming the posterior descending coronary artery. In a small portion of the population, the posterior descending coronary artery is supplied by the left circumflex artery.

RIGHT VENTRICULAR MYOCARDIAL INFARCTION

Right ventricular myocardial infarction is often a complication of inferior myocardial infarction as previously discussed. Right ventricular infarction must always be suspected in the presence of inferior myocardial infarction. A specific lead to the right ventricle is available, called V_4R (see Chapter 4), though it is not commonly applied as the diagnosis of right ventricular infarction can often be made on a clinical basis. However, the field use of V_4R is essential for early detection and appropriate therapeutic intervention. The diagnosis of right ventricular infarction is made in the presence of inferior myocardial infarction when hypotension is present along with signs of elevated right ventricular filling pressure (jugular venous distention) and clear lungs.

During right ventricular infarction the right ventricle does not effectively pump blood to the pulmonary vasculature. Blood then backs up into the systemic venous vessels, causing jugular venous distention. There is no evidence of pulmonary edema because the lungs are dry, that is, blood is not being pumped into the pulmonary system from the right ventricle. Cardiac output is subsequently decreased as left ventricular filling pressures fall and the left ventricle does not fill adequately during diastole (the pump is cavitating). Decreased cardiac output ultimately results in hypotension and shock.

Patients with right ventricular infarction are dependent on an elevated right ventricular filling pressure to maintain cardiac output. Caution must therefore be exercised when using preload reducing agents (nitrates, morphine, and diuretics) in the setting of right ventricular infarction. Preload reducing agents further reduce right ventricular filling pressure, causing the cardiac output to further decrease.

Cautious fluid boluses may be used to increase right ventricular filling pressure and cardiac output. Some patients may require up to several liters of normal saline or lactated ringers in order to maintain an adequate filling pressure. If signs of pulmonary congestion (rales, wheezes, difficulty breathing) develop, discontinue fluid therapy. Pressor agents such as dopamine or norepinephrine may also be required in the setting of right ventricular infarction to maintain cardiac output.

RECIPROCAL CHANGES

As you recall from Chapter 5, reciprocal changes on the ECG involve ST segment depression in the lead opposite to ST segment elevation (see Chapter 5, Figures 5–8 and 5–9). The presence of reciprocal changes increases the probability that the ECG is diagnostic for acute myocardial infarction. There are several theories regarding the origin of reciprocal changes. Reciprocal changes are attributed to an electrophysiologic phenomenon caused by displacement of the injury current vector away from the region of noninfarcting myocardium or distant ischemia/infarct extension. Most likely, reciprocal changes do represent additional ischemia or infarction rather than just an electrophysiologic phenomenon.

Reciprocal changes are associated with higher mortality rates because they are often associated with extensive myocardial necrosis. These patients tend to have lower ejection fractions (percent of blood in the left ventricle that is actually pumped out of the ventricle during systole), more extensive wall motion abnormalities (larger infarct), and a greater number of coronary arteries that are blocked. Further, these patients may benefit more from thrombolytic therapy. Reciprocal changes are most commonly found in patients with inferior wall myocardial infarction and may also be found in patients with anterior myocardial infarction.

ORGANIZED APPROACH TO 12-LEAD ANALYSIS

An organized method for interpreting 12-lead ECGs is essential. Each 12-lead ECG must be read consistently in the same order to ensure proper evaluation of all leads. A systemic approach to 12-lead ECG interpretation provides the emergency care worker the ability to detect patterns of myocardial ischemia/infarction, to screen for nonischemic but potentially life-threatening etiologies of chest pain, such as pericarditis or pulmonary embolism, to stratify the risk of adverse outcomes, and of course to determine criteria for the initiation of thrombolytic therapy. Most importantly, 12-lead ECG interpretation is used as an adjunct to support historical and physical examination findings.

Systematic Analysis

Step 1

Interpretation begins with determining the rate (Figure 6-9). The number of QRS complexes may be counted in a six-second strip and multiplied by ten to obtain the rate. The rate may also be estimated by counting the number of large boxes (5 mm) between QRS

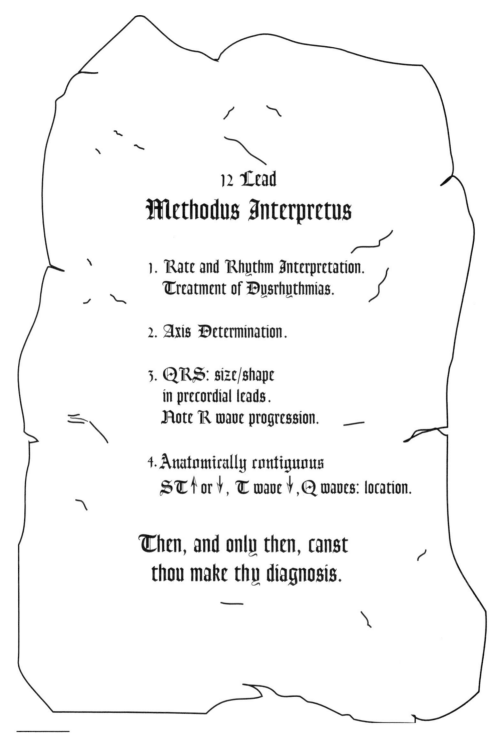

12 Lead
Methodus Interpretus

1. Rate and Rhythm Interpretation.
   Treatment of Dysrhythmias.

2. Axis Determination.

3. QRS: size/shape
   in precordial leads.
   Note R wave progression.

4. Anatomically contiguous
   ST↑ or↓, T wave↓, Q waves: location.

Then, and only then, canst
thou make thy diagnosis.

Figure 6–9.
Systematic analysis (methodus interpretus).

complexes. The rate is calculated by remembering the sequence of rates for each additional 5 mm between complexes (300, 150, 100, 75, 60, 50). Remember that rates faster than 100 beats per minute are termed tachycardia. Those rates slower than 60 beats per minute are termed bradycardia.

Step 2

The next step is to determine the heart rhythm. Begin by observing the ECG for an irregular rhythm or abnormal complexes. Look for a QRS complex after every P wave and a P wave before every QRS complex. P waves without QRS complexes indicate an AV block and QRS complexes without P waves indicate an ectopic rhythm (either AV nodal or ventricular). Check the intervals, that is, the PR interval and the duration of the QRS complex. This will allow detection of AV blocks and bundle branch blocks (see Chapter 7).

NOTE: Determination of cardiac rate and rhythm and the treatment of life-threatening dysrhythmias takes precedence over the acquisition of a 12-lead ECG and infarct recognition.

Step 3

Next, determine the QRS axis. An abnormal axis may indicate infarction or ventricular hypertrophy (enlargement of the ventricle). The axis may be grossly determined by observing the QRS complex in leads I and II (see Chapter 4, Table 4–5). The majority of the QRS complex will be above the baseline in both I and II if the QRS vector is normal. If the QRS complex is above the baseline in lead I and below the baseline in lead II then there is a left axis deviation. Conversely, if the QRS complex is below the baseline in lead I and above the baseline in lead II then right axis deviation exists. Finally, if the QRS complex of both leads I and II are below the baseline then intermediate axis or "no man's land" is present. The axis may also be determined in the precordial leads. Generally this is referred to as R wave progression. Normal R waves begin with small R waves in V_1 progressively becoming larger as V_6 is approached. The QRS complex is normally below the baseline in V_1, progressing to above the baseline in V_6. Abnormal R wave progression may also indicate infarction or hypertrophy.

Step 4

Observe the 12-lead ECG for evidence of ischemia or infarction. Each lead (except aVR) is evaluated for pathological (enlarged) Q waves, flat or inverted T waves, and ST segment elevation or depression. Remember that an isolated Q wave in lead III is not abnormal. The area of ischemia/infarction is then localized by the pattern of ischemic changes. Inferior ischemia is localized with leads II, III, and aVF, lateral ischemia with I, aVL, V_5, and V_6, and anterior ischemia with leads V_1 to V_4. Often, changes in V_1 and V_2 are referred to as septal ischemia. Posterior ischemia will produce large R waves and ST depression in leads V_1 to V_3. Inverting the 12-lead ECG and observing it in a mirror will make the posterior changes appear like the usual Q wave and ST elevation. Finally, note the progression of the R wave through the precordial leads. The loss of R wave progression in the presence of ischemic chest pain further signifies acute infarction.

SUMMARY

The 12-lead ECG provides the paramedic with a powerful tool for assessing chest pain and cardiac abnormalities. Detecting an acute myocardial infarction allows early notification of the emergency department that a patient with a life-threatening illness is en route. Early notification stimulates the rapid delivery of revascularizing therapies such as thrombolytic agents or angioplasty. Myocardial infarction patients with earlier intervention, especially within one hour of the onset of symptoms, have lower mortality rates and better outcomes after revascularization.

Localization of the area of ischemia will prepare the paramedic for cardiogenic shock and guide therapy for hypotension (i.e., fluids for inferior/right ventricular infarction and pressor agents for anterior infarction). Caution must, however, be exercised when interpreting the implications of a "normal" 12-lead ECG. A normal 12-lead ECG does not rule out a cardiac origin for chest pain.

KEY POINTS SUMMARY

Coronary Anatomy

1. The right and left coronary arteries arise from the base of the aorta just above the aortic valve. Both arteries provide the exclusive oxygenated blood supply to the myocardium and electrical conduction system.
2. The right coronary artery supplies the right atrium and ventricle, the inferoposterior wall of the left ventricle, the SA node in 60% of the population, and the AV node in 90% of the population.
3. The left coronary divides into two distinct divisions, the left anterior descending and circumflex arteries. The left anterior descending artery supplies the intraventricular septum and the anterior wall of the left ventricle, whereas the circumflex artery supplies the lateral wall of the left ventricle.

Coronary Artery Pathology

4. Coronary atherosclerosis is the main inciting event of myocardial infarction. Atherosclerosis results in the development of thick, hard atherosclerotic plaques and a loss of vessel elasticity, leading to luminal narrowing and subsequent clot formation. It is now recognized that 80 to 90% of AMIs are due to thrombotic occlusion.

Localization of Infarction

5. ST segment elevation and pathological Q waves are the major indicative ECG changes associated with myocardial infarction. Correlation of these findings with specific lead groups enables the examiner to localize the area of ischemic heart muscle and predict which coronary artery is occluded. Knowledge of such information provides the emergency worker with the ability to anticipate certain complications and improve treatment strategies.

Anterior Myocardial Infarction

6. Etiology: Occlusion of the left anterior descending coronary artery
7. Reflecting leads: V_1 through V_4
8. Reciprocal (ST depression) changes: Inferior leads II, III, and aVF
9. Complications: Cardiogenic shock and conduction abnormalities (Mobitz II and complete heart block)

Inferior Myocardial Infarction

10. Etiology: Occlusion of the right coronary artery
11. Reflecting leads: II, III, and aVF
12. Reciprocal (ST depression) changes: Lateral leads I and aVL
13. Complications: AV nodal heart blocks (typically of lower grade) and concomitant right ventricular infarction

Lateral Myocardial Infarction

14. Etiology: Occlusion of the circumflex artery
15. Reflecting leads: I, aVL, V_5, and V_6
16. Complications: Most often occurs as an extension of either anterior or inferior myocardial infarction

Posterior Myocardial Infarction

17. Etiology: Occlusion of the right coronary artery
18. Reflecting leads: Reciprocal ST depression and the presence of large R waves are evaluated in leads V_1 and V_2. These changes are analogous to ST segment elevation and pathological Q waves.
19. Complications: Most often occurs as an extension of either inferior or lateral myocardial infarction

Right Ventricular Infarction

20. Etiology: Right ventricular infarction complicates inferior wall infarction in up to 40% of cases. RVI is due to proximal right coronary artery occlusion.
21. Reflecting leads: V_3R through V_6R (V_4R is most sensitive for RVI)
22. Complications: Hypotension and cardiogenic shock
23. Treatment strategies: Fluid resuscitation and/or an inotrope

Systematic Analysis

24. An organized approach for interpreting the 12-lead electrocardiogram is essential to ensure proper evaluation of all leads. The following steps should be used when reading 12-lead ECGs.

- Determine the cardiac rate
- Determine the cardiac rhythm and treat life-threatening dysrhythmias
- Determine the QRS axis
- Examine the ECG leads for evidence of ischemia or infarction
- Localize the area of myocardial ischemia

BIBLIOGRAPHY

Albrich JM, Rothrock S, Salluzzo R. Acute myocardial infarction: Comprehensive guidelines for diagnosis, stabilization, and mortality reduction. *Emergency Medicine Reports.* 1994;15:51–62.

Davies MJ, Thomas AC. Thrombosis and acute coronary-artery lesions in sudden cardiac ischemic death. *New England Journal of Medicine.* 1984;310:1137–1140.

Davies MJ, Thomas AC. Plaque fissuring—The cause of acute myocardial infarction, sudden ischemic death, and crescendo angina. *British Heart Journal.* 1985;53:363–373.

DeWood MA, Spores J, Notske R, et al. Prevalence of total coronary occlusion during the early hours of transmural myocardial infarction. *New England Journal of Medicine.* 1980;303:897–902.

Dubin D. Rapid Interpretation of EKGs. 4th ed. Tampa, FL: Cover Publishing; 1989.

Falk E. Plaque rupture with severe pre-existing stenosis precipitating cortonary thrombosis: Characteristics of coronary atherosclerotic plaques underlying fatal occlusive thrombi. *British Heart Journal.* 1983;50:127–134.

Falk E. Unstable angina with fatal outcome, dynamic coronary thrombosis leading to infarction and/or sudden death: Autopsy evidence of recent mural thrombosis with peripheral embolization culminating in total vascular occlusion. *Circulation.* 1985;71:699–708.

Gibson RS. Non-Q-wave myocardial infarction: Pathophysiology, prognosis, and therapeutic strategy. *Annual Review of Medicine.* 1989;40:395–410.

Hedges JR, Kobernick MS. Detection of myocardial ischemia/infarction in the emergency department patient with chest discomfort. *Emergency Medicine Clinics of North America.* 1988;6:317–340.

Helfant RH, Vokonas PS, Gorlin R. Functional importance of the human coronary collateral circulation. *New England Journal of Medicine.* 1971;284:1277–1281.

Herr CH. The diagnosis of acute myocardial infarction in the emergency department; Part I. *Journal of Emergency Medicine.* 1992;10:455–461.

Herr CH. The diagnosis of acute myocardial infarction in the emergency department; Part 2. *Journal of Emergency Medicine.* 1992;10:591–599.

Hillis LD, Braunwald E. Myocardial ischemia (Part 1). *New England Journal of Medicine.* 1977;296:971–978.

Johns JA, Gold HK, Leinbach RC. Acute myocardial infarction. In: Eagle KA, Haber E, DeSanctis RW, Austen WG, eds. *The Practice of Cardiology.* 2nd ed. Boston, MA: Little, Brown and Company; 1989:403–453.

McQueen MJ, Holder D, El-Maraghi NRH. Assessment of the accuracy of serial electrocardiograms in the diagnosis of myocardial infarction. *American Heart Journal.* 1983;105:258–261.

Moore S. Platelet aggregation secondary to coronary obstruction. *Circulation.* 1976;53:166–171.

Pasternak RC, Braunwald E, Sobel BE. Acute myocardial infarction. In: Braunwald E, ed. *Heart Disease: A Textbook of Cardiovascular Medicine.* 4th ed. Philadelphia, PA: WB Saunders; 1992:1200–1291.

Phibbs B. "Transmural" versus "subendocardial" myocardial infarction: An electrocardiographic myth. *Journal of the American College of Cardiology.* 1983;1:561–564.

Rouan GW, Lee TH, Cook EF, Brand DA, Weisberg MC, Goldman L. Clinical characteristics and outcome of acute myocardial infarction in patients with initially normal or non-specific electrocardiograms (A report from the multicenter chest pain study). *American Journal of Cardiology.* 1989;64:1087–1092.

Stark ME, Vacek JL. The initial electrocardiogram during admission for myocardial infarction: Use as a predictor of clinical course and facility utilization. *Archives of Internal Medicine.* 1987;147:843–846.

Waller BF, Schlant RC. Anatomy of the heart. In: Schlant RC, Alexander RW, eds. *The Heart, Arteries and Veins.* 8th ed. Vol. 1. New York, NY: McGraw-Hill; 1994:84–91.

Zarling EJ, Sexton H, Milnor PJ. Failure to diagnose acute myocardial infarction: The clinicopathologic experience at a large community hospital. *Journal of the American Medical Association.* 1983;250:1177–1181.

Practice Exercises
In Localization

Using the following ECG strips, identify the location of myocardial infarction or ischemia in each.

Strip 1.

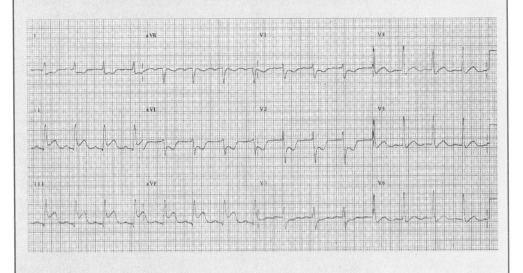

Strip 2.

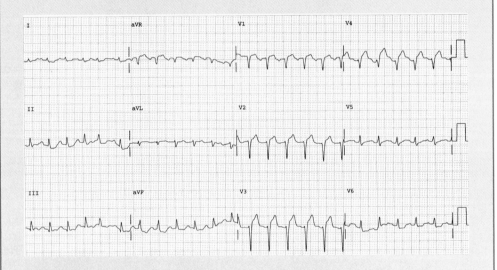

Strip 3.

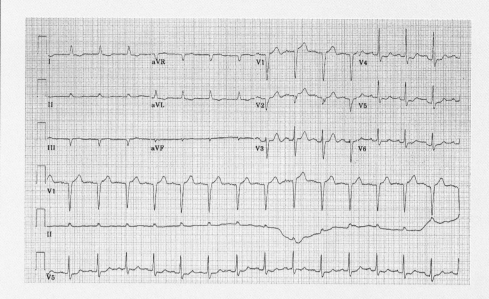

Strip 4.

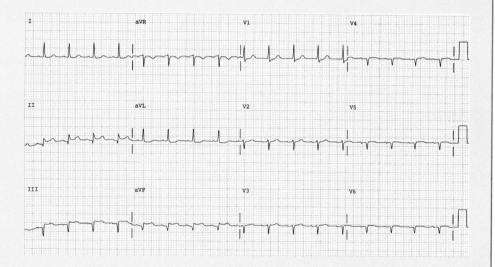

Strip 5.

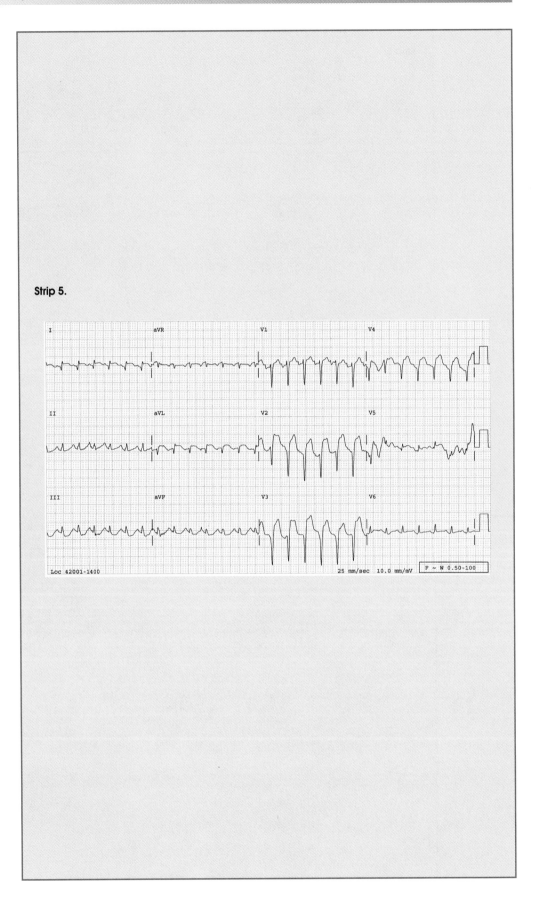

Loc 42001-1400   25 mm/sec 10.0 mm/mV   F ~ W 0.50-100

Strip 6.

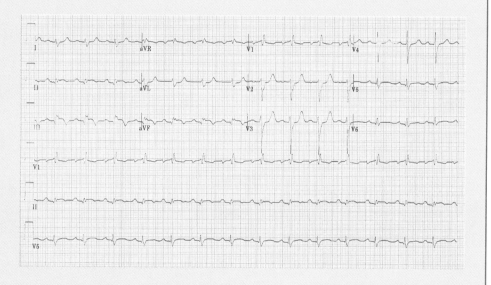

Strip 7.

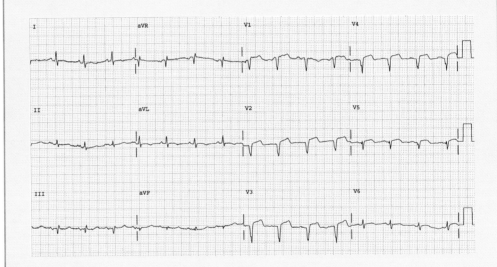

Chapter 6 Practice Exercises/Localization

1. Acute inferior wall myocardial infarction. Note the presence of ST segment elevation throughout the inferior leads (II, III, aVF) with reciprocal ST depression in leads I, aVL, V_1 and V_2.

2. Acute anterior wall myocardial infarction. Note the presence of ST segment elevation throughout the anterior leads (V_1, V_2, V_3, V_4) with the loss of R wave progression. Reciprocal ST depression and T wave inversion is found in the inferior leads.

3. Acute anteroseptal myocardial infarction. Note the presence of ST segment elevation isolated to the septal leads (V_1, V_2).

4. Acute inferior wall myocardial infarction. Note the presence of ST segment elevation and pathological Q waves throughout the inferior leads (II, III, aVF).

5. Acute anterolateral myocardial infarction. Note the presence of ST segment elevation throughout the anterior leads (V_1, V_2, V_3, V_4) with the loss of R wave progression. ST segment elevation and pathological Q waves are also present in lateral leads I, aVL, and V_5.

6. Acute inferior wall myocardial infarction. Note the presence of ST segment elevation throughout the inferior leads (II, III, aVF). In addition, reciprocal ST depression is present in leads I and aVL.

7. Acute anterior wall myocardial infarction. Note the presence of ST segment elevation throughout the anterior leads (V_1, V_2, V_3, V_4) with the loss of R wave progression.

7

Miscellaneous Conditions Mimicking Infarction and Other Cardiac Disorders

LEARNING OBJECTIVES

1. Describe the pathophysiological, historical, and objective findings of pericarditis.

2. Discuss benign early repolarization and identify the group of individuals most susceptible to this phenomenon.

3. Define left ventricular hypertrophy and discuss several clinical conditions responsible for this pathology.

4. List and describe the ECG characteristics of acute pericarditis, benign early repolarization, and left ventricular hypertrophy.

5. Identify acute pericarditis, benign early repolarization, and left ventricular hypertrophy on the electrocardiogram.

6. Differentiate acute pericarditis, benign early repolarization, and left ventricular hypertrophy from acute myocardial infarction.

7. Name and describe two formulas used for the diagnosis of left ventricular hypertrophy.

8. List the common causes of bundle branch block.

9. Describe the abnormal sequence of depolarization for right and left bundle branch block.

10. List and describe the ECG characteristics of right and left bundle branch block.

11. Name the steps required for "quickie block identification."

12. Identify and differentiate right and left bundle branch block on the electrocardiogram.

13. Define hemiblock and describe its two forms.

14. Describe the abnormal sequence of depolarization for left anterior and posterior fascicular block.

15. Describe the ECG characteristics of hemiblock and identify its two forms on the electrocardiogram.

16. Discuss the role of transcutaneous pacing for the treatment of heart block.

17. Describe the abnormal sequence of depolarization for wide complex tachycardias.

18. List the ECG characteristics of supraventricular tachycardia with aberration and ventricular tachycardia.

19. Differentiate supraventricular tachycardia with aberration from ventricular tachycardia.

20. Discuss the role of adenosine for the treatment of supraventricular tachycardias.

21. Define "accessory pathways" and list and describe the ECG characteristics of Wolff-Parkinson-White syndrome.

22. Discuss right and left atrial enlargement and describe their ECG characteristics.

23. List and describe the ECG characteristics of pulmonary disorders.

24. Define hypothermia and list the ECG findings associated with reduced body temperature.

25. Discuss the relationship between cerebral hemorrhage and the electrocardiogram.

26. Define hyperkalemia, hypokalemia, hypercalcemia, and hypocalcemia and describe the ECG characteristics of each.

INTRODUCTION

Acute myocardial infarction and its ischemic prodromes are not the only cause of ST segment and T wave changes. Abnormalities of ST-T waves have been exhaustively reviewed and have a virtually endless list of causes. Many of these pathologies can easily be confused with an evolving infarction, as can the clinical picture. The emergency care provider should note that when ST-T changes lack specific character or are scattered about the limb and precordial leads they are unreliable indicators of ischemic heart disease. This chapter will review some relatively common causes of ST-T abnormalities that are relevant to emergency medicine. These include pericarditis, benign early repolarization (BER), left bundle branch block (LBBB), and left ventricular hypertrophy (LVH). Other cardiac disorders that can substantially alter the normal pattern of the ECG are also introduced. In addition, exercises at the end of the chapter will give you an opportunity to practice differentiating true infarction from the conditions that mimic infarction.

NONISCHEMIC CAUSES OF ST-T WAVE ABNORMALITIES

Pericarditis

Pericarditis is the inflammation of the pericardial lining (sac) surrounding the heart. Although it may appear as a complication of acute myocardial infarction, pericarditis in ... is secondary to a more generalized disease process somewhere else in the ...arditis also involves the inflammation of the epicardium and the epicardial ...n (Figure 7–1). This inflammation creates changes in repolarization that are ... the ECG as ST segment elevation. Chest pain is a frequent subjective find-...nbined findings of chest pain and ST elevation may lead to an incorrect di-... acute myocardial infarction. A careful history, a complete physical exam, and ... review of the ECG will more likely lead to the correct diagnosis.

Cause of ST changes

...is is typically associated with other disease processes. It is often seen follow-...yocardial infarction (AMI) and cardiac or thoracic surgery. A recent or con-...ory of infectious disease (especially pulmonary infections), connective tissue ...ystemic lupus erythematosus), or neoplasms (especially metastatic thoracic ...nors) may also raise the index of suspicion. The chest pain associated with ...is similar to the pain of myocardial ischemia or infarction in that it can radi-...houlders or neck. It differs from the pain of AMI in that it is often described ... or sharp, is aggravated by deep inspiration (pleuritic) motion (twisting of ... or swallowing, and has no response to nitrate therapy (Table 7–1).

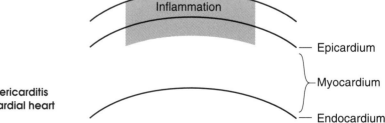

7–1.
...mmation of pericarditis
...to the epicardial heart

TABLE 7-1 • **Difference Between Pericarditis and Acute Myocardial Infarction**

	PERICARDITIS	AMI
Pain	Chest, radiates to the jaw or neck	Chest, radiates to the jaw, neck, arms
Quality	Sharp knifelike	Pressure, dull burning
Nitrate therapy	No response	Pain relief and reduced myocardial workload
Other	Aggravated by deep inspiration, swallowing, twisting of the trunk	Constant, unaffected by position

Objective Findings

A pericardial friction rub upon auscultation of the heart is the classic physical finding in pericarditis. Atrial systole, ventricular systole, and wall movement from diastolic filling will each produce a short squeak or rub (sounds like two pieces of sandpaper rubbing together), leading to a characteristic three-component friction rub of pericarditis. This sound is best heard along the lower left sternal border. Other signs depend on the degree of restriction created by the effusion of fluid into the pericardium. Signs of restrictive pericarditis include jugular vein distention, muffled heart sounds, decreased pulse pressure, hypotension, respiratory distress, and a paradoxical pulse (pulse strength increases with inspiration).

Electrocardiographic Criteria

ST segment elevation commonly accompanies pericarditis. Several significant differences exist between the ECGs of AMI and pericarditis patients. ST segment elevation in AMI is usually grouped into anatomically contiguous leads, such as II, III, and aVF with inferior wall infarction or V_1 and V_2 for septal infarction. This is in contrast to the more diffuse distribution seen in pericarditis. Pericarditis usually produces ST segment elevation in at least two limb leads and a number of precordial leads. Upward concavity (Figure 7–2) of the elevated ST segments is typical of pericarditis as is PR segment depression, low QRS voltage (due to effusion dampening the electrical output of the heart), and J-point notching (Table 7–2). Since the area of affected subendocardial muscle is

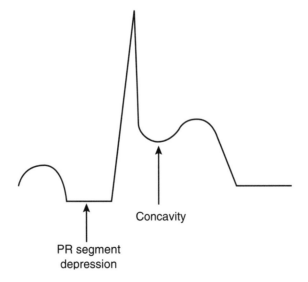

Concavity

PR segment
depression

Figure 7–2.
QRS complex demonstrating upward concavity of the ST segment along with PR segment depression commonly associated with pericarditis.

TABLE 7–2 • **ECG Findings of Pericarditis**
• Diffuse ST segment elevation (less than 5 mm) • Upward concavity of ST segments • PR segment depression • Low QRS voltage • Notching of the J-point • Pathological Q waves do not develop

usually relatively shallow, the ST elevation seen in pericarditis is usually no more than 3 mm. ST segment elevation over 5 mm virtually rules out pericarditis as a possible diagnosis. Also, pathological Q waves do not typically develop with pericarditis (Figure 7–3).

Tamponade

Pericarditis with significant effusion and life-threatening tamponade should be considered when pericarditis is recognized by ECG criteria and clinical evidence of effusion exists. The presence of total electrical alternans (alternately smaller P waves and QRS complexes appearing every second or third beat) is an uncommon, but reliable indicator of effusion with tamponade. This may represent a life-threatening situation requiring immediate pericardiocentesis (needle perforation and aspiration of blood and fluid from the pericardium).

Pericarditis

- Diffuse ST segment elevation that does not localize into right or left coronary artery distribution
- PR segment depression (always use the TP segment as a baseline for ST segment evaluation)

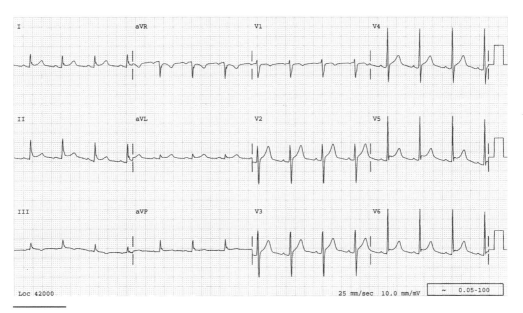

Figure 7–3.
12-lead ECG recording of pericarditis.
Note the widespread ST elevation and PR segment depression throughout the limb and precordial leads.

TABLE 7–3 • **ECG Findings of Benign Early Repolarization**

- ST segment elevation (most commonly V_3 through V_6)
- Upward concavity of ST segments
- J-point notching
- T waves appear taller
- Reciprocal changes are rare

- Sharp chest pain worsened by inspiration and movement
- Pericardial friction rub
- No response to nitroglycerin

Benign Early Repolarization (BER)

Benign early repolarization is most often discovered on routine physical examination. It creates a pattern of ST segment elevation that resembles acute myocardial infarction or acute pericarditis. Benign early repolarization is considered a harmless finding in asymptomatic patients. The exact mechanism of its etiology is unclear. Although it may occur in any race, sex, or age, BER occurs most frequently in young (25 to 35 years of age), thin-chested black males.

Electrocardiographic Findings in BER

The ECG findings of benign early repolarization closely resemble those of acute pericarditis and may also mimic AMI (Table 7–3). Slight (1 to 3 mm) ST segment elevation over the mid and left precordial leads (V_3 through V_6) is most typical, but ST segment elevation in a variety of lead combinations can occur. The elevated ST segments are upwardly concave as in pericarditis. Reciprocal (mirror-image) ST changes are rare. J-point notching often occurs and T waves may appear tall (Figure 7–4).

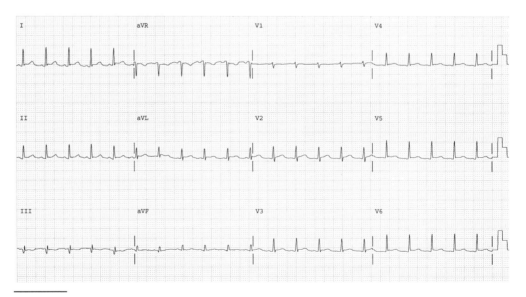

Figure 7–4.
12-lead ECG recording of a 30-year-old male demonstrating benign early repolarization.
Note the widespread and upwardly concave ST elevation (1 mm) throughout the tracing.

Benign Early Repolarization

- ST segment elevation often identified in the anterolateral leads
- Concave ST segments
- Tall T waves
- Most predominant in young black males
- No symptomology

Left Bundle Branch Block (LBBB)

Left bundle branch block is discussed in greater detail later in the chapter. This section is limited to the effects LBBB has on ST-T wave changes and other indicators of myocardial ischemia or infarction.

As you recall normal intraventricular conduction begins with septal depolarization from left to right and terminates with near simultaneous depolarization of the ventricles. In LBBB, the septum is depolarized from right to left, followed by depolarization of the right ventricle and finally the larger left ventricle. This alteration in the order and direction of depolarization has a major effect on the ECG that prevents the use of standard infarct recognition criteria.

Recognition of Left Bundle Branch Block

Left bundle branch block is recognized by a QRS width of 120 msec (0.12 sec) or greater and a primarily negative qS or rS pattern in V_1 with a fully positive R or RR pattern in V_6 (Table 7–4). Widening of the QRS is due to asynchronous depolarization of the ventricles. The morphological QRS changes result from the generalized leftward depolarization of the ventricles. The QRS in question must be activated by a supraventricular source (Figure 7–5).

Alteration of Q Waves

Pathological Q waves from left ventricular infarctions are lost in LBBB due to late activation of the left ventricle and the change of direction in septal depolarization. Traditional Q wave criteria for infarction cannot be used in the presence of left bundle branch block.

ST-T Wave Changes

Abnormal ST-T wave changes observed in the presence of left bundle branch block are secondary manifestations of the abnormal sequence and direction of ventricular depolarization. These changes are somewhat predictable and are not an indication of myocardial ischemia. The typical repolarization abnormality of LBBB is reflected on the ECG as ST segments and T waves being directed opposite the QRS complex. In any given lead, when the QRS is predominantly positive, the ST segment will be depressed and the T wave will be inverted. If the QRS is predominantly negative, the ST segment will be elevated and the T wave will be upright (see Figure 7–5). Traditional ST-T criteria for

TABLE 7–4 • **Left Bundle Branch Block**

- Evidence of a supraventricular source (p wave)
- QRS is $\geq$ 120 msec (0.12 sec)
- QS or RS pattern in V_1/MCL_1
- Fully positive R or RR' pattern in V_6/MCL_6

ST-T Changes with Left Bundle Branch Block

QRS negative: ST segment elevated
T wave upright

QRS positive: ST segment depressed
T wave inverted

A

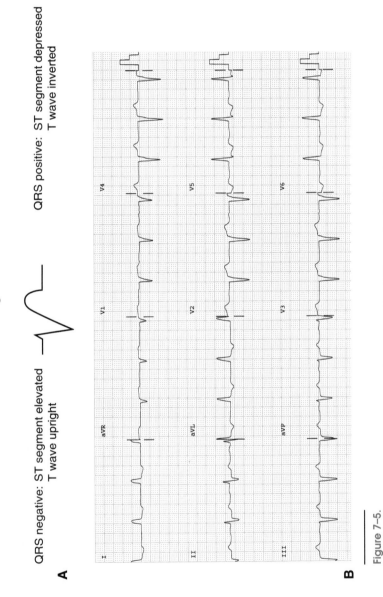

B

Figure 7-5.

(A) Graphic representation demonstrating a negative QRS complex in V_1 and a positive QRS complex in V_6. **(B)** 12-lead ECG recording of left bundle branch block.

Note ST elevation throughout the anterior leads (V_1 through V_4), a QRS of 120 msec, and a QS in V_1 and an R wave in V_6.

AMI cannot be used in the presence of left bundle branch block. However, in patients who present with clinical symptoms consistent with infarction (i.e., chest discomfort, dyspnea, hypoperfusion, etc.) cardiac ischemia must be considered. In fact, newly developed LBBB resulting from infarction often represents a significant complication.

Left Bundle Branch Block

- QRS complex width of 120 msec or greater
- ST segments and T waves are directed opposite the QRS complex
- QS complex in V_1 and a R or RR pattern in V_6
- ST segment elevation is commonly present in V_1 through V_3
- ECG evidence of infarction in the presence of LBBB is difficult to distinguish

Left Ventricular Hypertrophy (LVH)

Left ventricular hypertrophy is the abnormal dilation or thickening of the left ventricle which causes ST segment changes that can imitate acute myocardial infarction. LVH results from clinical conditions that either increase ventricular work or impose a volume overload on the ventricle. It is most often caused by hypertension and valvular disease, but can also accompany cardiomyopathy as well as disorders of the aorta.

The diagnosis of left ventricular hypertrophy requires a careful assessment of the QRS complex in many leads. Increased R wave amplitude or an exaggeration of the normal R wave progression in leads V_1 through V_6 forms the basis for the electrocardiographic diagnosis. A multitude of voltage (QRS height) criteria exist for LVH. ECG evidence of left ventricular hypertrophy is very specific; unfortunately it is not very sensitive. Most ECG methods identify left ventricular hypertrophy in less than 50% of the patients with echocardiographic evidence of LVH. Echocardiography (a noninvasive diagnostic method using ultrasound to visualize internal cardiac structures) has virtually replaced the ECG in the diagnosis of left ventricular hypertrophy. Although not sensitive, the ECG is very specific in the identification of LVH. LVH is actually present in nearly 100% of the cases with voltage criteria for left ventricular hypertrophy.

Most formulas for voltage criteria are too cumbersome for emergency use. This text presents two methods that are reasonably sensitive and specific while at the same time are simple to use.

Cornell Voltage Criteria

This method is recommended when leads aVL and V_3 are obtainable (Table 7–5). Simply add the *height* of the R wave in aVL to the *depth* of the S wave in V_3. If the sum equals > 28 mm in men or > 20 mm in women, left ventricular hypertrophy is diagnosed (Figure 7–6). This method is 42% sensitive and 98% specific.

TABLE 7–5 • **Cornell Voltage Criteria for Left Ventricular Hypertrophy**

- QRS height in aVL plus the QRS depth in V_3 equals
  > 28 mm in males
  > 20 mm in females
- LVH is diagnosed

Note: Proper calibration of the ECG signal is a must.

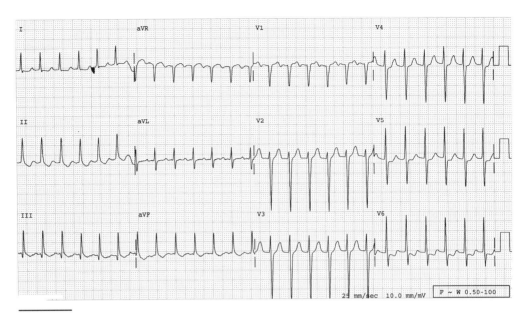

Figure 7–6.
12-lead ECG recording of LVH (increased QRS voltage).
Using the Cornell voltage criteria, add the height of the R wave in aVL (6 mm) to the depth of the S wave in V_3 (24 mm). This equals 30 mm; therefore, LVH is said to exist.

Sokalov and Lyon System

Since aVL cannot be obtained with a 3-wire cable system, an alternate method for 3-wire systems is necessary. The Sokalov and Lyon system utilizes the precordial V leads which can be obtained on a 3-wire cable system using the bipolar modified chest (MCL) leads. Use of MCL leads in place of V leads for the purpose of obtaining voltage criteria for LVH has not been scientifically studied. However, experience has shown that the MCL leads when properly placed and calibrated virtually duplicate the precordial V leads.

The Sokalov and Lyon method simply adds the depth of the S wave in V_1 to the height of the R wave in V_5 or V_6 (whichever is greater) (Table 7–6). If the sum amounts to > 35 mm LVH is diagnosed (Figure 7–7).

ST-T Wave Changes in Left Ventricular Hypertrophy

In addition to increased voltage, left ventricular hypertrophy is often accompanied by ST-T wave changes. The ST-T wave pattern seen in LVH is called a strain pattern and it should not be mistaken for evidence of AMI. In precordial leads with upright QRSs (usually leads V_5 and V_6) the ST segments become depressed, often showing upward convexity and tend to blend into asymmetrically inverted T waves (Figure 7–8). In precordial leads with negative QRSs (usually V_1 and V_2) the ST segments are elevated with an upward concavity. The T waves are upright in these leads. In limb leads with upright

TABLE 7–6 • **Sokalov and Lyon System of Voltage Criteria for LVH**

Depth of the S wave in V_1/MCL_1 + the height of the R wave in V_5/MCL_5 or V_6/MCL_6 (whichever is greater) is ≥ 35 mm, LVH is diagnosed

Note: Proper calibration of the ECG signal is a must.

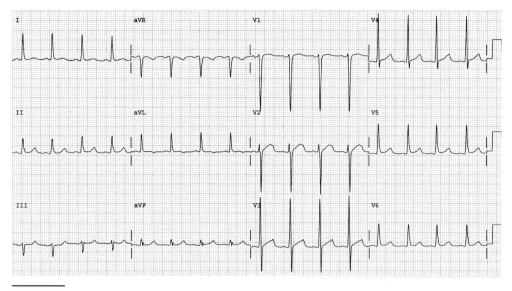

Figure 7–7.
12-lead ECG recording demonstrating LVH.
 Using the Sokalov and Lyon system, add the depth of the S wave in V_1 (28 mm) to the height of the R wave in the larger V_5 (15 mm). This equals 43 mm; therefore, LVH is said to exist.

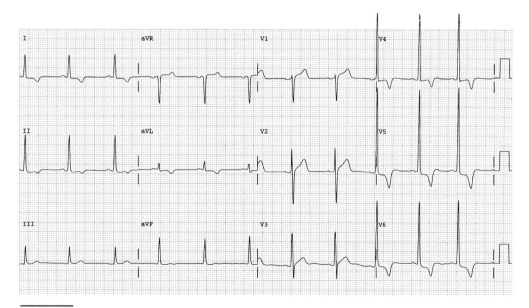

Figure 7–8.
12-lead ECG recording demonstrating LVH.
Note the depressed ST segments with inverted T waves in V_4 through V_6 along with ST elevation in V_1 and V_2.

complexes, the same changes seen in V_5 and V_6 will occur. In limb leads with negative QRS complexes, changes similar to V_1 and V_2 will occur. These changes are remarkably similar to the ST-T wave changes seen in LBBB. The criteria for LVH is used only in the absence of bundle branch block.

Left Ventricular Hypertrophy

* Pathology most often resulting from hypertension and valvular disease
* ECG clues are identified by changes in the QRS complex, ST segment, and T wave
* Increased QRS voltage in the chest leads; R wave grows taller and S wave deeper

OTHER CARDIAC DISORDERS

Intraventricular Conduction Defects

Understanding abnormal conduction through the ventricles is of vital importance to the emergency care provider. The ability to recognize the patterns of left and right bundle branch block will allow the provider to discover the origin of wide QRS tachycardia, predict the development of serious heart block, and aid in the recognition of a variety of other cardiac disorders.

Normal Intraventricular Conduction

Emerging from the AV node is the bundle of His. This structure bifurcates at the intraventricular septum into two distinct pathways called bundle branches. The left bundle branch (LBB) travels down the left side of the intraventricular septum and further divides into two fascicles (anterior and posterior). Purkinje fibers extend from the fascicles and reach deep into the septum and left ventricular myocardium. The right bundle branch (RBB) travels along the right side of the intraventricular septum. The right ventricular myocardium is reached by Purkinje fibers emerging from this branch (Figure 7–9).

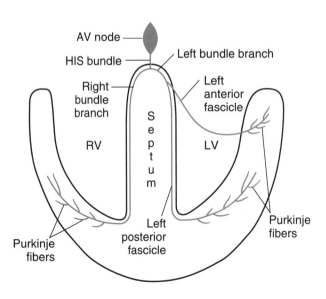

Figure 7–9.
Anatomical diagram of the electrical conduction system.
Branching off the His bundle are two bundle branches (left and right) that travel down the lateral aspects of the intraventricular septum. The LBB further divides into anterior and posterior branches (fascicles). Both the left and right bundle branches transmit the electrical wave of depolarization to the Purkinje fibers that spread throughout the ventricular myocardium.

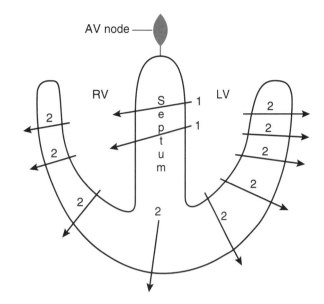

Figure 7–10.

Septal activation proceeds in a left-to-right direction.

Both ventricles are depolarized simultaneously.

1. Septal depolarization

2. Simultaneous ventricular depolarization from endocardium to epicardium

Normally the depolarization impulse emerges from the His bundle and as it reaches the bifurcation of the left and right bundles is conducted down both bundles. Conduction is somewhat preferential through the left bundle branch. This causes the septum to depolarize from left to right. Following septal depolarization is simultaneous depolarization of the ventricles. Since the bundle branches are on the endocardial surface of the heart, depolarization occurs from endocardium to epicardium. This entire sequence takes approximately 60 to 80 msec (Figure 7–10).

All leads record ventricular depolarization as a QRS complex which may contain virtually any combination of Q, R, or S waves. By selecting specific advantageously positioned leads the examiner can utilize morphological (shape) clues to determine the exact sequence and duration of depolarization across the septum, right ventricle, and free wall of the left ventricle. This data can be used to differentiate left from right bundle branch block. Lead V_1 (MCL$_1$) has its positive pole situated over the right ventricle and V_6 (MCL$_6$) is positioned over the left ventricle. These two leads are able to view the direction of depolarization through the septum and free ventricular walls (Figure 7–11).

Recall from Chapter 3 that as depolarization forces move toward a positive pole the stylus goes up and as depolarization forces move away from a positive pole the stylus will go down. Apply this principle to the position of the positive poles of V_1 and V_6 and it becomes evident that the duration and sequence of intraventricular depolarization can be recorded and studied.

Let's look at normal ventricular conduction once again, this time from the perspective of leads V_1 and V_6. As the depolarization impulse reaches the bifurcation at the end of the His bundle it is conducted down both of the bundle branches. Preferential conduction down the left bundle causes depolarization of the septum from left to right. The positive pole of V_1 will record this as a positive deflection (R wave) since the depolarization forces are moving predominately toward it. Lead V_6 would record this as a negative wave (Q wave) since the depolarization force is moving away from its positive

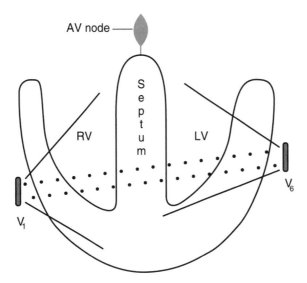

Figure 7–11.

V₁ is positioned over the right ventricle and V₆ over the left ventricle.

This location allows observation of the septum, right ventricle, and left ventricle.

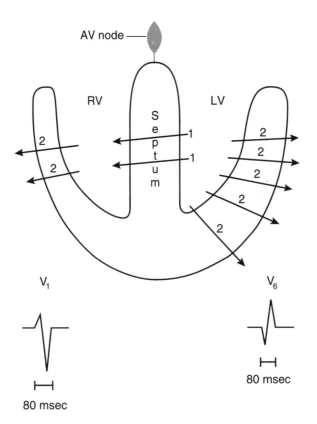

1. Septal depolarization
2. LV and RV depolarization

Figure 7–12.

Normal ventricular depolarization.

Septal depolarization occurs from left to right, inscribing a small r in V₁ and a small q in V₆. Depolarization of the right ventricle is canceled by the larger left ventricle, inscribing a deep S wave in V₁ and a tall R in V₆.

pole. Next, both ventricles are simultaneously depolarized from endocardium to epicardium. Since the left ventricle is approximately three to four times as thick as the right, a majority of the depolarization wave is moving across the left ventricle from endocardium to epicardium, away from V_1, creating a negative wave (S wave), and toward V_6, creating a positive wave (R wave) (Figure 7–12).

Bundle Branch Blocks (BBB)

Conduction through the bundle branches can be impeded for a number of reasons, ischemic heart disease being the most common cause of intraventricular conduction problems. Calcification or degeneration of the conduction system resulting from rheumatic heart disease, congenital deformity, systemic hypertension, or simply old age may cause BBB in the absence of ischemic heart disease.

Right Bundle Branch Block (RBBB)

When electrical block occurs in the right bundle branch, the septum depolarizes as usual from left to right. This inscribes the expected r in V_1 and q in V_6. The block impedes conduction into the right ventricle, allowing the free wall of the left ventricle to depolarize unopposed. This creates an S wave in V_1 and an R wave in V_6. These waves are often quite large due to the lack of opposing forces from the right ventricle (lack of cancellation). Finally, the impulse makes its way to the right ventricle and it is depolarized, creating a second r wave (R′) in V_1 and a terminal S wave in V_6 (Figure 7–13). Again, lack of depolarization from an opposing ventricle allows for a relatively large waveform. An rSR pattern in V_1 and a qRS pattern in V_6 with a QRS width of 120 msec (0.12 sec) is the classic pattern of RBBB (Figure 7–14).

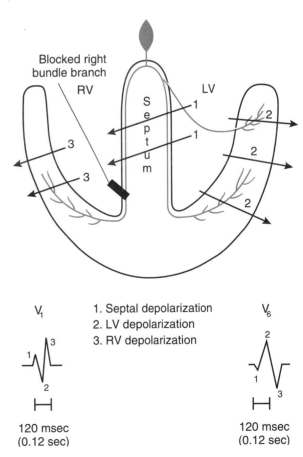

Blocked right
bundle branch

RV   LV

1. Septal depolarization
2. LV depolarization
3. RV depolarization

V_1

V_6

Figure 7–13.
Right bundle branch block.

120 msec
(0.12 sec)

120 msec
(0.12 sec)

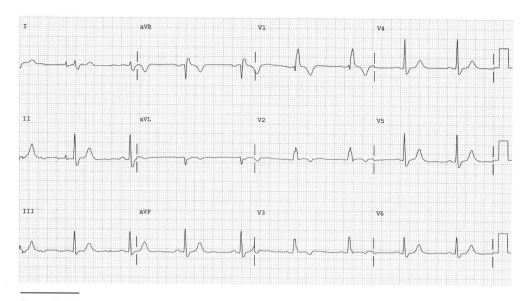

Figure 7–14.
12-lead ECG recording of RBBB.
Note the wide QRSs (> 0.12 sec) and the positive R wave pattern in V_1 and the qRS in V_6.

Left Bundle Branch Block (LBBB)

When the left bundle branch is blocked, the impulse no longer travels preferentially down the LBB. Instead, it proceeds down the RBB, depolarizing the septum from right to left. The thin right ventricle is then free to depolarize, followed by the left ventricle. Given that the septum and free wall of the left ventricle make up a vast majority of the depolarizing myocardium, the overall effect is depolarization with extreme leftward force. This leftward depolarization causes a completely negative QS wave in V_1 and a completely positive R or RR pattern in V_6 (Figure 7–15).

Atypical Bundle Branch Block Patterns

Not all bundle branch blocks will present with the patterns described above. Infarct, hemiblock (block of the anterior or posterior fascicle), medications, and other causes may disturb the picture of BBB. One way to determine left from right BBB is to use the terminal portion method. Once bundle branch block is recognized (evidence of supraventricular origin and a QRS width of 120 msec or more) (Figure 7–16), look at V_1 and locate the terminal portion (last wave) of the QRS complex (Figure 7–17). Determine the direction of the terminal portion (up or down). If the terminal portion of the QRS in V_1 is upright then RBBB exists (Figure 7–18). If the terminal portion of the QRS points down, LBBB is diagnosed (Figure 7–19). A simple analogy exists that may assist the paramedic when using the terminal portion method.

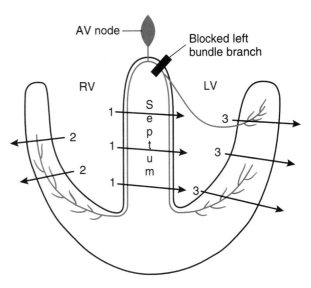

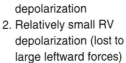

Figure 7–15.
(A) Left bundle branch block. (B) 12-lead ECG recording of LBBB. Note the wide QRSs (> 0.12 sec) and the completely negative QS wave in V_1 and the R wave in V_6. **A**

V_1

V_6

1. Right-to-left septal depolarization
2. Relatively small RV depolarization (lost to large leftward forces)
3. LV depolarization

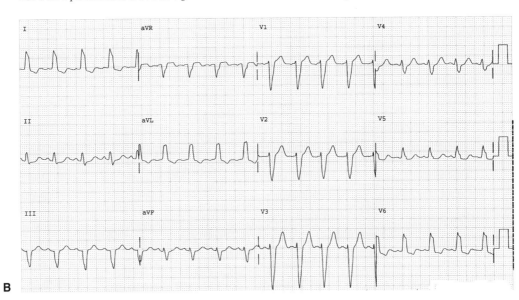

B

Figure 7–16.
Lead II example of bundle branch block. Note the presence of atrial activity (P wave) and a wide QRS complex (> 0.12 sec).

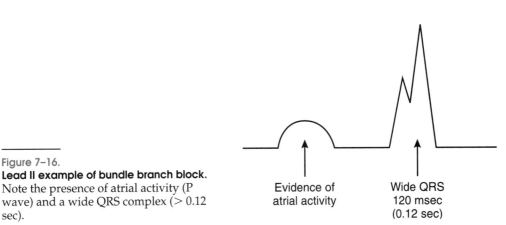

Evidence of atrial activity

Wide QRS 120 msec (0.12 sec)

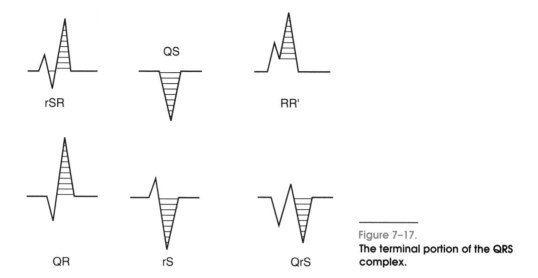

rSR   QS   RR'

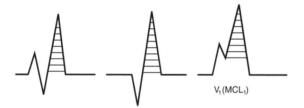

QR   rS   QrS

Figure 7–17.
The terminal portion of the QRS complex.

$V_1 (MCL_1)$

Figure 7–18.
Terminal portion of the QRS is positive in V_1/MCL_1. RBBB is present.

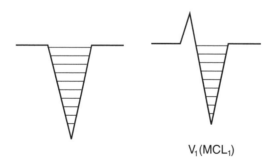

$V_1 (MCL_1)$

Figure 7–19.
Terminal portion of the QRS is negative in V_1/MCL_1. LBBB is present.

TABLE 7-7   •   **Important Points of BBB ECG Recognition**

Atrial Activity Is Present
  P Wave
    Indicates that the QRS is not of ventricular origin
QRS Width
  120 msecs (0.12 sec) or greater
  QRS aberration always present
RBBB
  V_1 is positive (often RSR deflection)
  V_6 is negative
LBBB
  V_1 is negative (QS deflection)
  V_6 is positive

Quickie Block Identification

* Locate the terminal portion of the QRS as previously described
* Identify its direction (up or down)
* Compare this to the turn signal of an automobile
* Up is for right turn and an upright terminal deflection is RBBB
* Down is for left turn and a downward terminal deflection is LBBB

The term nonspecific intraventricular conduction defect (NSIVCD) is used when a beat of supraventricular origin has a QRS width of 120 msec or greater, but does not meet satisfactory criteria for left or right bundle branch block.

The reader is encouraged to refer to (Table 7–7) for a summary of BBBs.

Hemiblocks

The left bundle branch has two electrocardiographically distinct divisions, the anterior and posterior fascicles. Blocks of the anterior and posterior fascicles can be recognized on the surface electrocardiogram and are traditionally referred to by the term hemiblock. The most common cause of hemiblock is septal (or anterior septal) infarction since both fascicles receive blood supply from the septal perforating branches of the left anterior descending artery. The posterior fascicle also receives blood from the nodal branch of the right coronary artery. Because the posterior fascicle has a dual blood supply, it is far less likely to block, and usually represents extensive myocardial damage when blocked.

Recognition of Hemiblock

The primary effect of hemiblock on the ECG is a radical shift of QRS axis. (See Chapter 4 for a review of axis deviation.) The term hemiblock implies that half of the left bundle branch is blocked. The two hemiblocks are identified by the fascicle involved. Left anterior fascicular block (LAFB) is used for block of the anterior fascicle and left posterior fascicular block (LPFB) identifies block of the posterior fascicle.

Left Anterior Fascicular Block (LAFB)

The anterior fascicle reaches upward in the left ventricle, terminating at the anterior papillary muscle of the mitral valve. When blocked, depolarization is directed initially downward, away from the block, then radically upward as the area normally served by the left anterior fascicle is depolarized. This causes an initial Q in leads I and aVL followed by a tall R in the same leads. Leads III and aVF display a small R wave followed by a deep S wave (Figure 7–20). Left axis deviation of −30 degrees or more will be present with LAFB.

Left Posterior Fascicular Block (LPFB)

The posterior fascicle travels downward, terminating at the posterior papillary muscle. When blocked, depolarization is directed initially upward, away from the block, then radically downward as the area normally served by the left posterior fascicle is depo-

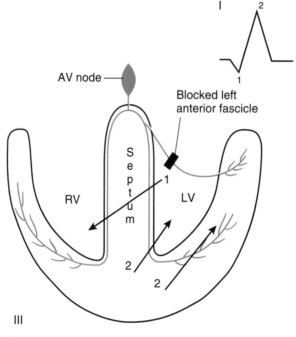

1. Initial depolarization directed "downward" (away) from the blocked anterior fascicle

2. Subsequent depolarization is directed "upward" to the area served by the left anterior fascicle

* q in I
* r in III
* Left axis deviation: -30° or more

Figure 7–20.
Left anterior fascicular block.

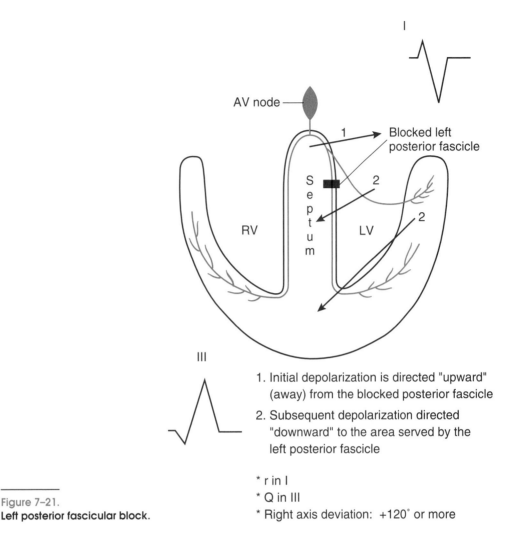

1. Initial depolarization is directed "upward" (away) from the blocked posterior fascicle

2. Subsequent depolarization directed "downward" to the area served by the left posterior fascicle

* r in I
* Q in III
* Right axis deviation: +120° or more

Figure 7–21.
Left posterior fascicular block.

larized. This causes an initial Q in leads III and aVF followed by a tall R wave. Leads I and aVL display a small R wave followed by a deep S wave (Figure 7–21). Right axis deviation of approximately 120 degrees or more will be present in LPFB.

Right Bundle Branch Block and Hemiblock Combinations

Right bundle branch block and anterior hemiblock occur together quite commonly (Figure 7–22). Right bundle branch and posterior hemiblock occur less often but usually indicate extensive heart disease. The term bifascicular block is used when RBBB and hemiblock exist at the same time.

Clinical Application

The emergency care provider can utilize his or her knowledge of bundle branch block and hemiblock to recognize pending complete heart block (CHB) in patients with anteroseptal infarct, determine the origin of wide QRS tachycardias (SVT versus VT), and provide supportive evidence of other serious medical disorders.

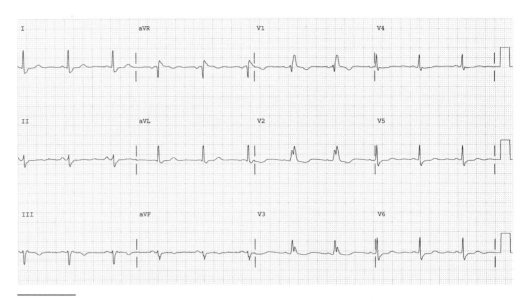

Figure 7–22.
12-lead ECG of bifascicular block: RBBB and LAFB.
RBBB is identified by the wide QRS complexes and the upward terminal force in V$_1$. LAFB is identified by a q in leads I and aVL followed by tall R waves. Leads III and aVF have small r waves with deep S waves.

Recognition of Pending Complete Heart Block

The left anterior descending artery (LAD) supplies the intraventricular septum and the left and right bundle branches that flank the septum. Occlusion of the LAD produces anteroseptal infarct and frequently affects the bundle branches. The development of bundle branch block in the setting of anteroseptal MI is an adverse prognostic indicator. The most serious problem associated with the development of bundle branch block in anteroseptal MI is not the block itself, but the extensive myocardial damage and pump failure that generally accompanies it. Electrocardiographically, the development of bundle branch block in anteroseptal infarct is a warning that the pathways of normal atrial-ventricular conduction are threatened.

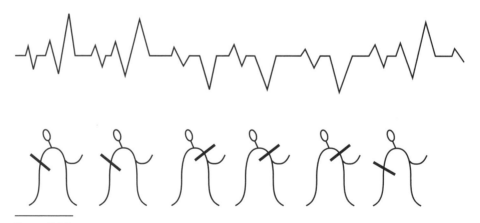

Figure 7–23.
Alternating right and left BBB.
This is a serious sign of impending complete heart block.

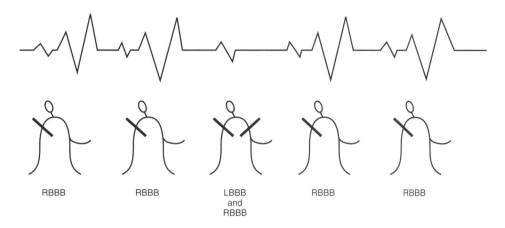

Figure 7–24.
Intermittent infranodal block.
When both bundles block intermittently, second-degree type II block exists. This is a serious warning of pending complete heart block.

When one bundle is blocked, the impulse can make its way down the remaining bundle and the ventricles will depolarize sequentially. When the second bundle becomes blocked, the supraventricular impulse will be unable to proceed to the ventricles. Sometimes the block of the second bundle is intermittent. This may present as either alternating left and right bundle branch block (Figure 7–23) or "dropped" QRS complexes (second-degree type 2 block) (Figure 7–24). Often the blocking of both bundles will become complete, resulting in a ventricular escape rhythm (CHB) (Figure 7–25). Since the block is below the AV node (infranodal) the escape pacemaker will be of ventricular origin and therefore very slow (20 to 40 per minute). Since the ventricles have little or no parasympathetic innervation, atropine is often ineffective for infranodal CHB. Transcutaneous pacing is the correct therapeutic choice in the emergency setting. Other warning signs of pending infranodal CHB include RBBB and alternating LAFB and LPFB (trifascicular block). The sudden development of a wide PR interval in the presence of a bundle branch block that occurs in the setting of infarct may be a warning of increasing resistance through the last remaining bundle or fascicle and indicate pending CHB. The American Heart Association *Advanced Cardiac Life Support* (ACLS) textbook recom-

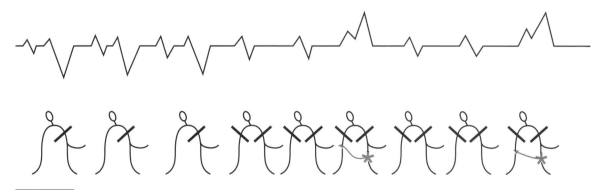

Figure 7–25.
Complete heart block.

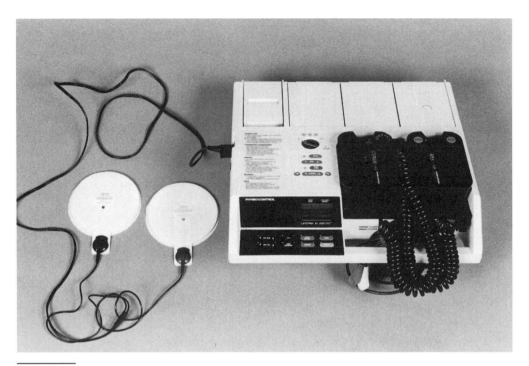

Figure 7–26.
An integral transcutaneous pacemaker-portable monitor/defibrillator.

mends that "Pacing be used in all (AMI) patients with right bundle branch block unless it is clear that the RBBB is old. The need for pacing is less clear in LBBB" (p. 5–2).

Transcutaneous Pacemakers (TCP) and Infranodal Block

Available as a component of most modern monitor/defibrillator units, TCP is readily available, noninvasive, and relatively inexpensive (Figure 7–26). It should be considered for standby use even in hemodynamically stable patients when signs of impending infranodal CHB are present. In the presence of acute anteroseptal MI, these signs include alternating left and right bundle branch block, trifascicular block, second-degree type 2 block, new bundle branch block, and sudden widening of the PR interval in the presence of bundle branch block (Table 7–8).

Wide QRS Tachycardia

Wide QRS tachycardias may emerge from either supraventricular (sinus, atrial, junctional) or ventricular (left or right ventricle) sites. They may be created by an ectopic foci or reentry.

TABLE 7–8 • **Warning Signs of Pending Infranodal Block**

- New BBB in the setting of anteroseptal MI
- Alternating left and right BBB
- Second-degree type 2 block
- Trifascicular block
- Sudden prolongation of the PR interval with BBB and anteroseptal MI

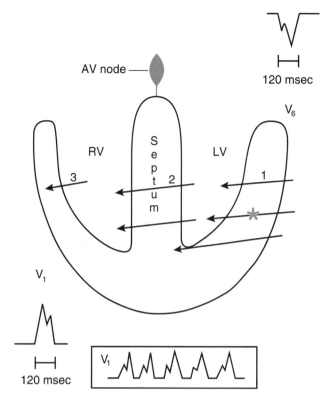

Figure 7–27.
Ventricular tachycardia (QRS morphology).

Abnormal depolarization focus beginning in the left ventricle (1) and spreading to the septum (2) and right ventricle (3)

In both ventricular tachycardia (VT) and wide supraventricular tachycardia (SVT) the cause of the widened QRS is the asynchronous depolarization of the ventricles. In VT, the focus starts in one ventricle and then spreads to the other ventricle. This takes approximately 120 msec (Figure 7–27). In wide SVT, the impulse arrives from above the ventricles, but finds one of the bundle branches is unable to accept the impulse. The ready ventricle is depolarized, followed by the remaining ventricle. This also takes approximately 120 msec (Figure 7–28). The supraventricular impulse arriving at the ventricle may find a bundle branch that is blocked from disease, or as is often the case in tachycardia, one that has simply not had enough time to recover from the preceding impulse. The right bundle branch normally repolarizes slower than the left. If the rate is fast enough, a supraventricular impulse will reach the ventricles before the right bundle branch has had time to recover, creating a physiological RBBB. This is often called aberration. (The left bundle branch will be the slowest to repolarize in some hearts, but this is relatively rare.) In rapid rates it is common to lose evidence of atrial activity (Ps become lost in the T waves of the preceding beats) and common to find wide QRS complexes (right bundle branch is refractory because it has not had time to recover). Use of elementary criteria for VT (no P wave, wide QRS) often leads to the wrong interpretation.

ECG Diagnosis of SVT with Aberration Versus VT

The most reliable criteria for accurately diagnosing supraventricular tachycardia with aberration from ventricular tachycardia is morphological (QRS shape) criteria. What this method does is attempt to identify patterns of LBBB or RBBB in the QRS. When a

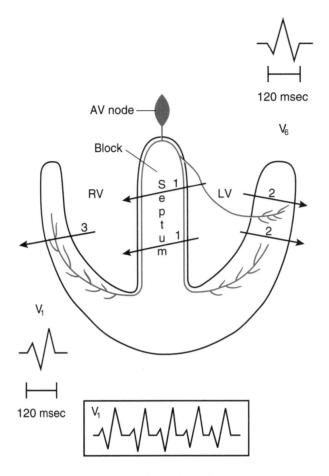

1. Left-to-right septal depolarization
2. LV depolarization preceding activation of the
   RV (asynchronus)
3. RV depolarization

Figure 7–28.
SVT with aberration.

pattern indicating bundle branch block is found, SVT with aberration is probably the cause of the wide QRS tachycardia. If no bundle branch block is found, then the assumption is that the wide QRS is of ventricular origin. A number of specific methods exist to accomplish this task, but most are quite complex and all have exceptions and limitations. For the paramedic or other emergency care worker, a quick and reasonably accurate method is best. Since a majority (80%) of aberrant SVTs result from right bundle branch aberration (remember, the RBB repolarizes slower than the left in most hearts), looking for RBBB patterns to prove aberration is most productive. Left bundle branch aberration in diseased hearts is virtually indistinguishable from right ventricular tachycardia. Using the following rules will allow for reasonable diagnostic accuracy for the emergency care provider.

If V_1 is triphasic with rSR' pattern, aberration is favored 10:1.
If V_6 or MCL_6 displays a qRs pattern, aberration is favored 20:1
    (Figure 7–29a).

Conversely, ventricular ectopy has some distinctive patterns as well.

If V_1 or MCL_1 has a RR' or qRR' with the first R taller than the second, left ventricular ectopy is favored 10:1.

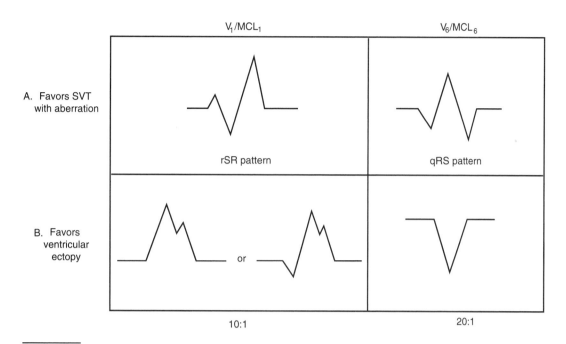

Figure 7–29.
Rules of thumb for quickly diagnosing (A) supraventricular tachycardia and (B) ventricular ectopy.

If V_6 or MCL_6 is completely negative (QS) pattern then ventricular ectopy is favored 20:1 (Figure 7–29b).

Although not perfect, these rules provide reasonable accuracy and are simple to commit to memory.

Premature Atrial Contractions with Aberration

These morphological clues also apply to individual early beats. Premature atrial contractions (PACs) frequently find the right bundle branch refractory to their early impulse. The PACs are then conducted with RBBB aberration, thus widening the QRS complex. Aberrant PACs are often mistaken for premature ventricular contractions (PVCs). When faced with an early wide beat that has no evidence of atrial activity, these morphological clues can aid in differentiating wide PACs from PVCs.

Role of Adenosine

The advent of adenosine for the treatment of SVTs has greatly reduced the need to differentially diagnose wide QRS tachycardias. Unlike verapamil, adenosine is short acting and therefore generally safe for most patients, regardless of the origin of the tachycardia. The ACLS algorithm for wide QRS tachycardias of uncertain type includes the use of lidocaine, adenosine, procainamide, and bretylium (Table 7–9).

Prehospital Significance

The emergency care provider has two critical responsibilities when treating wide QRS tachycardia. The first is to recognize unstable patients and treat them immediately with cardioversion regardless of the tachycardia's origin. The second is to gather sufficient data so that the correct diagnosis of the tachycardia can be made after the emergency is over.

TABLE 7–9 • **Prehospital Intervention Sequence of Wide-Complex Tachycardia (Uncertain Type)**
Lidocaine 1–1.5 mg/kg IV ↓
Lidocaine 0.5–0.75 mg/kg IV ↓
Adenosine 6 mg IV ↓
Adenosine 12 mg IV ↓
Procainamide 20–30 mg/min IV ↓
Bretylium 5–10 mg/kg IV

Modified from the *Textbook of Advanced Cardiac Life Support*, American Heart Association: Scientific Publishing, 1994.

Ideally, a diagnostic-quality 12-lead ECG should be recorded prior to conversion of the more stable patient. If a complete 12-lead ECG is not available, then leads I, II, and III should be obtained (for axis determination) and leads V_1, V_2, and V_6 (or their MCL equivalents) should be obtained for morphological criteria. If time allows for only one lead to be recorded, then MCL_1 is arguably the best choice. The pre- and postconversion recordings will provide useful information for the physicians determining the patient's definitive care.

Accessory Pathways

The atria are separated from the ventricles by the fibrous rings of the AV valves, called the annulus fibrosis. This cartilage-like structure normally insulates the atrium from the

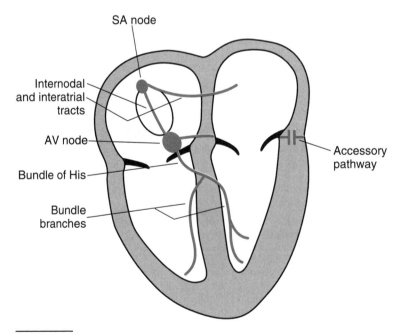

Figure 7–30.
Anatomical description of an accessory pathway created between the atria and ventricles.

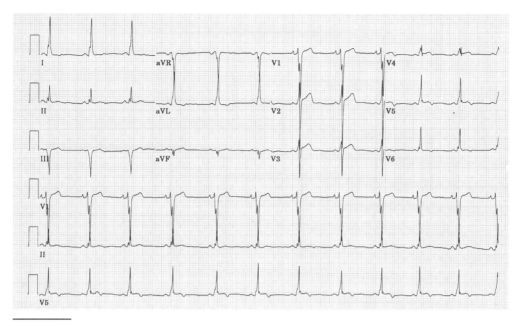

Figure 7–31.
12-lead ECG recording of Wolff-Parkinson-White syndrome.
Note the shortening of the P-R interval and the delta wave created on the
upstroke of the QRS complex.

ventricles, forcing all conduction from the atrium to the ventricles to pass through the AV node. On occasion, breaks in this insulation occur, creating extra or "accessory" pathways into the ventricles (Figure 7–30). Accessory pathways can shorten the PR interval and widen the QRS complex by preexcitation of the ventricle. The AV node conducts depolarization very slowly, allowing for adequate ventricular filling time. The accessory pathway conducts rapidly and bypasses the AV node. It reaches the ventricles before the polarization impulse makes its way through the AV node. The ventricle then begins to depolarize at the site of the accessory pathway, causing a widening of the first portion of the QRS (delta wave). Normal AV conduction then fuses with the preexcited myocardium, completing the QRS. Patients with this anomaly frequently suffer from episodes of reentrant SVTs. This is often referred to as Wolff-Parkinson-White syndrome (WPW) (Figure 7–31).

P Wave Abnormalities

The normal sinus P wave has a distinct pattern in leads II and V_1/MCL_1 (Figure 7–32). This pattern is predictably altered when either atrium is enlarged or when conduction occurs retrograde (backwards) through the atrium from a focus originating in the AV junction or one of the ventricles.

Right atrial enlargement (RAE) occurs most often from pulmonary disease. Since the SA node is in the right atrium, the initial forces of the P wave are exaggerated. This causes a peaked P wave in lead II and an exaggerated initial positive deflection in V_1/MCL_1 (Figure 7–33).

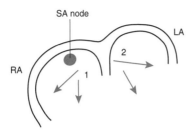

V₁/MCL₁   II

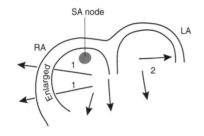

Figure 7–32.
Normal intraatrial conduction.
The P wave in V_1/MCL_1 is normally of +/− morphology. Lead II is normally upright and well-rounded. Because depolarization begins in the right atrium at the SA node, the initial portion of the P wave is depolarization of the right atrium and the terminal portion is depolarization of the left atrium.

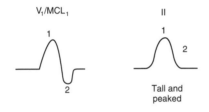

V₁/MCL₁   II

Tall and
peaked

1. RA depolarization
2. LA depolarization

A

Figure 7–33.
(A) In right atrial enlargement the initial portion of the P wave is enlarged. (B) 12-lead ECG recording of RAE.
Note the large (> 3 mm) peaked P wave in lead II and the exaggerated initial positive deflection in V_1.

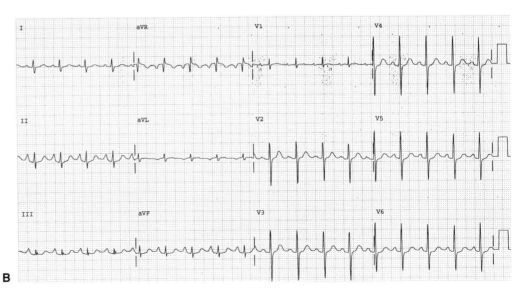

B

Left atrial enlargement (LAE) usually accompanies hypertension, mitral valve disease, and left ventricular hypertrophy. The terminal portion of the P wave is enlarged. In lead II, the P wave becomes notched (m-shaped), resembling the two humps of a camel. In lead V_1/MCL$_1$ the terminal negative portion of the P is exaggerated, sometimes creating an almost entirely negative P wave (Figure 7–34).

Retrograde conduction through the atria reverses the normal picture of the P wave. In lead II, the P wave becomes inverted, in V_1/MCL$_1$ it appears in a positive-negative configuration (Figure 7–35).

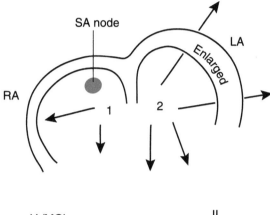

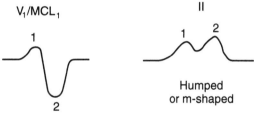

1. RA depolarization

2. LA depolarization

A

Figure 7–34.

(A) In left atrial enlargement the terminal portion of the P wave is enlarged. (B) 12-lead ECG recording of LAE.
Note the enlarged (> 3 mm) m-shaped P wave in lead II and the terminal negative P wave in V_1.

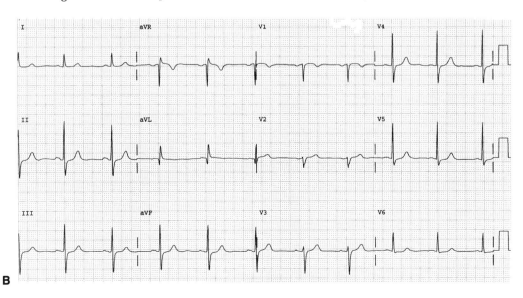

B

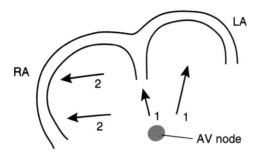

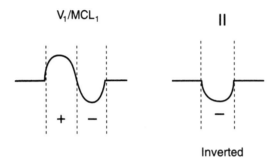

Inverted

1. Retrograde (backward) atrial depolarization
2. Atrial depolarization

Figure 7–35.
Retrograde (backward) conduction produces a negative P wave in lead II and a positive-negative P wave in V$_1$.

Pulmonary Disorders

ECG changes from chronic pulmonary disease usually occur long after the disease is otherwise apparent. Chronically distended alveoli and bronchial constriction lead to thoracic hypertrophy. Hypertrophy of the right ventricle occurs as a result of chronic overwork as the right ventricle struggles against resistant pulmonary circulation. The right atrium enlarges as blood from the failing right ventricle "backs up" into the atrium and vena cava. These structural changes each result in an electrocardiographic manifestation.

QRS amplitude is often diminished in patients with hypertrophic chests (barrel chests) due to the increased air-filled space between electrodes. The changes of right atrial enlargement are present and usually produce a tall, peaked P wave in lead II and a large initial positive portion of the P wave in lead V$_1$/MCL$_1$. The changes seen with right ventricular hypertrophy include a rightward swing of the QRS axis (> +110 degrees) and enlargement of the R waves in V$_1$ through V$_3$. The R wave of V$_1$ will be taller than its S wave (R:S ratio of > 1.0).

Hypothermia

Hypothermia is generally defined as a rectal temperature below 34°C (93°F). The American Heart Association defines severe accidental hypothermia as a body temperature below 30°C (86°F). ECG changes are expected below 34°C and become more pronounced and numerable as the temperature decreases. Prolongation of all intervals (PR, QRS, QT, and RR) is characteristic of hypothermia. The lengthening of the RR represents bradycardia, often profound at very low temperatures. The QRS will often develop a characteristic hump or notch (J-point or Osborne wave) at its terminal portion and elevate the ST segment where it meets this hump (Figure 7–36). This change is most prominent in the mid precordial leads (V$_3$ and V$_4$). Almost all profoundly hypothermic patients are bradycardic and about 50% develop atrial fibrillation at body temperatures below 32°C.

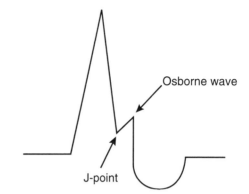

Figure 7–36.

The Osborne wave is a distinctive type of ST segment elevation that may be seen in hypothermia. It consists of an abrupt upward deflection at the J-point followed by a sudden plunge back to the baseline.

It is unlikely that hypothermia would be mistaken for AMI. History and physical exam (including body temperature) usually direct the examiner toward hypothermia. The ECG changes of hypothermia disappear as body temperature normalizes.

Brain Hemorrhage and the ECG

Emergency care providers should be aware that central nervous system catastrophes, such as intracerebral or subarachnoid hemorrhage, can cause dramatic changes in the ECG. Bradycardia is common as is the development of large U waves that seem to merge with wide prominent (sometime inverted) T waves, especially in the precordial leads (Figure 7–37a). The merger of T and U waves often gives the appearance of a prolonged QT interval. These changes are thought to occur from alterations within the autonomic nervous system.

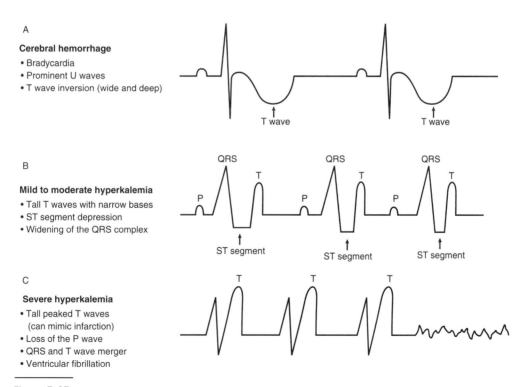

Figure 7–37.

ECG changes associated with (A) cerebral hemorrhage, (B) mild to moderate hyperkalemia, and (C) severe hyperkalemia.

Electrolyte Disturbances

Electrolyte imbalance can create a variety of dysrhythmias and other ECG changes. Paramedics should be alert to these changes in order to avoid misdiagnosis and untoward therapeutic actions.

Hyperkalemia (Serum Potassium Level above 5.5 mEq/L)

In the emergency setting, hyperkalemia is often the result of the excessive intake of potassium supplements or inadequate renal dialysis. Hyperkalemic patients commonly present with lethargy, weakness, and in severe cases, coma. Most have a history of diuretic therapy and concomitant potassium supplement intake and/or are renal dialysis patients.

Hyperkalemia produces a progressive evolution of changes in the electrocardiogram. The presence of ECG changes is often a better measure of clinically significant potassium toxicity than the serum potassium level. Changes associated with moderate hyperkalemia include tall narrow T waves, ST depression, and widening of the QRS (Figure 7–38b). Severe hyperkalemia will cause gross QRS widening, tall peaked T waves (this effect can easily be confused with peaked T waves of an acute myocardial infarction), loss of the P wave (from atrial paralysis), and eventually, ventricular fibrillation (Figure 7–38c). It should be noted that the peaked T waves of AMI are confined to the leads overlying the area of infarct, whereas in potassium intoxication the changes are diffuse.

Hypokalemia (Serum Potassium of Less Than 3.5 mEq/L)

Causes of hypokalemia seen in the emergency setting include diuretic therapy, noncompliance with potassium supplement therapy, liver disease, laxative abuse, or starvation (often seen in dieting teenage females), and prolonged episodes of vomiting. Hypokalemia is often present in the immediate postresuscitation period following cardiopulmonary arrest. Chief complaints include weakness, muscle tenderness, and drowsiness or lethargy. ECG changes associated with hypokalemia include enlarged P waves, PR interval prolongation, depression of the ST segment, decreased T wave amplitude, increased U wave amplitude, and in severe cases, QRS widening (Table 7–10). When the U wave amplitude exceeds T wave amplitude the potassium level is usually under 2.7 mEq/L. Severe hypokalemia is a relatively common and dangerous condition. Digitalis toxicity is worsened by hypokalemia and opens the door to a variety of dysrhythmias.

Hypercalcemia (Serum Calcium above 10.5 mg/dl)

Increased levels of calcium result from various carcinomas and renal disorders. Excessive doses of vitamin D increases the reabsorption of calcium from the intestines, while chronic thiazide diuretics inhibit calcium excretion. Both can lead to hypercalcemia. Lethargy, muscle weakness, fatigue, and increased urine output are common subjective

---

TABLE 7–10 • **Hypokalemia**

- Enlarged P waves
- PR interval prolongation
- ST segment depression
- Decreased T wave amplitude
- Increased U wave amplitude

TABLE 7–11 • **Hypercalcemia**

- Shortened QT interval
- Early proximal end of the T wave
- Increased QRS amplitude
- Possible J wave

TABLE 7–12 • **Hypocalcemia**

- Prolonged QT interval
- Normal-shaped T wave
- Possible T wave inversion

findings. ECG changes include a shortened QT interval with an abrupt proximal limb of the T wave (early peak of the T wave) (Table 7–11), widespread increase in QRS amplitude, and in severe hypercalcemia, a J-wave similar to that seen in hypothermia may appear.

Hypocalcemia (Serum Calcium Level below 8.5 mg/dl)

Large gastrointestinal losses of calcium via diarrhea and calcium losses due to diuretic therapy are common etiologies of hypocalcemia. Acute pancreatitis often leads to calcium deficiency as well. Signs and symptoms of hypocalcemia include lethargy, muscle tremors, and cramps, even with minor calcium level reductions. Tetany, seizures, and decreased cardiac output may occur with more severe reductions. Rarely does impairment of respiratory musculature and neuromuscular involvement cause respiratory distress with bronchospasms and respiratory arrest. Prolongation of the ST segment results in a long QT interval and a normal-shaped T wave (Table 7–12). T wave inversion occurs in about one-third of cases.

The reader is encouraged to refer to Table 7–13 for a review of the electrocardiographic changes associated with electrolyte disorders.

TABLE 7–13 • **Summary of ECG Changes Due to Electrolyte Disturbances**

COMPLEXES AND INTERVALS	HYPER-KALEMIA	HYPO-KALEMIA	HYPER-CALCEMIA	HYPO-CALCEMIA
P Wave	Lost	Enlarged		
PR Interval	Prolonged	Prolonged		
QRS Complex	Widening	Widening (less common)	Increase amplitude	
ST Segment	Depression	Depression	Shortening	Lengthening
T Wave	Tall, narrow	Low amplitude (possible inversion)	Short QT, early peaked T	Prolonged QT T wave inversion (1/3 of cases)
U Wave	None	Present, may be taller than T wave		
Other	Ventricular dysrhythmias	Multiple dysrhythmias in conjunction with digitalis toxicity	Atrial and ventricular dysrhythmias	Atrial and ventricular dysrhythmias

KEY POINTS SUMMARY

Nonischemic Causes of ST Segment Elevation

1. Acute pericarditis, benign early repolarization, left bundle branch block, and left ventricular hypertrophy are four nonischemic causes of ST segment elevation that often mimic acute myocardial infarction.

Bundle Branch Block

2. Conduction through the bundle branches can be impeded for a number of reasons. Electrical block of either the right or left bundle branch results in asynchronous depolarization of the ventricles.
3. ECG evidence of right bundle branch block
   - Atrial activity is present (P wave)
   - QRS duration is > 0.12 sec
   - rSR pattern in V_1 and a qRS pattern in V_6
4. ECG Evidence of left bundle branch block
   - Atrial activity is present (P wave)
   - QRS duration is > 0.12 sec
   - QS pattern in V_1 and a positive R or RR pattern in V_6

Hemiblocks

5. The term hemiblock refers to the electrical block of either the anterior or posterior fascicle of the left bundle branch. Left anterior fascicular block is a block of the anterior fascicle, while left posterior fascicular block is a block of the posterior fascicle.
6. ECG evidence of left anterior fascicular block
   - Q wave in leads I and aVL followed by a tall R wave
   - Small R wave followed by a deep S wave in leads III and aVF
   - Left axis deviation of −30 degrees or more is present
7. ECG evidence of left posterior fascicular block
   - Q wave in leads III and aVF followed by a tall R wave
   - Small R wave followed by deep S wave in leads I and aVL
   - Right axis deviation of 120 degrees or more will be present

Wide QRS Tachycardia

8. Wide complex tachycardias emerge from either supraventricular or ventricular sites. In both cases, the cause of the widened QRS is the asynchronous depolarization of the ventricles. In ventricular tachycardia, the ectopic impulse

originates in one ventricle and then spreads to the other ventricle. In supraventricular tachycardia the impulse arrives from above the ventricles, but finds one of the bundle branches (most commonly the RBB) refractory to that impulse.

9. Distinguishing supraventricular tachycardia with aberration from ventricular tachycardia involves identifying patterns of right bundle branch block. SVT with aberration usually presents with ECG criteria of RBBB, whereas V-tach does not.

Accessory Pathways

10. Accessory pathways are additional conductive pathways created between the atria and ventricles. Such pathways usually bypass the AV node and transmit electrical impulses with great velocity. Therefore, accessory pathways shorten the PR interval and widen the QRS by preexcitation of the ventricles. Wolff-Parkinson-White syndrome is an example of such a phenomena.

P Wave Abnormalities

11. Enlargement of the atria can result in morphological changes of the P wave. The P wave assumes an exaggerated form of greater than 3 mm in height and width. Enlargement of the right atria often occurs as a result of pulmonary disorders, while enlargement of the left atria usually accompanies hypertension, mitral valve disease, or left ventricular hypertrophy.

Pulmonary Disorders

12. ECG changes occurring from chronic pulmonary disorders are the result of both right atrial enlargement and right ventricular hypertrophy as the ventricle struggles against the resistant pulmonary circulation.

Hypothermia

13. Hypothermia is defined as a rectal temperature below 34°C (93°F). Prolongation of all intervals (PR, QT, and RR) is characteristic of hypothermia, as well as the development of an Osborne wave.

Electrolyte Disturbances

14. Electrolyte imbalances can create a variety of dysrhythmias and ECG changes. Hyperkalemia will produce tall narrow T waves, while hypokalemia will decrease T wave amplitude. Hypercalcemia will produce a shortened QT interval and an increase in QRS amplitude. Hypocalcemia results in a prolonged ST segment and a long QT interval.

BIBLIOGRAPHY

Conover MB. *Understanding Electrocardiography: Arrhythmias and the 12-Lead ECG.* St. Louis, MO: Mosby; 1992.

Huszar RJ. *Basic Dysrhythmias Interpretation and Management.* St. Louis, MO: Mosby; 1994.

Johnson R, Swartz MH. *A Simplified Approach to Electrocardiography.* Philadelphia, PA: WB Saunders; 1986.

Langer F. *12-Lead Electrocardiography: Advanced Dysrhythmias.* Orlando, FL: Florida Hospital Medical Center, 1992.

Lipman BC, Casio T. ECG *Assessment and Interpretation.* Philadelphia, PA: FA Davis Company; 1994.

Marriott HJL. *Practical Electrocardiography.* Baltimore, MD: Williams & Wilkins; 1988.

Marriott HJL, Conover MB. *Advanced Concepts in Arrhythmias.* 2nd ed. St. Louis, MO: Mosby; 1989.

Thaler MS. *The Only EKG Book You'll Ever Need.* Philadelphia, PA: JB Lippincott; 1988.

Practice Exercises
In Identification of Cardiac Disorders

Study the following ECG tracings and determine the underlying pathophysiology for each one. Some show infarctions, some show conditions mimicking infarction.

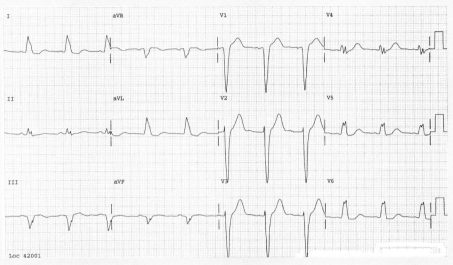

Exercise 7–1.

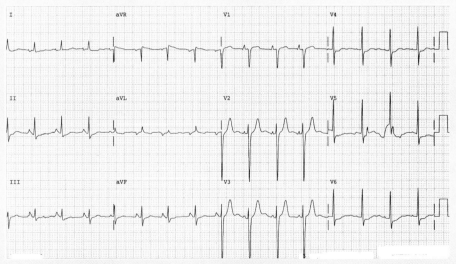

Exercise 7–2.

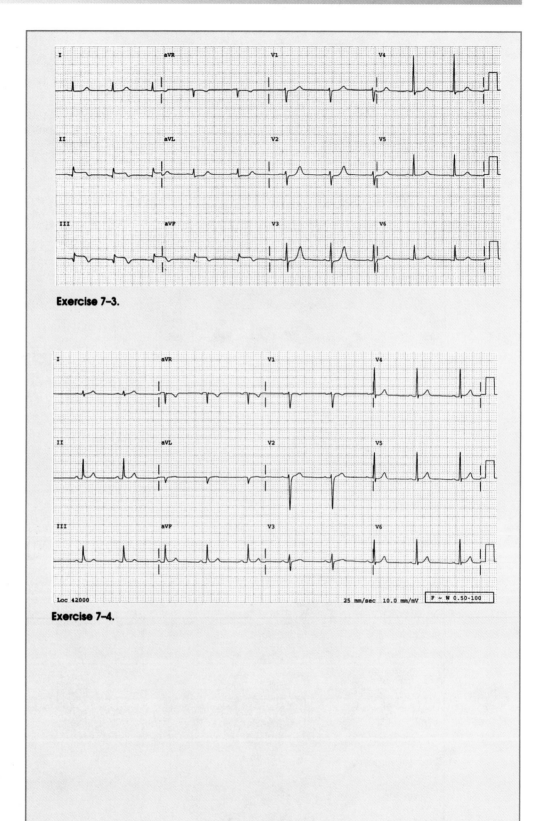

Exercise 7-3.

Exercise 7-4.

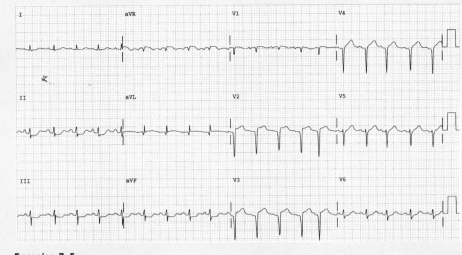

Exercise 7–5.

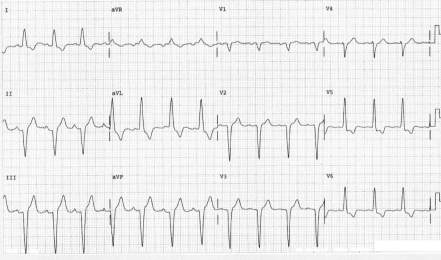

Exercise 7–6.

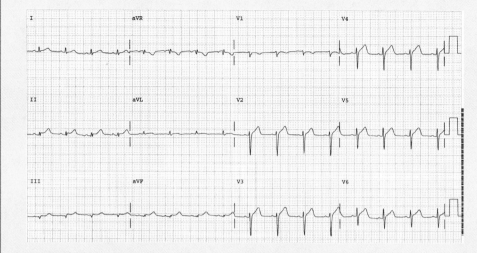

Exercise 7-7.

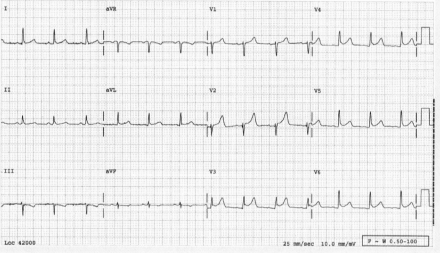

Exercise 7-8.

Answer Key

Chapter 7 Practice Exercises/Identification of Cardiac Disorders

Exercise 1. Left bundle branch block

Exercise 2. Left ventricular hypertrophy

Exercise 3. Inferior wall infarction

Exercise 4. Benign early repolarization

Exercise 5. Anterior wall infarction

Exercise 6. Left bundle branch block

Exercise 7. Pericarditis

Exercise 8. Anterolateral infarction

8

OUTLINE

The Pathophysiology and Clinical Manifestations of Ischemic Heart Disease

LEARNING OBJECTIVES

1. Describe the pathophysiology of coronary artery disease and list the effects of atherosclerosis.

2. List the major modifiable and nonmodifiable risk factors for coronary artery disease.

3. Discuss the pathophysiology of myocardial ischemia and infarction.

4. Explain the imbalance that exists between myocardial oxygen supply and demand that precipitates ischemia.

5. Define angina pectoris and describe its pathophysiological evolution.

6. List and describe the signs, symptoms, ECG characteristics, and clinical implications of stable angina, unstable angina, and Prinzmetal's angina.

7. Discuss the treatment of angina.

8. Describe the electrocardiographic evolution of myocardial infarction.

9. Outline the coronary circulation and list those vessels that perfuse the anatomical quadrants of the left ventricle and conduction system.

10. Name the leads that reflect anterior infarction, inferior infarction, lateral infarction, and posterior infarction.

11. Discuss the common conduction defects associated with anterior and inferior infarction.

12. List and describe the most common complications of infarction.

13. Discuss the pathophysiology of right ventricular infarction and describe its clinical symptoms, ECG characteristics, and treatment strategies.

14. List and describe the signs and symptoms of myocardial infarction.

15. Discuss the role of the electrocardiogram for the diagnosis of infarction.

16. Discuss the differential diagnosis of myocardial infarction and describe the following mimicking conditions: acute pericarditis, aortic dissection, pulmonary emboli, Boerhaave's syndrome, pneumothorax, musculoskeletal pain, and gastrointestinal/abdominal distress.

INTRODUCTION

Ischemic heart disease and its complications cause the greatest number of deaths each year in the United States. Nearly half of these deaths occur prior to arrival at the hospital, with lethal dysrhythmias (e.g., ventricular fibrillation) accounting for the overwhelming majority. While there are many processes which produce the imbalance between myocardial oxygen supply and demand that precipitate ischemia, the most common cause by far is atherosclerosis of the coronary arteries, commonly termed coronary artery disease. Knowledge of coronary artery disease and the nature of the myocardial response to oxygen deprivation (owing to progressive narrowing of the coronary arteries and subsequent hypoperfusion), will enhance the paramedic's ability to accurrately evaluate and diagnose the various syndromes of ischemic heart disease. This in turn will optimize patient management and further reduce the morbidity and mortality associated with this disease.

This chapter will address the pathophysiological evolution and clinical manifestations of myocardial ischemia and infarction, followed by a discussion of several pathological conditions that can mimic infarction.

CORONARY ARTERY DISEASE

Coronary Atherogenesis

Coronary atherosclerosis is a degenerative disease process characterized by progressive narrowing of the lumen of coronary arteries. It results from the accumulation of fatty deposits (lipids and cholesterol), platelets, macrophages (white blood cells), and cell debris throughout the tunica intima (innermost endothelial cell layer) and eventually into the tunica media (smooth muscle layer). This in turn results in the development of thick, hard atherosclerotic plaques which are most commonly found in areas of turbulent blood flow such as vessel bifurcations.

Although the exact pathogenesis of atherosclerosis is unclear, it is believed that the disease process is a result of the endothelial cells' response to chronic mechanical or chemical injury. According to this theory, after fat is deposited within the intimal layer of the artery, an injury response occurs in the vessel wall. With injury, endothelial cell integrity is breached and the permeability of endothelial cells to various plasma substances increases, allowing access to inside of the artery. Over time, plasma cholesterol, additional fats, and calcium are deposited, forming plaques that eventually extend into the tunica media. Small hemorrhages occur which in turn lead to scarring, fibrosis, and enlargement of the plaques. Partial or total obstruction of the involved artery or arteries results, either by additional plaques or by a blood clot (thrombus).

Effects of Atherosclerosis

Atherosclerosis has two major effects on the coronary blood vessels. First, the disease disrupts the intimal surface, causing a loss of vessel elasticity and an increase in thrombi formation. Second, plaque formation reduces the diameter of the vessel lumen and thus decreases blood perfusion. As a result, the diseased coronary artery is unable to transport adequate blood volume to the area of heart muscle it supplies, thereby precipitating myocardial ischemia. Common manifestations of coronary atherosclerosis include angina pectoris (chest pain due to partial vessel obstruction) and myocardial infarction (tissue death due to total vessel obstruction).

Major Risk Factors of Coronary Artery Disease

Coronary atherosclerosis appears to be part of the aging process and occurs to some extent in all middle-aged and older people and in some younger individuals. It seems to have a heritable component and is often seen at a younger age in men than in women.

TABLE 8–1 • **Risk Factors of Coronary Artery Disease**

MODIFIABLE	NONMODIFIABLE	OTHER
Cigarette smoking	Advanced age	Type A personality
Hypertension	Male gender	Sedentary lifestyle
Hypercholesterolemia	Family history	Obesity
	Diabetes mellitus	Use of oral contraceptives

Epidemiologic research has identified seven major (modifiable and nonmodifiable) risk factors that contribute to the onset and escalation of coronary artery disease (Table 8–1). Modifiable risk factors include cigarette smoking, hypertension, and hypercholesterolemia (high levels of circulating cholesterol). Nonmodifiable risk factors refer to those conditions that cannot be altered by persons wishing to decrease their risk of cardiovascular disease. These include advanced age, male gender, genetic predisposition (family history), and diabetes mellitus.

MYOCARDIAL ISCHEMIA

Pathophysiology

The coronary arteries normally supply sufficient blood flow to meet the demands of the myocardium as it labors under varying workloads. Oxygen extraction from these vessels occurs with maximal efficiency. If efficient exchange does not meet myocardial oxygen needs, healthy coronary arteries can dilate to increase the flow of oxygenated blood to the myocardium. However, if the coronary arteries are stiffened or narrowed with atherosclerosis and cannot dilate in response to an increased demand for oxygen, myocardial ischemia (inadequate blood supply and oxygen deprivation) occurs. Myocardial ischemia, therefore, represents an imbalance between myocardial oxygen supply and demand and occurs the moment blood supply to the myocardium is reduced. In the majority of cases, it is a temporary condition that resolves without any permanent structural damage to the heart muscle.

Anomalies of Myocardial Oxygen Supply and Demand

Myocardial ischemia occurs when coronary blood flow or the oxygen content of the blood is insufficient to meet the metabolic demands of myocardial cells. Imbalances between myocardial blood supply and demand can arise from a number of conditions (Table 8–2). Abnormalities in one or both of these factors may be present in an individual patient.

Coronary artery obstruction (due to an atherosclerotic lesion) and coronary artery spasm limiting myocardial perfusion are the most common causes of reduced myocardial oxygen supply. Other causes of reduced supply include hypotension, decreased blood volume (e.g., due to hemorrhage), anemia (decrease in red blood cells), severe anoxia, and hypoxemia caused by respiratory disease (e.g., chronic obstructive pulmonary disease).

Myocardial oxygen demand is increased by conditions that increase myocardial workload. The most common causes of increased workload are an elevation in heart rate and blood pressure (systemic vascular resistance). Other causes include thickening of the myocardium (e.g., left ventricular hypertrophy), which increases the total amount of muscle mass requiring oxygen, and any condition that heightens the myocardium's contractile response (e.g., exercise or sympathetic stimulation).

TABLE 8–2 • **Causes of Myocardial Ischemia**

DECREASED MYOCARDIAL OXYGEN SUPPLY
Coronary artery obstruction
Atherosclerosis
Arterial spasm
Hypoxemia
Systemic hypotension
Severe anemia
INCREASED MYOCARDIAL OXYGEN DEMAND
Myocardial hypertrophy
Increased workload
Increased afterload
Hypertension
Aortic stenosis
Tachycardia

CLINICAL MANIFESTATIONS OF MYOCARDIAL ISCHEMIA

The continuum of ischemic heart disease encompasses a variety of clinical syndromes, ranging from silent ischemia (unknown to the patient) through the various patterns of angina, acute myocardial infarction, to the complications of acute myocardial infarction and sudden death. Although all of these syndromes represent a cascade of the same disease process, they may present with quite different clinical pictures and ECG findings. Knowledge of such findings, as well as their various presentations, will ensure proper and efficient patient management.

Angina Pectoris

Angina pectoris or "choking chest" describes the severe pain originating from the heart that occurs in response to an inadequate oxygen supply of the myocardial cells compared to their oxygen demand. It is commonly caused by atherosclerotic narrowing of the coronary arteries and is the principle symptom of ischemic heart disease. The discomfort of angina results when the oxygen demands of the heart are transiently exceeded by the blood supply, resulting in an accumulation of lactic acid and carbon dioxide in ischemic myocardial tissues. These metabolites are responsible for activating nerve endings that produce anginal pain (see Chapter 9).

Angina pectoris is typically experienced as retrosternal (behind the sternum) chest discomfort, ranging from a sensation of heaviness, to pressure, to moderately severe pain. The pain often radiates to the neck, lower jaw, left arm, left shoulder, and epigastrium. It may occasionally radiate to the back or down the right arm. Secondary symptoms such as lightheadedness, nausea, and palpitations (abnormal awareness to one's own heartbeat) may also accompany the pain. Frequently seen objective anginal companions include pallor, diaphoresis, grimacing, and clutching of the chest (Table 8–3).

TABLE 8–3 • **Symptoms of Angina Pectoris**

• Retrosternal heaviness or pressure
• Neck, jaw, upper extremity, and epigastric discomfort
• Lightheadedness, nausea, and palpitations
• Pallor, diaphoresis, grimacing, and clutching of the chest

TYPES OF ANGINA

There are three types of angina: stable angina, unstable angina, and Prinzmetal's angina. All three are unique in their own right, presenting with distinct but often highly variable signs, symptoms, and clinical implications (Table 8–4).

Stable Angina (Exertional Angina)

When paroxysms of ischemic chest pain (or anginal equivalents such as dyspnea or severe weakness) accompany a somewhat predictable amount of exertion or emotional stress, stable angina is said to exist. The mechanism of stable angina is related to the narrowing of the coronary arteries (> 50% stenosis), to the point that they adequately perfuse the heart at rest or with mild exertion, but lack the required flow to meet the increased needs of the myocardium during exercise or stress.

The discomfort of stable angina usually lasts only a few minutes (5 to 10 minutes), and is typically relieved by rest and/or nitroglycerin. The prognosis for this condition is quite good, and usually no emergency treatment other than sublingual nitroglycerin is required. However, if unrelieved by either rest or nitrates, the individual may be progressing toward more severe ischemic syndromes. Furthermore, stable angina usually involves ischemia to the subendocardial portion of the heart; rarely is it transmural. An ECG taken during an acute attack will demonstrate ST segment depression and/or T wave inversion (Figure 8–1). These changes will resolve once the myocardium is no longer ischemic, making early (prehospital) detection an important diagnostic finding.

Unstable Angina (Preinfarction Angina)

Unstable angina represents a clinical state between stable angina and acute myocardial infarction. It is seen in patients with prolonged periods of ischemic chest pain, but who at the same time do not demonstrate evidence of infarction (i.e., ST elevation and pathological Q waves). Unstable angina is therefore more serious than stable angina and often precedes acute infarction by hours, days, or weeks.

The pathogenesis of unstable angina is thought to be due to the progression and extent of coronary atherosclerosis (often exceeding 90% obstruction) in the affected arteries. Current evidence suggests that coronary artery spasm or incomplete coronary thrombosis at the site of a fixed arterial lesion may also play a role in its occurrence. Diagnostically, unstable angina is differentiated from stable angina by one or more of the following: (1) a noticeable decrease in the exertion or stress required to initiate the event; (2) an increase in the frequency, duration, and/or intensity of the discomfort; and (3) an

TABLE 8–4 • **Anginal Conditions and Their Variations**

	STABLE	UNSTABLE	PRINZMETAL'S
Exertional onset	Yes	Yes	No
Rest onset	No	Yes	Yes
Duration < 15 min.	Yes	No	On occasion
Relieved with rest and/or nitroglycerin	Yes	Yes	Yes
ST depression/T wave inversion	Yes	Yes	No
ST elevation	No	On occasion	Yes
Pathological Q waves present	No	No	No
ECG changes resolve	Yes	Yes	Yes

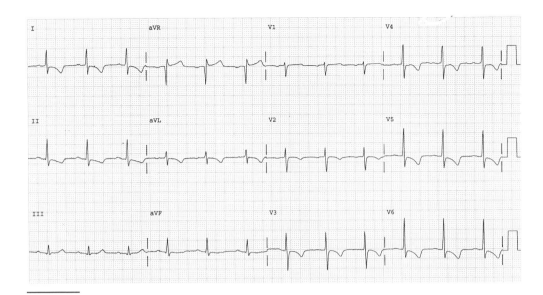

Figure 8–1.
A 12-lead ECG recording of an acute anginal attack.
Note the widespread presence of ST segment depression and T wave inversion throughout the anterolateral leads. This pattern is consistent with myocardial ischemia.

increase in the amount of rest or nitroglycerin needed to terminate the event. Furthermore, the ischemia associated with unstable angina is more likely to be transmural than with stable angina. Electrocardiographic evidence of the attack is demonstrated by ST segment depression (subendocardial ischemia) and on occasion, ST elevation (transmural ischemia).

Prinzmetal's Angina (Variant or Vasospastic Angina)

Prinzmetal's angina is an ischemic myocardial condition resulting from coronary artery spasm. It differs from stable and unstable angina in a number of ways. The chest discomfort of Prinzmetal's angina occurs primarily at rest and without provocation. There is a tendency for attacks to recur at similar times of the day (often at night) and are frequently associated with dysrhythmias (tachydysrhythmias and atrioventricular blocks) and sometimes syncope. Furthermore, spasm of the coronary arteries causes transmural ischemia and may appear in patients with relatively clean coronary arteries. The transmural ischemia associated with Prinzmetal's angina produces ST segment elevation, duplicating the pattern seen in acute myocardial infarction. Differential diagnosis is accomplished in most cases when nitroglycerin (or Procardia) administration rapidly resolves both the symptoms and the electrocardiographic changes. It is necessary then to record an ECG before pain relief whenever possible, otherwise the diagnosis may be missed.

ELECTROCARDIOGRAPHY AND THE TREATMENT OF ANGINA

Electrocardiography is an essential tool for the diagnosis of myocardial ischemia. Because many individuals demonstrate normal electrocardiograms in the absence of pain, diagnosis requires that electrocardiography be performed during an anginal attack. Remember that transient ST segment depression and T wave inversion are characteristic signs of subendocardial ischemia and are often demonstrated with stable and unstable angina, while ST elevation, indicative of transmural ischemia, is seen in patients with Prinzmetal's angina.

Increasing coronary blood supply while decreasing myocardial oxygen demand is the goal of therapy for acute myocardial ischemia and all forms of angina. This is best accomplished with rest and the use of nitroglycerin. Rest allows the heart to pump out less blood (decreased stroke volume) at a slower rate. This reduces the work of the heart, thereby reducing its oxygen requirements. Nitroglycerin acts as a potent dilator of the venous system, decreasing venous return of blood to the heart. A decreased venous return reduces ventricular filling pressure, allowing the heart to decrease stroke volume. Nitrates also dilate the arterial system, reducing the afterload against which the heart must pump and increase coronary blood flow. Both rest and nitroglycerin greatly reduce the inequalities of oxygen demand versus supply and will be discussed in further detail in the next chapter.

MYOCARDIAL INFARCTION

Pathophysiology

If ischemia is severe and prolonged, irreversible myocardial damage (myocardial infarction) will occur. Myocardial infarction represents the culminating response to unresolved myocardial ischemia and occurs the moment one of the coronary arteries becomes totally obstructed. The underlying pathogenesis in almost all cases is progressive narrowing of the coronary arteries by atherosclerosis.

The primary mechanism for acute myocardial infarction is that of acute coronary thrombosis resulting from abnormal platelet aggregation (see Chapter 6, Figure 6–2). Recent evidence indicates that the rupturing of atherosclerotic plaques stimulates platelet aggregation, platelet-thrombus formation, and abnormal vessel tone. Dislodgment of such plaques obstructs blood flow to the entire area of myocardium supplied by that vessel, resulting in cellular necrosis. Infarction may also occur if a thrombotic lesion adhering to a damaged coronary artery becomes large enought to totally obstruct blood flow, or if the heart chamber becomes so abnormally enlarged (ventricular hypertrophy) that it is unable to meet its oxygen demands.

Electrocardiographic Review of Infarction

When a clot forms in a coronary artery, the myocardial tissue distal to the clot becomes ischemic. This ischemic process is dynamic, changing its characteristics as the event progresses. In order to understand the process of infarction and the electrocardiographic changes that accompany it, we will review a typical progression model of the acute myocardial infarction process. In our model, an electrode will be placed directly over the epicardium on an area of myocardium supplied by our sample artery (Figure 8–2a).

With adequate myocardial perfusion, the ST segment is isoelectric (equal to the baseline) and the T wave upright. When the coronary artery is initially blocked, the tissue most distal to the artery (the endocardial surface) becomes ischemic. This causes inversion of the T wave and/or ST depression (Figure 8–2b). If perfusion is not restored, ischemia will often extend to the epicardial surface. This results in transmural ischemia and produces ST elevation in the investigating lead (Figure 8–2c). Although no actual injury or death has occurred at this point, the term injury pattern is commonly used. If the area is immediately reperfused, all with return to normal. However, if the area is not reperfused, infarction will likely ensue. Furthermore, if ischemic chest pain is present and is unrelieved by rest and nitroglycerin, and the ST segments remain elevated, an acute infarct is likely in progress. The term infarct is used loosely here, since no actual

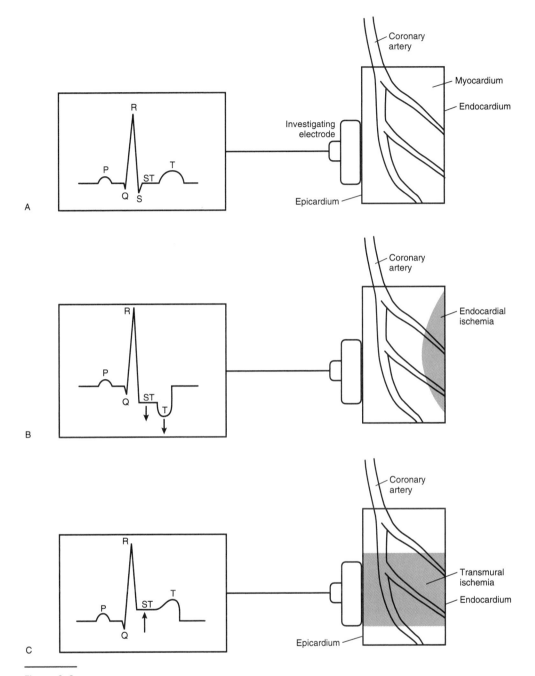

Figure 8-2.
(A) The normal ECG with adequate myocardial perfusion. (B) Endocardial is-chemia as evidenced by ST segment depression and/or T wave inversion. (C) Transmural ischemia as evidenced by ST segment elevation (the acute in-jury/infarction pattern).

evidence of tissue death exists. The reasonable assumption is that infarction will follow if definitive therapy (i.e., thrombolytic therapy) is not rapidly achieved.

Recall that when the tissue actually infarcts, it becomes electrically silent. This cre-ates a window beneath our electrode that allows one to see the opposing wall of the my-ocardium depolarizing from endocardium to epicardium. In the undisturbed heart, the

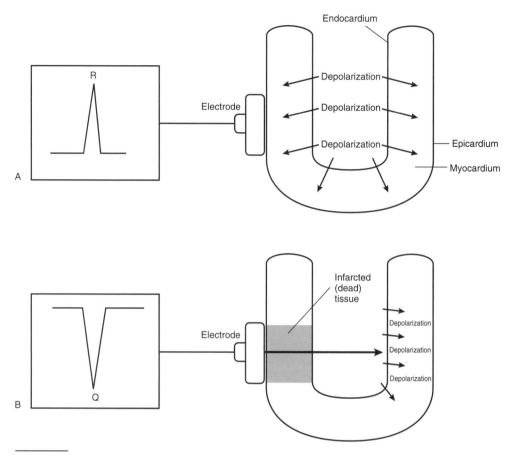

Figure 8–3.
(A) In the undisturbed heart, an electrode overlying the epicardial surface will record a positive R wave on the ECG as the net depolarization force is directed toward it. (B) An electrode overlying infarcted tissue looks through the dead area and records a negative Q wave as the impulse moves away from its positive pole.

electrode views the depolarization force as coming towards the epicardial surface and records it as a positive wave (R wave) (Figure 8–3a). With infarction, the electrode looks through the electrically dead tissue and sees the opposing wall depolarizing away from the positive electrode. This creates a negative Q wave on the ECG (Figure 8–3b).

Our example utilized an epicardial electrode in order to simplify the concept. In the field or other emergency-setting, a surface electrode (placed on the limbs or chest) will be utilized. Due to the distance of the surface electrode from the myocardium, a larger area of tissue will be observed in comparison to our model epicardial electrode. During the course of infarction, the surface electrode is subject to viewing a number of the electrical changes that occur simultaneously in the same general region.

Finally, the electrocardiographic patterns of subendocardial ischemia, transmural ischemia, and infarction as described above often occur concurrently due to the anatomical location and extent of myocardial tissue damage. The infarcted myocardium (zone of infarction) is surrounded by a zone of hypoxic injury, which may progress to necrosis or return to normal. Adjacent to the zone of hypoxic injury is a zone of reversible ischemia (Figure 8–4). Evidence of these zones are simultaneously displayed on the ECG as enlarged (pathological) Q waves, ST elevation, and T wave inversion.

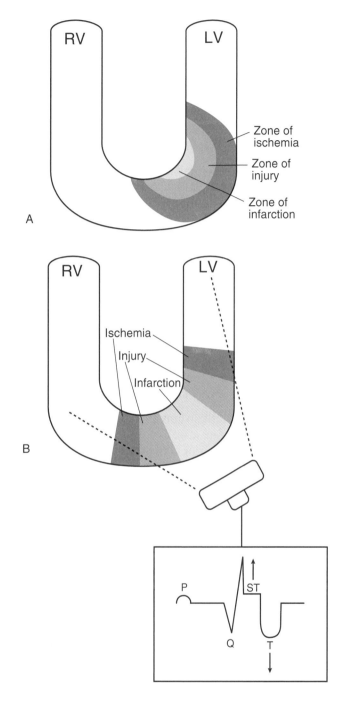

Figure 8–4.
(A) Schematic of the left ventricle identifying the zones of myocardial ischemia, injury, and infarction that are responsible for the evolutionary ECG patterns of infarction. (B) The simultaneous presence of the characteristic ECG changes of infarction.

LOCALIZATION AND CLINICAL PATTERNS OF INFARCTION

ST segment elevation and pathological Q waves are the major indicative ECG changes seen with acute myocardial infarction. Correlation of these findings with specific groups of leads enables the examiner to localize the infarct and predict, with reasonable certainty, which coronary artery is occluded. Knowledge of such information is important because the incidence and significance of complications vary with the site. For example, inferior wall myocardial infarction (right coronary artery occlusion) may affect the autonomic nervous system, manifested by enhanced vagal tone and subsequent bradycardia, whereas anterior wall myocardial infarction (left coronary artery occlusion) may directly damage the electrical conduction system, producing significant atrioventricular block (i.e., Mobitz II or complete heart block). Familiarity with coronary artery distribution and infarct localization is an essential element of 12-lead ECG interpretation and will be reviewed.

Coronary Artery Distribution

As you recall from previous chapters, two large coronary arteries (right and left) emerge from the base of the aorta just above the aortic valve (see Figure 2–6). Approximately 5% of the cardiac output is directed into these arteries, providing the myocardium with oxygenated blood. Both arteries are essentially superficial (i.e., located on the epicardial surface) and reach inward toward the endocardium. The following descriptions are commonly accepted, but one should keep in mind that coronary anatomy may vary from patient to patient.

The right coronary artery (RCA) travels in the groove (atrioventricular sulcus) between the right atrium and the right ventricle and branches off to supply blood to the posterior portions of the heart, including the posterior intraventricular septum and the inferior surface of the left ventricle. In most individuals, the right coronary artery also supplies blood to two important electrical sites of the heart: the sinoatrial (SA) node and the atrioventricular (AV) node (Table 8–5).

Summary of RCA Distribution

* Right atrium and right ventricle
* Inferior wall of the left ventricle
* Posterior wall of the left ventricle

The left coronary artery (LCA) originates from the aorta and passes behind the pulmonary artery, emerging onto the myocardium as the left main coronary artery. The left main coronary artery quickly bifurcates into two distinct branches, the left anterior descending artery (LAD) and the circumflex artery. The LAD artery travels down the anterior portion of the septal groove between the right and left ventricles and branches several more times to supply blood to the anterior portion of the septum and to the anterior muscle mass of the left ventricle. The circumflex artery runs between the left atrium and ventricle and supplies blood to the lateral wall of the left ventricle.

TABLE 8–5 • **Coronary Artery Distribution and Structures Supplied**

	LCA	RCA
SA node		X
AV node		X
Septal wall	X	
Anterior wall	X	
Lateral wall	X	
Inferior wall		X
Right ventricle		X
RBB	X	
LBB anterior division	X	
LBB posterior division		X

X = Most likely supplied by.

Summary of LCA Distribution

- Septal wall of the left ventricle
- Anterior wall of the left ventricle
- Lateral wall of the left ventricle

Anterior Wall Myocardial Infarction

Occlusion of the left anterior descending artery will cause ST segment elevation and eventually Q waves in the anterior leads V_1 through V_4. Reciprocal ST depression occurs in leads II, III, and aVF. In addition, the septum is flanked by the left and right bundle branches. These branches are often affected by anteroseptal wall infarction and conduction disturbances, such as second-degree type II block and complete heart block, may occur. Patients with complete heart block are at risk for profound bradycardia because the escape ventricular pacemaker is often slow and unreliable. Furthermore, higher degrees of block are usually associated with large infarctions and carry a grave prognosis. Immediate (transcutaneous) pacing is indicated for symptomatic patients (i.e., hypotension, chest pain, dyspnea, etc.) with anterior wall myocardial infarction, whereas standby pacing is warranted for asymptomatic patients and those with new onset bundle branch block (especially RBBB) (see Chapter 9). An excessive sympathetic response (e.g., tachycardia), pump failure, and cardiogenic shock may also occur if the infarct is extensive.

Inferior Wall Myocardial Infarction

Right coronary artery occlusions are the most common cause of inferior wall infarctions. Indicative ECG changes will be seen in leads II, III, and aVF, with reciprocal changes in leads I and aVL. The right coronary artery also supplies the AV node, so AV nodal heart blocks are often associated with this type of infarct. AV blocks occurring as a result of inferior infarction are typically of lower grade (e.g., first-degree and second-degree type I), and are associated with excessive vagal tone characterized by bradycardia and hypotension that is usually responsive to atropine and fluid therapy (see Chapter 9). Furthermore, considering the right ventricle is also supplied by the right coronary artery, the presence of inferior wall infarction should cause the examiner to rule out concomitant right ventricular infarction using the right-sided chest leads (especially V_4R).

Lateral Wall Myocardial Infarction

Occlusion of the circumflex artery is most often associated with lateral wall infarction. Indicative ECG changes are identified in leads I, aVL, V_5, and V_6. In a small minority of patients (10%), the circumflex artery extends to the posterior descending artery and feeds the inferior wall of the left ventricle. A patient with indicative changes in the lateral (I, aVL, V_5, V_6) and inferior (II, III, aVF) leads should be suspected of being left dominant.

Posterior Wall Myocardial Infarction

Posterior wall infarctions are most commonly extensions of either inferior or lateral infarcts; rarely do they occur as an isolated event. Since the standard 12-lead ECG does not include a direct view of the posterior wall, reciprocal changes must be evaluated in leads V_1 and V_2. The ST elevation of acute posterior infarction will present itself in leads V_1 and V_2 as ST depression, and the Q wave as an enlargement of the typical small r in V_1 and V_2. These changes are subtle and are usually difficult to separate from other causes.

TABLE 8–6 • **Complications of Acute Myocardial Infarction**

DYSRHYTHMIAS
Sudden death (ventricular fibrillation)
Sinus bradycardia (inferior wall MI)
Tachydysrhythmias

CONDUCTION DISTURBANCES
First-degree AV block (inferior wall MI)
Mobitz I (inferior wall MI)
Mobitz II (anterior wall MI)
Complete (third-degree) heart block (anterior wall MI)

PUMP FAILURE
Left ventricular failure and pulmonary edema
Right ventricular failure and hypotension
Cardiogenic shock

They are best viewed over a series of tracings, and if one is so inclined, the use of leads V_8 (left midscapular line) and V_9 (left paraspinal border) are probably better suited for emergency identification of posterior infarction.

COMPLICATIONS OF INFARCTION

Any number of complications may present during the course of myocardial infarction (Table 8–6). Some of these complications are more likely to occur early in the infarct process (e.g., ventricular fibrillation), while others are specific to the site of infarction (e.g., atrioventricular blocks). The number and severity of postinfarction complications depends on the location and extent of necrosis, the patient's physical condition prior to infarction, and the availability of swift therapeutic intervention (i.e., thrombolytic therapy). Common complications of acute myocardial infarction include dysrhythmias, conduction disturbances, and some form of left ventricular pump dysfunction. In addition, hypotension and reduced cardiac output often occur as a result of right ventricular infarction accompanying inferior wall MIs.

Dysrhythmias

Dysrhythmias are the most common complication of acute myocardial infarction, affecting 90% of individuals. The out-of-hospital mortality in AMI is almost entirely due to dysrhythmias. In fact, the incidence of lethal dysrhythmias is greatest in the prehospital setting, making early detection and treatment by EMS personnel paramount to a more favorable outcome. Dysrhythmias can be caused by ischemia, autonomic nervous system imbalance, lactic acidosis, electrolyte abnormalities, and a host of other disorders. Dysrhythmias may originate from the atria, ventricles, nodal region, or conductive tissue, and may be rapid or slow depending on their site of origin or pathological mechanism. The seriousness of dysrhythmias depends on their hemodynamic consequences. For example, tachydysrhythmias (such as PSVT) have a profound effect on heart rate and may further exacerbate the imbalance between myocardial oxygen supply and demand while reducing cardiac output. As a result, tachydysrhythmias usually require immediate suppression. On the other hand, those dysrhythmias that do not significantly alter heart rate or ventricular contraction are usually well tolerated and require no treatment.

Conduction Disturbances

Damage to the conduction system as a result of acute myocardial infarction often favors the development of atrioventricular blocks. These blocks range from first degree to third degree, and as previously discussed, are generally dependent upon the location of the infarct. First-degree atrioventricular block and Mobitz I (Wenckebach) are usually due to increased vagal tone impairing (slowing) AV nodal conduction and are frequently seen with inferior wall myocardial infarction. Progression to complete heart block rarely occurs, but if it does, a stable infranodal (below the AV node) pacemaker with narrow QRS complexes and a reasonable rate is usually maintained.

Mobitz II second-degree atrioventricular block and complete heart block are usually due to structural damage to the infranodal conduction tissue and are generally seen with anterior wall myocardial infarction. Mobitz II and complete heart blocks may occur suddenly, with only a slow, unstable ventricular escape rhythm available for cardiac activity. Both rhythms are an indication for prophylactic pacemaker placement and eventual treatment. Infarctions which cause these dysrhythmias are usually large, and even with pacemaker treatment many patients die of pump failure.

Left Ventricular Pump Failure and Cardiogenic Shock

Acute myocardial infarction is usually accompanied by some degree of left ventricular failure (congestive heart failure), which is characterized by pulmonary congestion and reduced myocardial contractility. Mortality from acute infarction and subsequent left ventricular failure is directly related to a reduction in stroke volume caused by the infarcted ventricle. If cardiac output is insufficient to maintain normal arterial blood pressure and/or to perfuse vital organs, cardiogenic shock develops. Cardiogenic shock characteristically develops if 40% or more of the left ventricular myocardium is infarcted. It may be fatal at the time of the infarct, or may cause death or disability days or weeks later.

Right Ventricular Infarction and Hypotension

As you recall from Chapter 6, right ventricular infarctions complicate inferior wall infarctions in up to 40% of cases. Right ventricular infarction is due to proximal right coronary artery obstruction, nearly always transmural, and almost always associated with left ventricular damage. Its presence is quite significant because it not only indicates a larger infarction, but also signifies that infarction involves both ventricles. Recognition of right ventricular infarction is important because patients are at great risk for hypotension and decreased cardiac output. In order to recognize and properly manage right ventricular infarction, we will review both its ECG and clinical manifestations.

As discussed in Chapter 4, electrocardiographic evidence of right ventricular infarction is obtained with the use of right-sided chest leads (V_3R through V_6R). These leads are applied to the right side of the chest in the same anatomical position as their left-sided counterparts (see Figure 4–12). Leads V_3R through V_6R look directly at the right ventricle, and if infarction is present, will demonstrate ST segment elevation. In the field, the sole use of V_4R is all that is necessary to evaluate the right ventricle. Research has shown that V_4R is by far the most sensitive and specific indicator of right ventricular infarction (Figure 8–5). To obtain V_4R, detach the lead wire from V_4 (left side of chest) and reconnect it to an additional electrode applied to the right side of the chest at the fifth intercostal space midclavicular line. The ECG is again recorded and the right ventricle can now be observed.

Clinical evidence of right ventricular infarction includes a triad of hypotension, jugular venous distention, and clear (dry) lungs. The presence and significance of these

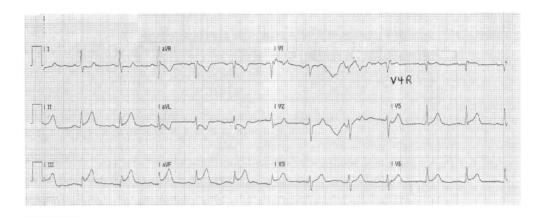

Figure 8–5.
A 12-lead ECG recording of an acute inferior wall myocardial infarction with the simultaneous presence of a right ventricular infarction.
Note the ST segment elevation in leads II, III, and aVF (inferior leads) and V_4R (right ventricular lead).

findings are based on the degree of damage created by the infarction. Recall from Chapter 2 that the function of the right ventricle is to pump blood to the lungs for oxygenation. Once oxygenated, the blood is delivered to the left atrium. From the left atrium, blood fills the left ventricle and is forcefully ejected into the systemic circulation. In the setting of right ventricular infarction, the right ventricle loses its ability to effectively pump blood into the pulmonary circuit. As a result, right atrial pressure rises and venous return exceeds the ventricular output (manifested by jugular venous distention). Hypotension occurs as the amount of blood entering the lungs and left ventricle is reduced. Remember, the left ventricle can only pump as much blood as it receives, and if less blood enters the ventricle, both stroke volume and cardiac output are decreased. Finally, because the left atrial pressure is normal or slightly decreased (less blood volume entering the left heart) in right ventricular infarction, blood does not back up from the left ventricle into the lungs. Therefore, pulmonary edema does not occur and the lungs remain clear.

Treatment of right ventricular infarction involves elevating the right ventricular filling pressure in an attempt to maintain cardiac output. Both judicious fluid therapy and/or the use of inotropic agents, such as dopamine or dobutamine, are effective strategies. Volume infusions of lactated ringers or normal saline are delivered in increments of 200 to 500 cc, followed by the evaluation of breath sounds (for crackles) and blood pressure. If the hypotension is not completely corrected with fluid therapy or the risk of pulmonary edema exists, an inotrope is then necessary. Furthermore, because patients with right ventricular infarction are preload dependent, the use of nitrates and morphine (preload reducers) should be administered with extreme caution or avoided altogether. The reader is encouraged to review Table 8–7 for a complete summary of right ventricular infarction.

EVALUATION AND DIAGNOSIS OF ACUTE MYOCARDIAL INFARCTION

Distinguishing acute myocardial infarction from other disease processes in the prehospital environment is often a difficult and challenging process. Because timely diagnosis and therapy are crucial to achieving a more favorable outcome, it is essential that the

TABLE 8–7 • **Right Ventricular Infarction**

- Etiology: Results from proximal right coronary artery occlusion
- Incidence: Occurs in combination with inferior wall myocardial infarction in up to 40% of all cases
- Reflecting leads: V_3R through V_6R (V_4R is best suited for prehospital use)
- Clinical symptoms: Hypotension, jugular venous distention, clear lung sounds
- Complications: Hypotension and decreased cardiac output
- Treatment: Fluid challenge (200 to 500 cc) and/or an inotrope (dopamine/dobutamine)

paramedic be familiar with not only electrocardiographic evidence of infarction, but also its clinical symptoms. The diagnosis of acute myocardial infarction is made primarily on the basis of typical complaints (e.g., chest pain, dyspnea, syncope, etc.), with the ECG lending confirmation to these findings.

Clinical Symptoms of Infarction

Although some individuals do not demonstrate any obvious signs of acute myocardial infarction (e.g., silent MI in the elderly or diabetic patient), significant clinical features usually occur. The majority of infarcts can be determined simply by the recognition of unrelieved ischemic chest pain (anginal pain), lasting longer than 15 to 30 minutes.

As with angina, the chest discomfort associated with myocardial infarction is typically described as pressure, tightness, heaviness or fullness, usually midline, behind the sternum, and often radiates to the arm(s), jaw, or epigastrium (refer to Table 8–3). Diagnostically, if ischemic chest pain subsides in short order with rest or nitroglycerin, the chance of infarction is not as likely. However, if the pain does not resolve with rest or nitroglycerin, then acute myocardial infarction should be strongly suspected even with a normal electrocardiogram. Remember that indicative electrocardiographic changes may not occur for hours following the infarct, and in some cases never develop. Therefore, *Do not use the ECG to rule out myocardial infarction.* Other symptoms associated with myocardial infarction are usually due to autonomic nervous system imbalances or result from complications of infarction, such as pump failure and dysrhythmias. Table 8–8 lists some of the more common subjective and objective findings accompanying acute myocardial infarction.

Role of Electrocardiogram

The electrocardiogram is an objective component of the physical examination. It should *not* be relied upon as the sole determinant for the diagnosis of acute myocardial infarction, and should *never* be used to rule out infarction. Patients presenting with physical and historical indications of acute myocardial infarction should be treated as potentially infarcting, even when the ECG appears normal. Conversely, if a patient presents atypically or his/her symptoms do not outwardly appear to be of cardiac origin, but the ECG demonstrates evidence of infarction, AMI protocol (i.e., oxygen, IV access, pulse oximetry, etc.) should be initiated until further study provides a more definitive diagnosis. It is more prudent, especially in the prehospital phase, to err on the side of treatment rather than to allow the patient with cardiac chest pain to go untreated. The electrocardiogram is a useful tool, but should not replace the history and physical exam in the diagnosis and treatment of ischemic heart disease.

TABLE 8-8 • **Symptoms of Acute Myocardial Infarction**

CARDIAC SYMPTOMS
- Palpitations
- Abnormal heart sounds (S_3 and S_4)
- Cardiac murmurs (papillary muscle dysfunction)
- Irregular pulses
- Dysrhythmias
- Hypotension
- Jugular venous distention
- Dependent edema

RESPIRATORY SYMPTOMS
- Dyspnea
- Cough (pink sputum)
- Crackles (rales)
- Use of accessory muscles of respiration

CENTRAL NERVOUS SYSTEM SYMPTOMS
- Syncope
- Confusion
- Irritability

GASTROINTESTINAL SYMPTOMS
- Nausea
- Vomiting
- Abdominal cramping

INTEGUMENTARY SYMPTOMS
- Pallor
- Cool and clammy
- Diaphoresis

DIFFERENTIAL DIAGNOSIS OF CHEST PAIN

Not all chest pain results from ischemic heart disease. A number of conditions can mimic ischemic heart disease, and must be considered in order to provide appropriate care and avoid catastrophes. Some of these conditions present with signs and symptoms similar to that of acute myocardial infarction, but lack the specific ECG findings. Others mimic both the exam and the ECG, making the diagnosis extremely difficult. A careful history and physical exam, coupled with a 12-lead ECG, will usually clarify the distinction between infarction and other various mimicking conditions. We have selected a number of the more common imitators of ischemic chest pain; however, this list is not complete (Table 8-9).

Pericarditis

As you recall from Chapter 7, pericarditis is inflammation of the fluid-filled pericardial sac surrounding the heart. Although frequently idiopathic, pericarditis is also caused by infection, connective tissue disease, or neoplasm. With disease or infection, inflammation of the pericardial membranes causes fluid to accumulate in the interstitial space. If left untreated, compression of the heart due to excessive fluid accumulation occurs and diastolic filling is impaired, reducing stroke volume and cardiac output.

TABLE 8–9 • **Conditions Mimicking Myocardial Infarction**
Pericarditis
Aortic dissection
Pulmonary embolism
Boerhaave's syndrome
Pneumothorax
Musculoskeletal pain
Gastrointestinal/abdominal distress

Symptoms of pericarditis include a sudden onset of sharp (pleuritic) chest pain that worsens with respiration, cough, or changes in position. Although the pain may radiate to the back, it is generally felt in the anterior chest and may certainly be confused initially with the pain of acute myocardial infarction. The chest pain, however, is frequently lessened when the individual sits up and leans forward.

Physical examination often discloses low-grade fever and sinus tachycardia. Friction rub, a short, scratchy, grating sensation similar to the sound of sandpaper, may be heard at the cardiac apex (fifth intercostal space) and left sternal border. The sound is caused by roughened pericardial membranes rubbing against each other and may be intermittently heard and transient. In addition, electrocardiographic changes usually reflect the inflammatory process through diffuse ST segment elevation without pathological Q waves.

Aortic Dissection

Long-standing hypertension is the most common factor predisposing patients to dissection of the aorta. The dissection process begins as a tear in the aortic intima, allowing blood to seep between the other aortic layers. About 50% of aortic aneurysms are in the ascending aorta, 30% occur in the arch, and 20% in the descending aorta. The dissections may extend proximally, distally, or both, and the specific signs will vary depending on the site of the aneurysm.

The chest pain associated with aortic aneurysms is ripping or tearing in nature, is often most severe at its onset, and usually radiates or migrates to the back or abdomen. Radial and carotid pulses may be unequal, and the lower extremities may be pulseless and/or paralyzed. A marked difference in systolic blood pressure (> 20 mmHg) between arms is often reflective of aortic dissection. Unfortunately, the ECG is not a useful or reliable tool for diagnosing aortic aneurysms, so one must rely exclusively on historical and physical examination findings. In addition, infarct and/or tamponade may occur concurrently and further complicate the clinical picture.

Pulmonary Embolism

Obstruction of the pulmonary arteries by a blood clot causes chest pain and ECG changes that may mimic acute myocardial infarction. Approximately 90% of the emboli reaching the pulmonary arteries originate in the popliteal or ileofemoral veins and are the result of deep vein thrombophlebitis (DVT). Any condition that gives way to prolonged immobility and subsequent venous stasis places an individual at risk for DVT. Other sites and causes of pulmonary emboli include mural emboli from the right heart, fat from damaged bone and tissue, and amniotic fluid.

The clinical presentation of pulmonary emboli is greatly dependent on the site(s) of occlusion, the preexisting condition of the lungs and heart, and the patient's general physical condition. Dyspnea and unilateral pleuritic chest pain are the most common subjective complaints, whereas tachypnea, tachycardia, hemoptysis, petechiae over the thorax and upper arms, cyanosis, and shock are common objective findings. Crackles and/or a pleural friction rub may also be present. Changes in consciousness, anxiety, and a sense of impending doom often occur with massive pulmonary emboli.

The ECG signs of pulmonary emboli are not always diagnostic and are often obscured by prior cardiac disease. Certain changes on the ECG, however, may raise suspicion, allowing the diagnosis via an emergency echocardiogram (a noninvasive technique that uses ultrasound to visualize internal cardiac structures). If the acute phase of a pulmonary emboli is recognized and promptly treated, death can be prevented in an estimated 75% of patients who otherwise would have died. The following describes the ECG changes in acute pulmonary embolism:

- Right axis deviation
- Right bundle branch block pattern (may be incomplete)
- Q waves in III, aVF, and V_1
- S waves in I and aVL
- ST elevation in leads III, aVR, and V_1
- Dysrhythmias: sinus tachycardia, atrial flutter, and atrial fibrillation

Boerhaave's Syndrome

Esophageal perforation secondary to forceful vomiting is known as Boerhaave's syndrome. Because the esophagus has no serosal covering, esophageal perforations provide direct entry of contaminated and caustic esophageal contents into the mediastinum. More than 80% of these cases involve middle-age males following excessive intake of food or alcohol. Since chest pain is a nearly universal symptom of this condition, it is often misdiagnosed as acute myocardial infarction.

Pain from Boerhaave's syndrome is often localized in the epigastrium and substernal area of the back. The pain typically worsens with time and tends to migrate from the abdomen to the chest. Unfortunately, this description is not unlike that of acute myocardial infarction. A history of forceful emesis prior to the onset of chest discomfort may suggest esophageal rupture, but is either not present or not clearly described in over half of the cases. Signs and symptoms that differentiate Boerhaave's syndrome from acute myocardial infarction include subcutaneous emphysema (usually found at the root of the neck), a nasal quality in the patient's voice, or the presence of a systolic "crunch" that can be auscultated as air surrounds the heart (Hammond's crunch). If undiagnosed and untreated, cardiopulmonary collapse, sepsis with fever, and signs of hypoxia will occur. The ECG plays no specific role in the diagnosis of esophageal rupture.

Pneumothorax

Pneumothorax occurs when air accumulates in the pleural space compressing the lung beneath it. Pneumothorax may be the result of injury, rupture of a bleb or superficial lung abscess (commonly seen in COPD), or occur spontaneously. Rarely, is this condition confused with myocardial infarction because trauma to the chest is the most common etiology. Classic physical findings of pneumothorax include unilateral pleuritic chest pain, increasing dyspnea, and unilateral diminished or absent-breath sounds. Careful auscultation can reveal early, small pneumothoracies when breath sounds are absent or diminished above the clavicle on the affected side. Aside from sinus tachycardia, no significant ECG changes appear with pneumothorax.

Musculoskeletal Pain

Costochondritis, muscle strains, rib fractures, and other musculoskeletal thoracic problems are differentiated from acute myocardial infarction by careful history (especially prodrome) and physical exam. Pain that is reproducible or increases on palpation or movement, such as twisting of the trunk or leaning forward, is rarely of cardiac origin.

Gastrointestinal/Abdominal Distress

A virtually endless list of gastrointestinal disorders can cause pain similar to that of acute myocardial infarction. Typically, gastrointestinal distress involves subdiaphragmatic organs such as the gallbladder, pancreas, and stomach. Often there is a history of the pain occurring for days to months to years. Fortunately, no true ECG changes occur with gastrointestinal or abdominal problems. Careful history and examination usually reveal specific gastrointestinal symptoms (e.g., coffee-ground emesis, bloody stools, etc.), and/or a tender bloated or rigid abdomen. It should be noted, however, that a normal ECG in the presence of gastrointestinal symptoms does not rule out acute myocardial infarction. Many cases of gas or stomachache turn out to be myocardial infarction.

KEY POINTS SUMMARY

Coronary Artery Disease (Atherosclerosis)

1. Coronary atherosclerosis is a degenerative disease process characterized by the progressive narrowing of the lumen of coronary arteries. It results from the accumulation of fatty deposits, platelets, WBCs, and cell debris throughout the innermost and smooth muscle layer of the artery. As a result, the diseased coronary vessel is unable to transport adequate blood volume to the area of heart muscle it supplies.

Risk Factors of Coronary Artery Disease

2. Research has identified seven major (modifiable and nonmodifiable) risk factors that contribute to the development of coronary artery disease. These include cigarette smoking, hypertension, hypercholesterolemia, advanced age, male gender, genetic predisposition (heredity), and diabetes.

Clinical Manifestations of Myocardial Ischemia

3. Myocardial ischemia encompasses a variety of clinical syndromes. Ischemic heart disease ranges from silent ischemia through the various patterns of angina and acute myocardial infarction.

Angina Pectoris

4. Angina pectoris describes the chest pain originating from the heart that occurs in response to an imbalance between myocardial oxygen supply and demand. The chest discomfort of angina is experienced as retrosternal heaviness or pressure, and often radiates to the neck, jaw, left arm or shoulder, and epigastrium. Other symptoms such as lightheadedness, nausea, palpitations, and pallor may also accompany the discomfort.

Stable Angina (Exertional Angina)

5. Mechanism: Stable angina occurs during physical activity or emotional stress. It is due to narrowing of the coronary arteries to the point that they adequately perfuse the heart at rest, but lack the required flow to meet the exertional needs of the myocardium. The discomfort of stable angina is usually short lived.

6. ECG criteria: ST segment depression and/or T wave inversion as a result of subendocardial ischemia.

Unstable Angina (Preinfarction Angina)

7. Mechanism: Unstable angina represents a clinical state beyond that of stable angina. It is characterized by an increase in the frequency, duration, and intensity of chest discomfort.
8. ECG criteria: ST segment depression and/or T wave inversion as a result of subendocardial ischemia.

Prinzmetal's Angina (Vasospastic Angina)

9. Mechanism: Prinzmetal's angina is an ischemic myocardial condition resulting from coronary artery spasm. The chest discomfort occurs primarily at rest and without provocation.
10. ECG criteria: ST segment elevation as a result of transmural ischemia mimicking the pattern of infarction.

Myocardial Infarction

11. Mechanism: Myocardial infarction occurs when blood flow to the myocardium is abruptly decreased and irreversible cell damage ensues. The underlying pathogenesis in almost all cases is acute coronary thrombosis.
12. ECG criteria: ST segment elevation and development of pathological Q waves.

Localization and Clinical Patterns of Infarction

13. Anterior wall myocardial infarction
    - Reflecting leads: V_1 through V_4
    - Complications: High-degree heart blocks (Mobitz II and third degree) and cardiogenic shock
    - Treatment: Immediate transcutaneous pacing for the symptomatic patient and standby pacing for the asymptomatic patient
14. Inferior wall myocardial infarction
    - Reflecting leads: II, III, aVF
    - Complications: AV nodal blocks (first degree and Mobitz I) and concomitant right ventricular infarction
    - Treatment: Atropine and pacing for symptomatic bradycardia and volume challenge for right ventricular infarction

Complications of Infarction

15. Common complications of infarction include dysrhythmias, conduction disturbances, and left ventricular pump failure.
16. Dysrhythmias are the most common complication of AMI. They can originate anywhere in the atria, ventricles, or conduction system, and may be rapid or slow depending on their site of origin.
17. Conduction disturbances are usually in the form of atrioventricular blocks that occur as a result of infarction. These blocks range from first degree to complete heart block.
18. Left ventricular pump failure almost always accompanies AMI and is characterized by pulmonary congestion and reduced myocardial contractility.

Evaluation and Diagnosis of Acute Myocardial Infarction

19. Diagnosis of acute myocardial infarction is made primarily on the basis of historical findings, with the physical exam and ECG lending confirmation to the diagnosis. It is essential to remember that the ECG should never be relied upon as the sole indicator for the diagnosis of infarction. *A normal ECG does not exclude the diagnosis of acute myocardial infarction.*

Differential Diagnosis of Chest Pain

20. Not all chest pain results from myocardial ischemia and infarction. The differential diagnosis of chest pain must take into account an extensive list of nonischemic causes of discomfort that may mimic infarction both electrically and clinically. Some of the more common imitators of infarction include pericarditis, aortic dissection, pulmonary emboli, Boerhaave's syndrome, pneumothorax, musculoskeletal pain, and gastrointestinal distress.

BIBLIOGRAPHY

Bledsoe BE, Porter RS, Shade BR. *Paramedic Emergency Care.* Englewood Cliffs, NJ: Prentice-Hall Inc; 1994.

Bresler MJ, Gilber WB. Acute myocardial infarction: Subtleties of diagnosis in the emergency department. *Annals of Emergency Medicine.* 1990;19(suppl.):1–15.

Caroline NL. *Emergency Care in the Streets.* Boston, MA: Little, Brown and Company; 1995.

Conover MB. *Understanding Electrocardiography: Arrhythmias and the 12-lead ECG.* St. Louis, MO: Mosby; 1992.

Copstead LE. *Perspectives on Pathophysiology.* Philadelphia, PA: JB Lippincott; 1996.

Foster DB. 12-Lead Electrocardiography for the ACLS Provider. Philadelphia, PA: WB Saunders; 1996.

Hagley MT. Emergency intervention for acute myocardial infarction: Thrombolytic agents and adjuvant therapy. *Emergency Medical Reports.* 1993;14:9–15.

Huszar RJ. *Basic Dysrhythmias: Interpretation and Management.* St. Louis, MO: Mosby; 1994.

Johnson R, Swartz MH. *A Simplified Approach to Electrocardiography.* Philadelphia, PA: WB Saunders; 1986.

Lipman BC, Casio T. *ECG: Assessment and Interpretation.* Philadelphia, PA: FA Davis Company; 1994.

Marriot HJ. *Practical Electrocardiography.* 8th ed. Baltimore, MD: Williams & Wilkins; 1988.

Martini FH. *Fundamentals of Anatomy and Physiology.* 3rd ed. Englewood Cliffs, NJ: Prentice-Hall, Inc.; 1995.

Price SA, Wilson LM. *Clinical Concepts of Disease Processes.* 4th ed. St. Louis, MO: Mosby; 1992.

Sanders MJ. *Mosby's Paramedic Textbook.* St. Louis, MO: Mosby; 1994.

Thaler MS. The Only EKG Book *You'll Ever Need.* Philadelphia, PA: JB Lippincott; 1988.

Tortora GJ, Grabowski S. *Principles of Anatomy and Physiology.* New York, NY: Harper Collins; 1996.

9

Prehospital Evaluation and Therapy for Acute Myocardial Ischemia and Infarction

LEARNING OBJECTIVES

1. Discuss the pathophysiology of myocardial ischemia and infarction.

2. Explain the relationship between myocardial oxygen supply and demand.

3. Describe the pathological origin of ischemic chest pain.

4. Discuss the evaluation of acute chest pain and list six conditions other than myocardial ischemia that can imitate infarction.

5. List and describe the most common characteristics of ischemic chest pain.

6. Describe the role of the physical exam for the diagnosis of myocardial ischemia.

7. Describe the ECG criteria diagnostic of myocardial ischemia/infarction and explain the limitations of the electrocardiogram.

8. Describe appropriate history and physical assessment goals for the infarcted patient.

9. Describe the out-of-hospital therapy for acute myocardial infarction.

10. Describe the pathophysiology and management for the following special patient conditions: significant bradycardia, hypotensive and hypoperfusing, left ventricular failure, and tachydysrhythmias in the setting of acute myocardial ischemia.

11. Discuss the role of volume resuscitation for the infarcted patient.

12. Describe the mechanism of action, indications, contraindications, dosages, and precautions for the following cardiovascular medications: oxygen, aspirin, nitroglycerin, morphine, nalbuphine, lidocaine, bretylium, procainamide, adenosine, atropine, verapamil, diltiazem, epinephrine, dopamine, dobutamine, norepinephrine, isoproterenol, metoprolol, esmolol, propranolol, nifedipine, nitroprusside, furosemide, magnesium, and thrombolytic therapy.

13. Describe the indications, technique, and application for external cardiac pacing.

INTRODUCTION

Coronary artery disease causes one-third to one-half of all deaths in patients age 36 to 64 years old in the United States. Each year, approximately 1.7 million patients nationwide are admitted to cardiac and other intensive care units for episodes suspected to represent acute ischemic heart disease. Far more patients yearly are evaluated in the prehospital setting, complaining of acute chest pain. Yet the evaluation of these patients is not precise. For example, up to 13% of middle-aged men have significant coronary artery disease, much of it unrecognized. Many patients with known coronary artery disease remain clinically asymptomatic until infarction or sudden death prompts their first medical evaluation. The complexity of the evaluation of chest discomfort and other symptoms suspicious for myocardial ischemia or infarction is amplified in the prehospital setting. Decision making prior to hospital arrival requires reliance on a limited and unpredictable amount of historical and physical examination findings. A careful consideration of the various presentations consistent with myocardial ischemia and infarction is necessary to assure early and optimal management of these patients. To that end the pathophysiology of myocardial ischemia and infarction along with the appropriate clinical signs and symptoms will be reviewed, followed by a discussion of the appropriate therapeutic interventions.

PATHOPHYSIOLOGY OF MYOCARDIAL ISCHEMIA AND INFARCTION

Cardiac ischemia develops when there is an imbalance such that myocardial oxygen supply is inadequate for the heart's metabolic demand. Myocardial infarction occurs when ischemia is prolonged and severe enough to lead to irreparable damage to heart cell structural integrity. Thus, the treatment of myocardial ischemia and infarction is tightly correlated, especially in the prehospital setting where it is often impossible to discern whether the ischemia has progressed to the point that cell death has occurred. Myocardial infarction is not an all-or-none condition, but rather a progressive, dynamic disease process. A short period of severe cardiac ischemia may damage only a few cells, while prolonged coronary hypoperfusion (inadequate blood and oxygen delivery) may destroy all of the myocardial cells in the distribution of the involved coronary artery. Interruption of myocardial ischemia at the earliest moment is the best method to limit cardiac cellular damage.

Coronary Atherosclerosis

Coronary patency is under most circumstances the main determinant of myocardial oxygen supply, and disorders that affect coronary patency are the main inciting events for myocardial ischemia and infarction. The coronary arteries are subject to various disease processes over our lifetimes. The most important arterial disease process is atherosclerosis, which involves fatty tissue deposition along with subsequent scarring and calcification in the wall of the artery, narrowing the lumen. Atherosclerosis is a disease process which has several risk factors (Table 9–1), and represents the primary problem predisposing individuals to myocardial ischemia today. On top of these fixed atherosclerotic lesions, the coronary arteries, like other arteries in the body, have the ability to dilate and contract in response to various stimuli. Vasoconstriction of the coronary arteries decreases blood flow and if this occurs in an atherosclerotic vessel with a fixed lesion, this may lead to significant myocardial ischemia.

TABLE 9–1 • **Risk Factors for Atherosclerosis**

MODIFIABLE RISKS

Tobacco use
Hypertension
Elevated cholesterol
Lack of exercise
Obesity

NONMODIFIABLE RISKS

Diabetes mellitus (good control reduces risk)
Advanced age
Male gender
Family history of heart disease and atherosclerosis

Myocardial Oxygen Supply and Demand

The heart extracts nearly 70% of the oxygen available in the coronary circulation under normal circumstances. Increased demand normally leads to coronary vasodilation and an increased supply. If a fixed lesion limits an increase in blood flow despite increased cardiac demand, this may precipitate myocardial ischemia. Increased myocardial demand with a limit to supply is the common mechanism of angina pectoris (see Chapter 8), which is usually resolved when demand is reduced by rest or medications. Unstable angina pectoris occurs when this pain pattern occurs more frequently, with less cardiac demand, or requires longer or more medications to resolve. There is sometimes difficulty distinguishing prolonged angina pectoris from myocardial infarction, and to a great extent they represent a continuum of disease process. Prinzmetal's angina or vasospastic angina is due to abnormal spasm of the coronary arteries leading to myocardial ischemia and resultant chest pain. This type of angina commonly occurs at rest and produces ECG changes characteristic of infarction. This form of angina, as well, is often difficult to distinguish from myocardial infarction in the prehospital environment.

Coronary Thrombosis

Most cases of prolonged myocardial ischemia and/or infarction are precipitated by a blood clot, or thrombus that forms on a predisposing atherosclerotic lesion. The cause of this thrombus is multifactorial, but usually occurs secondary to an atherosclerotic lesion already causing 75% or more stenosis (narrowing) of the coronary vessel. The most effective intervention for acute myocardial infarction to date is early thrombolytic therapy, which acts to dissolve the clot and partially reopen the occluded coronary vessel, restoring perfusion to the involved myocardial tissue. Optimally, this occurs prior to significant cell damage and death.

Origin of Ischemic Chest Pain

When myocardial oxygen demands exceed supply, changes are created in the myocardium which stimulate pain transmission in sympathetic nerves of the autonomic nervous system. The discomfort of myocardial ischemia is transmitted primarily via sympathetic nerves and ganglia (masses of nerve cell bodies) to the lower cervical as well as upper five thoracic roots of the spinal cord. These fibers eventually synapse (electrically connect) with the cerebral cortex. In addition, nerve fibers originating from the upper thorax and upper extremities, as well as visceral fibers from various internal chest structures, send information to the same cord levels. Unfortunately, the brain is not capable of recognizing where this message of pain originated, only at what level of the spinal cord it occurred. The cerebral cortex often misinterprets the origin of the pain and may thus register chest discomfort and pain radiation from any of the thoracic structures as indistinguishable from that resulting from myocardial ischemia. This is why ischemic chest pain is often referred to the arm, neck or jaw, or epigastric area, and also why chest pain is often difficult to recognize as clearly myocardial-related. In addition, aging and diseases which affect the autonomic nervous system (e.g., diabetes mellitus) may lead to minimal or no recognizable chest pain even in the setting of acute myocardial ischemia.

EVALUATION OF ACUTE CHEST PAIN

The evaluation of acute chest pain must take into account an extensive differential diagnosis list which includes many life-threatening clinical problems (Table 9–2). Consideration of such entities as pulmonary embolus, aortic dissection, pericarditis, pneumonia, and pneumothorax is important (see Chapter 8). In addition, various musculoskeletal and gastrointestinal diseases may present with symptoms and signs not unlike those of myocardial ischemia. The correct treatment requires making a reasonably precise diagnosis, as misdiagnosis may lead to disastrous consequences. For example, thrombolytic therapy for pericarditis or aortic dissection may rapidly lead to death.

Historical Description of Chest Pain

Conventional wisdom states that the historical description of chest pain by the patient is the most important feature in determining whether acute myocardial ischemia is present. Unfortunately, the description of chest discomfort is often misleading. In one important multicenter chest pain study, only 54% of those who described their chest discomfort as crushing, pressure, tightness, or heaviness had ongoing myocardial ischemia; 44% of those with complaints of burning or indigestion had acute ischemia; 22% of those with sharp or stabbing chest discomfort were having acute ischemia. Thus, the character of the pain is not always a reliable discriminator for acute myocardial ischemia. Additionally, it was recognized that substernal chest discomfort accompanied by pain in the neck, jaw, shoulder, or arm greatly increases the risk of myocardial infarction. Likewise, similar discomfort radiating to the right shoulder was found in patients with infarction. To make matters more complex, patients may either underrepresent or overrepresent their degree of chest discomfort and associated symptoms. Ultimately, complaints like nausea, shortness of breath, anxiety or apprehension, syncope, weakness, diaphoresis, and others do not exclusively distinguish myocardial ischemia or infarction from other disease processes. Thus, historical determination as to

TABLE 9–2 • **Differential Diagnosis List of Acute Chest Pain**

GENERAL CLASSIFICATION OF CHEST PAIN	SPECIFIC PATHOLOGIES
Cardiac	Myocardial infarction
	Angina pectoris
	Pericarditis
	Aortic dissection
Respiratory	Pulmonary emboli
	Pneumothorax
	Pneumonia
Gastrointestinal	Esophageal and abdominal disorders
Musculoskeletal	Spasms, strains, costalgia

the origin of chest pain is too imprecise to always be reliable, and used alone allows probability for misdiagnosis.

The Physical Exam

The physical examination rarely contributes to the diagnosis of acute myocardial ischemia. Those patients with acute ischemia have a slightly higher incidence of abnormal heart sounds, but not enough to be helpful and not commonly appreciated in the out-of-hospital setting. Similarly, although crackles on pulmonary exam are twice as common in acute myocardial ischemia as in nonischemic chest pain, the incidence is not high enough to be discriminatory. Furthermore, chest wall tenderness reproducing the patient's pain has been viewed as representing clear evidence of a musculoskeletal problem, but is frequently coincident in patients with ongoing myocardial ischemia.

Although historical and physical examination evidence of acute myocardial ischemia may be quite helpful when there are multiple positive findings, the majority of patients do not present with fully typical clinical features. In fact, atypical presentations in patients with acute myocardial infarction are frequent. Common features among patients with missed myocardial infarction include younger age and atypical complaints. Often these patients do not even receive serious consideration because the clinical evaluation does not suggest myocardial ischemia as a likely cause. In an era where widespread use of cocaine, amphetamines, and other substances of abuse may predispose younger people to myocardial ischemia and infarction, prehospital providers need to be particularly attentive.

Diagnostic ECG Evaluation of Myocardial Ischemia

The electrocardiogram is the most time-honored test for the evaluation of acute myocardial ischemia. It is used to screen chest pain patients with atypical presentations not clearly suggestive of ischemia, to evaluate nonischemic causes of chest pain (e.g., pericarditis), to stratify the risk of acute myocardial ischemia in patients with suggestive chest pain, and to evaluate therapeutic intervention options. New ST segment elevation (greater than 1 mm in two related limb leads or 2 mm in consecutive precordial leads) suggesting acute myocardial infarction in the appropriate clinical setting is the key parameter for initiating thrombolytic therapy. However, the initial ECG is diagnostic of infarction in only 25 to 50% of patients subsequently confirmed to have AMI. Not only do many patients have a totally normal ECG or nonspecific ST-T changes, but at least 10% have left bundle branch block, paced rhythm, or other findings making interpretation difficult. Furthermore, if chest pain resolves prior to obtaining an ECG, ischemic changes may have resolved.

Acquisition of a diagnostic electrocardiogram in the prehospital setting may help to optimize the early care of the infarcted patient. The 12-lead ECG has been demonstrated to improve diagnostic accuracy in recognizing myocardial ischemia and infarction when compared to single-lead telemetry. A quality tracing can be obtained in almost all patients in the prehospital environment. In addition, the prehospital 12-lead electrocardiogram can improve treatment, triage, and transport prioritization of chest pain patients. In conjunction with appropriate training and base-station physician support in rural areas with prolonged transport times, a prehospital 12-lead electrocardiogram will benefit a number of patients with obvious ECG criteria for thrombolytic therapy. Even with short transport times, a transmitted 12-lead ECG can alert the receiving hospital to ready the cardiac resuscitation team and prepare thrombolytic therapy for patients who meet criteria. This certainly has the potential to greatly decrease the door-to-drug time in certain clinical environments. The field use of the 12-lead electrocardiogram is rapidly becoming the standard of care for early detection of myocardial ischemia and infarction. EMS systems throughout the country will undoubtedly find utility in its use.

TREATMENT OF MYOCARDIAL ISCHEMIA AND INFARCTION

The therapy of myocardial ischemia and infarction involves improving myocardial oxygen supply in relation to demand, and preventing or treating complications. Appropriate prehospital intervention may mean the difference between life and death for these patients (Table 9–3). As always, airway, breathing, and circulation must be evaluated and determined to be adequate, or necessary interventions undertaken. Pulse oximetry units should be considered for all patients with acute chest pain suggestive of myocardial ischemia. Supplemental oxygen is necessary in all patients who are not already nearly 100% oxygen saturated on oximetric monitoring, and should always be used if monitoring is not available, preferably by high-flow mask. If ventilation is not adequate, respiration should be supported with a bag-valve mask using 100% oxygen. If endotracheal intubation is deemed necessary, it should preferably be done by the oral route, as nasotracheal intubation greatly increases the risk of epistaxis, which may complicate future thrombolytic therapy and sometimes prevent its use. Intravenous access should always be secured if possible, and two IV sites are necessary in these patients. Continuous cardiac monitoring is always important in this setting. A prompt hemodynamic evaluation of heart rate, blood pressure, and perfusion should next be accomplished. Patients with normal or high heart rate, normal or elevated blood pressure, and with adequate perfusion represent the ideal patients for therapeutic intervention.

Special Patient Considerations

The hypotensive, hypoperfusing patient needs attention to two particular details in the prehospital setting. First, in the setting of significant bradycardia, usually with rates less than 60 beats per minute, slow heart rate may in itself be responsible for decreased cardiac output and hypoperfusion. In that case, intervention to increase heart rate with atropine, atrioventricular (transcutaneous) pacing, or vasopressor agents such as epinephrine or dopamine may be necessary (Table 9–4). (*Remember that slow heart rates are not dangerous and do not require treatment unless there is hypotension or evidence of hypoperfusion.*) If hypotension occurs in the setting of suspected acute myocardial infarction and slow heart rate is not the problem, then aggressive intravenous volume challenge with isotonic crystalloid solutions such as lactated ringers or normal saline is appropriate. One important cause of acute hypoperfusion with apparent heart failure, but absent pulmonary congestion, is right ventricular infarction (see Chapters 6 and 8). Approximately one-third of patients with acute inferior wall infarction have right ventricular involvement, which leads to inadequate pulmonary perfusion and low left ventricular priming. They present with hypotension and other evidence of right-sided pump dysfunction. Right-sided chest leads, particularly V_4R, may provide further evi-

---

TABLE 9–3 • **Prehospital Management of Myocardial Infarction**

Ensure adequate airway, ventilation, and circulation
Administer oxygen and monitor delivery with pulse oximetry
Evaluate vital signs
Apply the cardiac monitor, identify, and treat any dysrhythmias
Establish intravenous access
Administer aspirin, nitroglycerin, and provide pain relief with narcotics (morphine)
Acquire a 12-lead ECG
Prescreen for thrombolytic therapy
Initiate a cardiac alert
Initiate thrombolytic agents (prehospital or emergency department)

TABLE 9–4 • **Symptomatic Bradycardia Intervention Sequence**
Atropine 0.5–1.0 mg IV
↓
Transcutaneous (external) pacing
↓
Dopamine 2–20 µg/kg/min IV infusion
↓
Epinephrine 2–10 µg/min IV infusion
↓
Isoproterenol 2–10 µg/min IV infusion

dence of right ventricular infarction. In this setting, massive volume infusion may be required to provide adequate preload to the left ventricle.

Left Ventricular Failure

Left ventricular pump failure occurs with a large infarction involving at least 25% of left ventricular muscle mass. Cardiogenic shock consists of the triad of hypotension, pulmonary congestion, and decreased peripheral perfusion. In the setting of acute myocardial infarction, approximately 40% of myocardial ventricular mass is damaged before cardiogenic shock ensues, and acute mortality is up to 80% in this group. Field treatment of cardiogenic shock begins with expeditious transport to the hospital and the administration of dopamine or dobutamine to improve left ventricular pump function.

Volume Resuscitation

Volume or fluid challenge is almost always indicated in the hypotensive, hypoperfusing patient without bradycardia and should only be withheld in the prehospital setting if severe pulmonary edema is present. Even in the setting of pulmonary edema, evidence of hypoperfusion may prompt a small aliquot fluid challenge of 200 to 500 cc, as any improvement in blood pressure may improve coronary perfusion and thus pump function. The fluid challenge may be indicated because the acute precipitating event may have caused pulmonary edema while depleting intravascular volume, and a small trial of isotonic fluid may improve preload and cardiac output. However, if volume challenge is ineffective, then contractile agents such as dopamine can be used. Improvement of cardiac pump function while minimizing myocardial oxygen requirements are the main interventions indicated with hypotension and concomitant pulmonary edema.

Tachyarrhythmias in the Setting of Acute Myocardial Ischemia

Tachyarrhythmias are also common in the setting of acute myocardial ischemia. If a 12-lead electrocardiogram is available, this is optional for deciding whether the tachycardia is wide-complex or narrow-complex (see Chapter 7). Wide-complex tachycardia in the setting of ongoing myocardial ischemia is assumed to be ventricular in origin and should be treated with rapid cardioversion, although lidocaine may be administered initially under certain circumstances (Table 9–5). Defibrillation is indicated for ventricular fibrillation, with the resuscitation protocol clearly established. Narrow-complex tachycardia may be secondary to a supraventricular tachydysrhythmia, and should be treated either with adenosine or prompt cardioversion (Table 9–6). If the rhythm is felt to be si-

TABLE 9–5 • **Prehospital Intervention Sequence of Wide-Complex Tachycardia of Ventricular Origin**	
STABLE PATIENT	**UNSTABLE PATIENT**
Lidocaine 1–1.5 mg/kg ↓ Lidocaine 0.5–0.75 mg/kg ↓ Procainamide 20–30 mg/min ↓ Bretylium 5–10 mg/kg ↓ Synchronized cardioversion	Synchronized cardioversion 100, 200, 300, 360 joules (Premedicate if possible) ↓ Lidocaine 1–1.5 mg/kg ↓ Procainamide 20–30 mg/min ↓ Bretylium 5–10 mg/kg

Unstable Patient Criteria: Chest pain, shortness of breath, decreased level of consciousness, hypotension, shock, pulmonary congestion, congestive heart failure, acute myocardial infarction

TABLE 9–6 • **Prehospital Intervention Sequence of Narrow Complex Tachycardia**

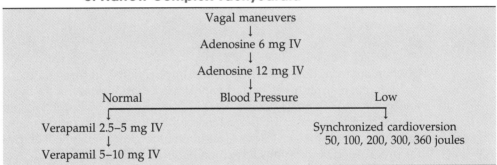

nus tachycardia, adequate volume resuscitation, pain relief, anxiety improvement, and sometimes beta blocker therapy may be appropriate.

SPECIFIC PHARMACOLOGIC AND ELECTRICAL INTERVENTIONS

Oxygen

Mechanism of Action and Therapeutic Implications. Oxygen delivery is an essential component of cardiac resuscitation and emergency cardiac care. It is required to enable body cells to break down glucose into a usable energy form. Oxygen is a colorless, odorless, tasteless gas, essential to respiration. The administration of oxygen elevates arterial oxygen tension (PaO_2), increasing hemoglobin saturation. This improves tissue oxygenation when circulation is adequately maintained.

Indications. Oxygen administration is used

• To treat all patients with acute chest pain that may be due to cardiac ischemia

- To treat hypoxemia from any etiology
- To treat cardiopulmonary arrest

Contraindications. None in the emergency setting.

Dosage. Several devices, including masks and nasal cannulas, can be used to administer oxygen to spontaneously breathing patients. Positive pressure ventilation devices (e.g., bag-valve mask) and volume regulated ventilators are used to deliver oxygen to nonbreathing (intubated) patients or to support respiration in the spontaneously breathing patient with poor exchange. Some of the more common oxygen devices and their delivery capacity include

- Nasal cannula: 24 to 40% at flow rates of 1 to 6 L/min
- Simple face mask: 40 to 60% at flow rates of 8 to 10 L/min
- Nonrebreathing face mask (oxygen reservoir): 60 to 100% at flow rates of 8 to 12 L/min

Precautions. Caution should be used when administering oxygen to patients with chronic obstructive pulmonary disease (e.g., pulmonary emphysema). Oxygen therapy may reduce the respiratory drive in these patients, and if this occurs it may be necessary to assist ventilation. However, if oxygen is indicated, it should never be withheld. Even 100% oxygen is not hazardous to the patient during the minutes required for clinical resuscitation.

Aspirin

Mechanism of Action and Therapeutic Implications. In the setting of acute myocardial infarction, aspirin has been demonstrated to reduce mortality by 21% in patients who presented within 24 hours of onset of symptoms. This reduction in mortality is increased to 39% when aspirin is combined with a thrombolytic agent. Aspirin therapy results in rapid antiplatelet effects, thus augmenting thrombolytic therapy by decreasing the progression of thrombus formation.

Indications. Accepted prehospital uses of aspirin include

- Suspected myocardial infarction
- Unstable angina pectoris

Contraindications. Do not administer aspirin to patients with

- Hypersensitivity to the drug (including asthma, COPD with known intolerance)
- Relatively contraindicated in patients with active ulcer disease

Dosage. 162 mg (two children's aspirin or one-half of an adult-sized tablet) should be administered to all patients with suspected myocardial ischemia.

Precautions. Caution should be used in patients with a history of ongoing gastrointestinal bleeding.

Nitroglycerin (Nitrostat, Nitrospray)

Mechanism of Action and Therapeutic Implications. Organic nitrates increase coronary blood flow by relaxing vascular smooth muscle. At low doses, nitrates appear to be preferential venodilators and thus are highly beneficial in decreasing blood return to the heart (preload). Nitrates rapidly reduce pulmonary pressure and provide effective improvement of pulmonary edema. At higher doses, nitrates dilate arterial resistance vessels and reduce systemic vascular resistance (afterload) for both ventricles, thus improving myocardial pump function while reducing oxygen consumption. Coronary artery vasodilation also improves myocardial oxygen supply, increasing perfusion to the ischemic myocardium (anti-anginal).

Indications. Accepted prehospital uses of nitroglycerin include

- Angina pectoris, both exertional and nonexertional angina (Prinzmetal's angina)
- Acute myocardial infarction
- Pulmonary edema

Contraindications. Do not administer nitroglycerin to patients with

- Hypersensitivity to the drug
- Increased intracranial pressure
- Hypotension
- Hypovolemia

Dosage. For prehospital use, nitroglycerin tablets of (0.3, 0.4, or 0.6 mg) or spray should be delivered sublingually every 3 to 5 minutes. Sublingual administration will have an onset or action within 2 minutes and lasts approximately 20 minutes. Intravenous nitroglycerin may be given by continuous infusion (initial 10 to 20 μg/minute, titrate to effect) with the advantage of improved titratability for optimal control in patients with ongoing myocardial ischemia or borderline perfusion. Alternatively, nitroglycerin ointment (12.5 mg/inch, 30 minute onset) may be given along with sublingual nitroglycerin in more stable patients.

Precautions. Prolonged nitrate therapy leads to drug tolerance which requires increasing the dosage. Headache is a common side effect of nitroglycerin, resulting from vasodilation of cerebral vessels. Hypotension appears to be the most common complication to nitrate therapy, and these agents should generally be avoided in the patient with a low blood pressure. If hypotension should occur, it is best initially treated by laying the patient down, elevating the legs, and administering isotonic fluids (lactated ringers or normal saline).

Opiates/Analgesics

Morphine Sulfate

Mechanism of Action and Therapeutic Implications. Morphine is a potent CNS depressant that possesses a number of hemodynamic properties that make it extremely useful in emergency medicine. This narcotic increases venous capacitance, pooling blood and decreasing blood return to the heart, thereby reducing pulmonary congestion. Morphine also decreases systemic vascular resistance, reducing myocardial workload. Furthermore, through reduced systemic cathecholamines, morphine decreases cardiac contractility and myocardial oxygen consumption.

Indications. Morphine is used to treat

- Pain and anxiety associated with acute myocardial infarction
- Cardiogenic pulmonary edema

Contraindications. Morphine should not be used in patients with

- Hypersensitivity to the drug
- Hypotension (systolic BP < 90) or volume depletion
- Respiratory depression not associated with pulmonary edema
- Head injury
- Undiagnosed abdominal pain

Dosage. Morphine is administered intravenously in slow repetitive 1 to 3 mg doses titrated to the desired analgesic or hemodynamic effect.

Precautions. Morphine must be used judiciously in patients with impaired respiratory drive, primarily in the severe COPD patient. Because morphine can induce sedation and hypoventilation, it is wise to have naloxone (Narcan), a narcotic antagonist, immediately available.

Nalbuphine (Nubain)

Mechanism of Action and Therapeutic Implications. This partial narcotic agonist-antagonist is equally effective in pain relief at equivalent doses when compared to morphine in the setting of ongoing myocardial ischemia. It produces an agonist effect by binding to opiate receptors in the central nervous system and produces partial antagonistic effects by competitive inhibition at these receptors. The hemodynamic properties of nalbuphine are less well understood and it is therefore an analgesic of second choice compared to morphine.

Indications. Moderate to severe pain.

Contraindications. Same as those of morphine or any narcotic.

Dosage. 5 to 10 mg intravenously. Repeat with 2 mg doses if needed

Precautions. Respiratory depression and hypotension may occur from the administration of nalbuphine. Narcan and isotonic fluids should be readily available to treat these potential complications.

Antiarrhythmics

Antiarrhythmic drugs are used in three clinical situations: (1) to terminate an acute arrhythmia, (2) to prevent arrhythmia recurrence, and (3) to prevent a life-threatening arrhythmia for which the patient is perceived to be at risk. All antiarrhythmic agents should be used with caution as they can exert proarrhythmic effects and potentially exacerbate underlying arrhythmias.

Lidocaine

Mechanism of Action and Therapeutic Implications. Lidocaine is a cell membrane anesthetic which suppresses ventricular arrhythmias. It works by decreasing the excessive spontaneous activity (automaticity) of ectopic pacemaker sites in the His-Purkinje fibers and ventricular tissue. In therapeutic doses, lidocaine has little effect on contractility, atrioventricular conduction, or blood pressure. Lidocaine is the antiarrhythmic of choice for the management of ventricular ectopy, ventricular tachycardia, and ventricular fibrillation.

Indications. Accepted indications for lidocaine use in the prehospital setting with ongoing myocardial ischemia/infarction include:

- Frequent premature ventricular contractions (> 6/min)
- Closely coupled premature ventricular contractions
- Multifocal premature ventricular contractions
- Runs of three or more premature ventricular contractions (short runs of ventricular tachycardia)
- Ventricular tachycardia
- Ventricular fibrillation

Contraindications. Do not administer lidocaine to patients with
- High-degree heart block
- Wolff-Parkinson-White syndrome
- Stokes-Adams syndrome (decreased level of consciousness due to inadequate cardiac output)

Dosage. Lidocaine is administered as a 1 to 1.5 mg/kg bolus followed by subsequent boluses of 0.5 to 0.75 mg/kg every 5 to 10 minutes until the arrhythmia is resolved or a total of 3 mg/kg is reached. The initial bolus should be reduced by 50% in patients 70 years of age or older. Lidocaine is always indicated after resuscitation from ventricular tachycardia or fibrillation. Maintenance infusions are given at 2 to 4 mg/minute and are commonly prepared as either 1 gm/250 cc or 2 gm/500 cc of D_5W.

Precautions. Lidocaine can in high doses worsen high-grade atrioventricular block, and may slow or extinguish ventricular escape rhythms. Central nervous system reactions such as decreased level of consciousness, irritability, confusion, and seizures are all well recognized complications of lidocaine administration.

Bretylium Tosylate (Bretylol)

Mechanism of Action and Therapeutic Implications. Bretylium is a compound with adrenergic (sympathetic) blocking effects and potent antiarrhythmic activity. It causes an initial transient increase in norepinephrine release from adrenergic nerve terminals, followed by long-term inhibition of adrenergic activity. Therefore, bretylium's first effect may result in hypertension, tachycardia, and possibly an increase in cardiac output, while its later effects are just the opposite. The cellular mechanism of bretylium's antiarrhythmic activity are not well understood. It is equally effective compared to lidocaine in the setting of ventricular fibrillation, but side effects relegate it in most clinical settings to a second line of therapy after lidocaine.

Indications. Bretylium is recommended in the treatment of ventricular tachycardia and fibrillation in the following situations

- When defibrillation, epinephrine, and lidocaine have failed to convert ventricular fibrillation
- When lidocaine and procainamide have failed to control ventricular tachycardia

Contraindications. None, when used for life-threatening arrhythmias.

Dosage. When used for ventricular fibrillation, the dose is 5 mg/kg intravenously repeated in 5 minutes at 10 mg/kg. After that, bretylium can be repeated twice at 5 to 30 minute intervals to a maximum dose of 35 mg/kg. Maintenance therapy is 1 to 2 mg/minute following the initial bolus therapy.

Precautions. Bretylium may cause gastrointestinal distress (vomiting) in the conscious patient and postural hypotension after resuscitation. It is relatively contraindicated in the patient thought to have digitalis toxicity.

Procainamide (Pronestyl)

Mechanism of Action and Therapeutic Implications. Procainamide is a type I antiarrhythmic drug. Like lidocaine, it suppresses the automaticity of ectopic pacemakers and slows conduction velocity through the bundle of His. Procainamide may be effective in a variety of both supraventricular and ventricular arrhythmias, but is rarely a drug of first choice due to the relatively prolonged time required to achieve therapeutic levels.

Indications. Accepted uses of procainamide include

- Premature ventricular contractions refractory to lidocaine
- Ventricular tachycardia refractory to lidocaine
- Wide-complex tachyarrhythmias of uncertain type
- Paroxysmal supraventricular tachycardia

Contraindications. Procainamide should be avoided in patients with severe conduction system disturbances (high-degree block), and in any patient with preexisting QT prolongation and torsades de pointes (polymorphic ventricular tachycardia).

Dosage. 20 to 30 mg/minute by intravenous infusion until

- The arrhythmia is suppressed
- Hypotension ensues
- The QRS complex widens by 50% of its original width
- A total dose of 17 mg/kg has been administered

Maintenance infusion of procainamide is 1 to 4 mg/minute, with this dose reduced in the setting of renal insufficiency of congestive heart failure.

Precautions. Use caution in administering procainamide to patients who may be experiencing myocardial infarction, digitalis toxicity, and renal failure. Hypotension is possible with a rapid infusion rate. Constant monitoring of the ECG and blood pressure is essential.

Adenosine (Adenocard)

Mechanism of Action and Therapeutic Implications. Adenosine is a naturally occurring substance present in all body cells. It is used to slow conduction and interrupt reentry pathways through the AV node. Adenosine causes a concentration-dependent slowing of atrioventricular conduction, but is essentially devoid of effects on ventricular contractility. It has proven to be highly effective for the intravenous treatment of narrow complex tachyarrhythmias (PSVT), with conversion rates in excess of 90%.

Indications. Adenosine is used to convert narrow-complex supraventricular tachycardias (including that associated with Wolff-Parkinson-White syndrome) refractory to vagal maneuvers. Adenosine is not an effective therapeutic agent for atrial fibrillation or flutter, but may allow better recognition of these arrhythmias by temporarily slowing rapid ventricular conduction.

Contraindications. Adenosine is contraindicated in patients experiencing second- or third-degree AV block, sick sinus syndrome, or those hypersensitive to the drug.

Dosage. The recommended initial dose of adenosine is 6 mg given as a rapid intravenous bolus over 1 to 3 seconds. Ideally, adenosine is pushed in a proximal vein followed by a fluid bolus to ensure rapid delivery to cardiac tissue. It has an onset of action of 5 to 20 seconds, but its duration of effect is less than one minute. If no effect is achieved within 2 minutes, a 12 mg bolus flushed rapidly into the vein may be attempted. If rhythm conversion is not attained, it should be reassessed and another therapeutic modality employed.

Precautions. Side effects related to adenosine are common, and include flushing, dyspnea, chest discomfort, dizziness, and headache, with hypotension a rare effect. Transient periods of sinus bradycardia and ventricular ectopy are common after termination of supraventricular tachycardia. Prolonged periods of asystole lasting 15 seconds or more have been reported. All symptoms resolve rapidly without treatment. Theophylline and other methylxanthines antagonize the effects of adenosine, while dipyridamole (Persantine) potentiates its effects.

Parasympatholytics

Atropine Sulfate

Mechanism of Action and Therapeutic Implications. Atropine is a parasympatholytic drug which reduces vagal tone, thus increasing conduction through the atrioventricular node. It blocks acetylcholine receptors, thereby inhibiting the effects of the parasympathetic nervous system. Atropine is useful for the treatment of symptomatic sinus bradycardia and atrioventricular block. Although also used in asystole and idioventricular rhythm, its therapeutic efficiency in this setting is not well demonstrated.

Indications. Accepted uses of atropine include

- Hemodynamically significant sinus bradycardia or atrioventricular block
- Asystole
- Pulseless electrical activity (PEA) where the underlying rhythm is a bradycardia

Contraindications. None in the emergency setting.

Dosage. For symptomatic sinus bradycardia and atrioventricular block the recommended dose is 0.5 to 1 mg IV bolus, repeated every 3 to 5 minutes to a maximum dose of 0.04 mg/kg (3 mg). For treating asystole, the initial dose is 1 mg to a total of 3 mg. Little therapeutic effect is likely with total atropine doses above 2 mg. Atropine can also be given via the endotracheal tube at 2 to 2.5 times the intravenous dose.

NOTE: A total of 3 mg of atropine causes full vagal blockage.

Precautions. Doses of atropine less than 0.5 mg in an adult may have a paradoxical parasympathomimetic effect, actually slowing heart rate further, and should be avoided. Atropine may increase heart rate excessively, increasing myocardial oxygen consumption and potentially exacerbating ischemia. Also the potential for ventricular arrhythmias exists. External cardiac pacing is a potentially effective alternative for hypoperfusing bradyarrhythmias not adequately responsive to atropine.

Calcium Channel Blockers

Verapamil (Calan, Isoptin) and Diltiazem

Mechanism of Action and Therapeutic Implications. Verapamil and diltiazem are calcium channel blockers that inhibit the transport of calcium into cardiac and vascular smooth muscle. Both medications have drug-specific negative inotropic (contraction), chronotropic (rate), and dromotropic (conduction) effects. Verapamil and diltiazem reduce cardiac contractility, decrease both preload and afterload, while dilating the coronary arteries and reducing myocardial oxygen consumption. In addition, both drugs exert an electrophysiological effect of slowing conduction through the sinus and atrioventricular nodes, reducing ventricular response (rate).

Indications. Verapamil has become the agent of second choice after adenosine for the control of regular supraventricular tachyarrhythmias thought secondary to a reentrant pathway. Diltiazem, although sometimes also used for reentrant tachyarrhythmias, has emerged as the drug of first choice for rapid control of atrial flutter or fibrillation with a rapid ventricular response (Table 9–7).

Contraindications. Do not administer these agents to patients with

- Hypersensitivity to the drugs
- Bradyarrhythmias
- Severe CHF
- Wolff-Parkinson-White syndrome
- Significant hypotension
- Wide complex tachycardia that is possibly ventricular in origin

Dosage. Verapamil is dosed at 2.5 to 5 mg IV over 5 minutes. If necessary, repeat doses at 1 to 2.5 mg IV can be administered every 5 to 10 minutes to a total of 20 mg. In adults, diltiazem is given as a 20 mg intravenous bolus over 2 to 3 minutes, with a repeat 25 mg bolus if adequate rate control is not achieved in 10 to 15 minutes.

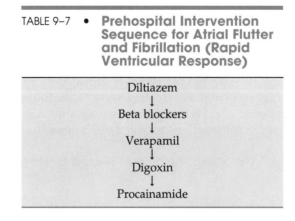

TABLE 9–7 • **Prehospital Intervention Sequence for Atrial Flutter and Fibrillation (Rapid Ventricular Response)**

Diltiazem
↓
Beta blockers
↓
Verapamil
↓
Digoxin
↓
Procainamide

Precautions. Hypotension is the most significant complication of calcium channel blockade. If this should become a concern, isotonic fluids and calcium chloride administration can reverse the decreasing blood pressure.

Sympathomimetics and Other Inotropic Agents

Epinephrine (Adrenaline)

Mechanism of Action and Therapeutic Implications. Epinephrine is a catecholamine that stimulates both alpha and beta adrenergic receptors (Table 9–8). Stimulation of alpha receptors causes an increase in peripheral and systemic vascular resistance raising arterial blood pressure resulting in increased myocardial and cerebral blood flow during CPR. The beta effects increase automaticity, heart rate, and cardiac contractile force, all resulting in an increase in cardiac output. Because of its strong inotropic and chronotropic properties, epinephrine greatly increases cardiac output. Therefore, when administering epinephrine in the emergency setting the myocardium must be adequately oxygenated.

Indications. Epinephrine is the drug of first choice for all forms of cardiopulmonary arrest, including

* Ventricular fibrillation
* Pulseless ventricular tachycardia
* Pulseless electrical activity (PEA)
* Asystole

Epinephrine may also be used for

* Symptomatic bradycardia refractory to atropine, external cardiac pacing, and dopamine

Contraindications. None during cardiopulmonary arrest. Otherwise do not administer epinephrine to patients hypersensitive to sympathomimetic amines.

Dosage. For emergency cardiac resuscitation, epinephrine is administered in bolus doses of 1.0 mg repeated every 3 to 5 minutes until the patient is resuscitated. If this approach fails, the following options can be used

* Intermediate dosage: 2 to 5 mg by IV bolus every 3 to 5 minutes
* Escalating dosage: 1 mg-3 mg-5 mg by IV bolus 3 minutes apart
* High dosage: 0.1 mg/kg by IV bolus every 3 to 5 minutes

For symptomatic sinus bradycardia IV infusion of 2 to 10 μg/min titrated to effect may be indicated. To prepare the infusion, add 1 mg (1 cc) of 1:1000 epinephrine solution to 250 cc of D_5W or sodium chloride.

TABLE 9–8   •   **Epinephrine's Cardiovascular Effect**

Increased systemic vascular resistance
Increased systolic and diastolic blood pressures
Increased electrical activity in the myocardium
Increased coronary and cerebral blood flow
Increased strength of myocardial contractility
Increased cardiac output
Increased myocardial oxygen consumption

Precautions. Administer epinephrine with caution to elderly patients and those with heart disease, diabetes, and hypertension. Epinephrine can be deactivated by alkaline solutions, such as sodium bicarbonate. Because of this, it is essential to flush the IV line between the administration of these two agents.

Dopamine (Intropin)

Mechanism of Action and Therapeutic Implications. Dopamine is a naturally occurring catecholamine that is a norepinephrine precursor. It is one of the most commonly used agents in the treatment of hypotension associated with cardiogenic shock. Dopamine has a dose-dependent effect on peripheral vascular tone and acts in a dose-dependent fashion, increasing myocardial contractility and heart rate (Table 9–9). Dopamine stimulates both alpha and beta receptors along with dopaminergic receptors, increasing blood pressure, cardiac output, and improving renal perfusion. At a dose of 1 to 2 µg/kg/min, dopamine stimulates primarily dopaminergic receptors in renal and mesenteric vessels, causing increased blood flow through a vasodilatory effect. At doses of about 2 to 10 µg/kg/min, dopamine acts primarily on beta receptors, exerting a positive inotropic effect on the heart. As the dosage of dopamine exceeds 10 µg/kg/min, its alpha effects predominate, resulting in peripheral vasoconstriction.

Indications. Dopamine is used to treat

- Cardiogenic shock
- Hemodynamically significant hypotension in the absence of hypovolemia

Contraindications. Do not administer dopamine to patients with

- Tachyarrhythmias
- Hypovolemia not fully fluid resuscitated
- Pheochromocytoma (tumor of the adrenal medulla), as dopamine may precipitate hypertensive crisis

Dosage. Dopamine is administered by intravenous infusion at an initial rate of 2 to 5 µg/kg/min. The infusion rate may be increased until a therapeutic effect is achieved. A final dosage range of 5 to 20 µg/kg/min is recommended. The standard infusion preparation of dopamine is to mix 400 mg of the drug into 250 cc of D_5W, yielding a concentration of 1600 µg/cc.

Precautions. Dopamine will increase heart rate and may worsen supraventricular or ventricular rhythms. Myocardial oxygen consumption will increase at higher doses due to vasoconstriction and increased afterload. This may induce or exacerbate myocardial

TABLE 9–9 • **Dopamine's Dose-Dependent Effects**

DOSE	RECEPTORS STIMULATED	RESPONSE
1–2 µg/kg/min	Dopaminergic	Vasodilation of renal, mesenteric, and coronary arteries
2–10 µg/kg/min	Beta	Increased heart rate, contractility, and cardiac output
10–20 µg/kg/min	Alpha	Renal, mesenteric, and peripheral vasoconstriction

ischemia. The dose of dopamine should be reduced in patients taking monoamine oxidase inhibitors (a type of antidepressant), as these medications potentiate dopamine's effects. Finally, dopamine is inactivated in alkaline solutions, such as sodium bicarbonate.

Dobutamine (Dobutrex)

Mechanism of Action and Therapeutic Implications. Dobutamine is a synthetic catecholamine structurally related to isoproterenol (Isuprel). It is mainly a beta-1 receptor agonist with some beta-2 and alpha agonist activity. Dobutamine acts by increasing cardiac contractility and stroke volume while having relatively little effect on heart rate. Unlike dopamine, dobutamine does not stimulate the heart indirectly by releasing norepinephrine from nerve endings. This and perhaps other reasons allow dobutamine to have minimal effects on heart rate, allowing the rate to be maintained near pretreatment levels. Dobutamine is presently the agent which produces the most potent contractile action with the least amount of undesirable heart rate and blood pressure effects. It is therefore, the inotropic agent of choice in acute myocardial ischemia or infarction with left ventricular dysfunction, as it most safely improves cardiac performance without overtly worsening myocardial ischemia.

Indications. Dobutamine is used to treat

- Pulmonary congestion and low cardiac output
- Hypotensive patients with pulmonary congestion who cannot tolerate vasodilator drugs

Contraindications. Dobutamine should not be used as the sole agent in hypovolemic shock, unless fluid resuscitation is well under way.

Dosage. Dobutamine is usually begun at 2 μg/kg/min and titrated upward according to hemodynamic effect. Two ampules of dobutamine, each containing 250 mg should be added to 250 cc of D_5W or sodium chloride.

Precautions. Use dobutamine with caution with patients who might be experiencing myocardial infarction. Dobutamine may cause tachycardia and arrhythmias, provoking myocardial ischemia.

Other Catecholamines: Norepinephrine (Levophed) and Isoproterenol (Isuprel)

Norepinephrine and isoproterenol are other catecholamines on occasion employed in treating emergency cardiac patients. Norepinephrine has similar cardiac effects as epinephrine, but its net vasoconstricting effects predominate. Therefore, norepinephrine causes arterial and venous constriction, relegating it as an agent to be used to elevate blood pressure. Isoproterenol is a pure beta adrenergic agent with potent vasodilating and cardiac stimulation effects. Because isoproterenol greatly increases myocardial oxygen consumption, it is contraindicated in patients with ischemic heart disease, limiting its role in the emergency setting.

Sympathetic Beta Blockers

Beta Blockers (Metoprolol, Esmolol, Propranolol)

Mechanism of Action and Therapeutic Implications. Beta adrenergic blocking agents block sympathetic activity at the beta receptor. This blockade reduces heart rate, blood pressure, and myocardial contractility, thus decreasing cardiac oxygen demand. Furthermore, reducing myocardial wall tension and prolonging time in diastole, myocardial blood flow may also be improved. These actions explain their effectiveness in the treatment of hypertension, angina pectoris, and for early intervention in acute MI. The clinical efficacy of beta blocker therapy in the setting of acute myocardial ischemia and infarction has been repeatedly studied. They appear to decrease infarct size and analgesic needs, and may reduce mortality if given early.

Indications. Beta blockers are commonly used for

- Angina pectoris
- Myocardial infarction
- Hypertension
- Control of recurrent ventricular tachycardia and fibrillation not responsive to other therapies
- Control of supraventricular tachyarrhythmias

NOTE: Beta blockers are most effective in the hyperadrenergic patient who is appropriately volume resuscitated.

Contraindications. There are multiple contraindications to the use of beta blocker therapy. These include

- Hypersensitivity to the drug
- Bradycardia or hypotension
- Atrioventricular conduction disturbances more severe than first-degree block
- Reactive airway diseases such as bronchial asthma or chronic obstructive pulmonary disease
- Congestive heart failure

Dosage. Metoprolol (Lopressor) is a beta-1-selective blocking agent which therefore has more specific cardiac effects and is recommended. It is given in 5 mg intravenous boluses every 5 minutes to a total of 15 mg, or significant side effects. Esmolol (Brevibloc) is a nonselective beta-blocking agent with a therapeutic half-life of about 8 minutes. It has the advantage of titratability, and discontinuation will rapidly reduce toxic effects if significant side effects occur. A loading dose of 0.5 mg/kg is recommended, with maintenance therapy at 50 to 200 mcq/kg/minute. Because of esmolol's rapid onset and short duration of effect, it is an attractive prehospital medication. Propranolol (Inderal) is a nonselective beta-blocking agent with a very long therapeutic half-life. One mg intravenous doses can be repeated every 5 minutes to a total of 3 mg, but it offers no particular advantage over the other agents.

Precautions. Use caution in administering beta blockers to patients with coronary insufficiency, because it may precipitate congestive heart failure. Caution should be exercised in critically ill patients who may be dependent on beta adrenergic receptor support. Furthermore, the administration of beta blockers to diabetic patients can mask the symptoms of hypoglycemia.

Antihypertensive Agents

Nifedipine (Procardia, Adalat)

Mechanism of Action and Therapeutic Implications. Nifedipine is a calcium channel blocker in widespread emergency use. It dilates both systemic and coronary arteries, making it an effective agent for the treatment of hypertensive emergencies and angina pectoris. Nifedipine decreases peripheral vascular resistance, reducing systemic blood pressure and afterload. By reducing afterload, nifedipine decreases myocardial oxygen consumption.

Indications. Accepted uses of nifedipine include

• Severe hypertension
• Angina pectoris

Contraindications. Do not administer nifedipine to patients who are hypersensitive to the drug or those with hypotension.

Dosage. One 10 mg capsule punctured and placed under the tongue for absorption. Alternatively, the capsule can be bitten by the patient and swallowed.

Precautions. Hypotension or a significant drop in blood pressure are the greatest adverse effects of nifedipine. Thus, blood pressure monitoring is essential with its use. Case reports of severe, unresponsive hypotension leading to myocardial infarction or stroke have been attributed to nifedipine. Nifedipine should be used with caution in patients with congestive heart failure, as it may worsen the condition.

Nitroprusside (Nipride)

Mechanism of Action and Therapeutic Implications. Nitroprusside is a potent peripheral vasodilator with effects on both the arterial and venous smooth muscle. It greatly increases the capacity of the venous circulation and reduces blood pressure by decreasing peripheral vascular resistance. The effects of nitroprusside are seen almost immediately and cease within minutes following termination of its infusion.

Indications. Nitroprusside is used in the treatment of

• Hypertensive crisis (medication of first choice)
• Acute left ventricular failure
• Cardiogenic shock

Contraindications. None in the treatment of life-threatening hypertensive crisis.

Dosage. Begin IV infusion at 0.1 μg/kg per minute titrated to the desired effect. The average therapeutic dose ranges from 0.5 mg to 8 μg/kg per minute. To prepare the infusion, add 50 mg of nitroprusside to 250 cc of D_5W or sodium chloride. Once prepared, immediately wrap the solution in aluminum foil or other opaque material, as nitroprusside may deteriorate upon exposure to light.

Precautions. Hypotension is the most common adverse reaction seen with the administration of nitroprusside. Frequent blood pressure monitoring is essential during its use. Caution should also be used when administering nitroprusside to patients with renal or liver disease. Excessive doses can produce cyanide toxicity which can exacerbate any side effects that may develop.

Diuretics

Furosemide (Lasix)

Mechanism of Action and Therapeutic Implications. Furosemide is a potent diuretic that inhibits the reabsorption of sodium and chloride in the kidneys (proximal loop of Henle). It is a drug used to treat pulmonary edema and to lessen blood pressure. Intravenous furosemide causes venous dilation which decreases venous return to the heart.

This effect is seen before the onset of diuresis and occurs within 5 minutes. Furosemide's diuretic effect begins roughly 10 minutes following IV administration.

Indications. Furosemide is given for the emergency treatment of pulmonary congestion associated with inadequate ventricular function.

Contraindications. Do not administer furosemide to patients with

- Hypovolemia
- Hypotension
- Hypokalemia

Dosage. 0.5 to 1 mg/kg IV pushed slowly over 1 to 2 minutes (average dose of 40 mg).

Precautions. Dehydration and hypotension may result from overzealous use of furosemide.

Other Treatment Options for Acute Myocardial Ischemia

Magnesium Sulfate

Mechanism of Action and Therapeutic Implications. Magnesium is one of the major cations (positive-charged ions) of the body. This electrolyte has important effects on a tremendous number of biochemical mechanisms in the body. It has been proposed as adjuvant therapy for a wide variety of ventricular and supraventricular tachyarrhythmias. Magnesium reduces magnesium-deficient states, which are associated with arrhythmias and sudden cardiac death. Furthermore, magnesium improves the movement of potassium into the cell, which may be important as many arrhythmias are thought to result from intracellular hypokalemia, especially in the setting of myocardial ischemia.

Indications. Magnesium is indicated to correct hypomagnesemia in the following

- Torsades de pointes
- Severe refractory ventricular fibrillation

Contraindications. Do not administer magnesium to patients with hypocalcemia and atrioventricular block. As magnesium is renally excreted, it is relatively contraindicated in severe renal insufficiency.

Dosage. Dilute 1 to 2 grams in 100 cc of D_5W and infuse intravenously over 2 minutes.

Precautions. Use caution when administering magnesium to patients with decreased renal function.

Thrombolytic Therapy

In true cases of ongoing myocardial infarction, especially with symptom duration lasting less than an hour but with some benefit up to 4 to 6 hours or more, opening the acute coronary occlusion provides the best method of preserving myocardial tissue. The adage "Time is muscle" is very important here, as delays in recognition and treatment of myocardial infarction severely limit the ability to salvage myocardium. The decision process concerning who should receive thrombolytic therapy, which agent has greatest efficacy, and whether prehospital administration is a good idea requires cost-benefit analysis. This and other issues will be addressed in the upcoming chapter.

The reader is encouraged to refer to (Table 9–10) for a summary of all phamacologic agents.

TABLE 9–10 • **Summary of Pharmacologic Interventions**

MEDICATION	INDICATION(S)	MECHANISM	DOSAGE
Oxygen	Chest pain of any etiology	Elevates arterial oxygen tension and content, improving tissue oxygenation	Nasal cannula: 4–6 L Nonrebreather: 12 L
Aspirin	Suspected myocardial infarction	Antiplatelet effects inhibiting reocclusion	162 mg (2 children's aspirin) PO
Nitroglycerin	Angina pectoris Myocardial infarction Pulmonary edema	Arterial and venodilators. Reduce preload, afterload, and pulmonary pressure	0.4 mg sublingually every 3–5 minutes 10–20 µg/minute via IV infusion Titrate to effect
Morphine	Myocardial infarction Cardiogenic pulmonary edema	Narcotic analgesic. Decreases preload, afterload, and myocardial oxygen consumption	1–3 mg IV titrated to the desired analgesic or hemodynamic effect
Nalbuphine	Moderate to severe pain (Ischemic chest pain)	Narcotic agonist/antagonist binding to opiate receptors	5–10 mg IV
Lidocaine	PVCs in the setting of myocardial ischemia and infarction Ventricular tachycardia Ventricular fibrillation	Decreases automaticity of ectopic pacemaker sites in the Purkinje fibers and ventricle	1–1.5 mg/kg IV followed by half doses every 5 minutes to a total of 3 mg/kg Maintenance infusion: 2–4 mg/min
Bretylium	PVCs in the setting of myocardial ischemia and infarction Ventricular tachycardia Ventricular fibrillation	Initial effect is the release of catecholamines. Later effect is sympatholytic	5–10 mg/kg IV, not to exceed 35 mg/kg
Procainamide	PVCs Ventricular tachycardia Ventricular fibrillation PSVT	Suppresses automaticity of ectopic pacemakers and slows condition velocity through the bundle of His	20–30 mg/min IV not to exceed 17 mg/kg
Adenosine	PSVT	Slows conduction and interrupts reentry pathways through the AV node	6 mg rapid IV No effect, then 12 mg rapid IV
Atropine	Symptomatic bradycardia	Parasympatholytic, accelerating the rate of sinus node discharge and improving atrioventricular conduction	0.5–1 mg IV every 3–5 minutes Total vagolytic dose is 3 mg
Verapamil	Supraventricular tachydysrhythmias	Calcium channel blocker Slows conduction in the AV node	2.5–5 mg slow IV
Diltiazem	Controls ventricular rate in atrial fibrillation and flutter	Calcium channel blocker Slows conduction through the sinus and atrioventricular nodes	20 mg IV over 2–3 minutes
Epinephrine	Ventricular fibrillation or pulseless ventricular tachycardia Pulseless electrical activity (PEA) Asystole Symptomatic bradycardia	Alpha and beta adrenergic receptor stimulator	1 mg IV every 3–5 minutes Bradycardia: 2–10 µg/min IV infusion
Dopamine	Cardiogenic shock	Dopaminergic, alpha, and beta adrenergic receptor stimulator	2–20 µg/kg/min IV infusion
Dobutamine	Hypotension with pulmonary congestion Cardiogenic shock	Beta 1 receptor agonist with little effect on heart rate	2–20 µg/kg/min IV infusion
Nifedipine	Severe hypertension Angina pectoris	Calcium channel blocker dilating both systemic and coronary arteries	10 mg capsule bitten and swallowed or punctured and placed sublingually
Nitroprusside	Hypertensive crisis	Potent peripheral venous and arterial dilator	0.1 µg/kg/min IV infusion titrated to effect
Furosemide	Cardiogenic pulmonary edema	Loop diuretic inhibiting the reabsorption of sodium and chloride Venous dilator	0.5–1.0 mg IV (40 mg average dose)
Magnesium	Torsades de pointes Refractory ventricular fibrillation	Reduces magnesium deficient states associated with arrhythmias	1–2 gm IV over 2 minutes

External Cardiac Pacing

External cardiac pacing or transcutaneous pacing (TCP) refers to the delivery of an electrical stimulus through electrodes applied to the anterior and posterior chest walls. Designed for emergency use, this form of pacing is the method of first choice due to the speed at which it can be delivered and because it is the least invasive technique currently available. Transcutaneous pacing is indicated for the treatment of symptomatic bradycardias (i.e., hypotension, decreased mentation, and angina) that have not responded to atropine therapy or when atropine therapy is not immediately available (Table 9–11). In the conscious patient with hemodynamically stable bradycardia, TCP is usually not necessary. However, it is advisable to attach the electrodes to such patients and leave the unit in the standby mode against the possibility of future deterioration. This should always be performed on patients with new type II second- and third-degree atrioventricular block, especially in the setting of myocardial ischemia or infarction. Additionally, transcutaneous pacing may be used to restore electrical activity in asystole and to accelerate an underlying electrical rate of less than 60 in pulseless electrical activity (PEA). TCP may cause discomfort in the conscious patient. If this should occur, administer diazepam (Valium) for treatment of anxiety and muscle contractions and morphine for analgesia.

Equipment for External Cardiac Pacing

Several manufacturers currently market defibrillator/monitors incorporated with external pacing capabilities. Some models use a special pacing cassette inserted into a receptacle on the defibrillator. Still others display the pacing controls on the front of the unit alongside the defibrillation controls. No matter which type of unit is used, all transcutaneous pacemakers have similar basic features. Most allow cardiac rate selection between 30 to 180 beats per minute. Current output is usually adjustable from 0 to 200 milliamps (mA). Paramedics should become completely familiar with the pacemaker unit they are subject to working with. Manufacturer operating manuals are beneficial in this regard.

Technique of Transcutaneous Pacing

The procedure for initiating transcutaneous pacing is quite simple (Table 9–12). Two large pacing electrodes are attached to the patient's thorax (Figure 9–1). The anterior electrode is placed to the left of the sternum and centered as close as possible to the point of maximal cardiac impulse (fifth intercostal space). The posterior electrode is placed directly behind the anterior electrode, just under the scapula to the left of the thoracic spinal column. A pacing cable then runs from the pacing pads to the defibrillator/monitor. ECG leads are also attached to the patient at the conventional sites, and the ECG signal is delivered directly to the machine through a separate patient cable. Pacing pa-

TABLE 9–11 • **Indications for Transcutaneous Pacing**

Symptomatic bradycardias
  Sinus bradycardia
  Junctional rhythms
  Atrioventricular (heart) blocks
  Idioventricular rhythms
Asystole
Pulseless electrical activity (electrical rate < 60)

TABLE 9-12 • **Procedural Guideline for External Cardiac Pacing**

Place the patient in the supine position
Initiate intravenous access, oxygen, and ECG monitoring
Confirm symptomatic bradycardia
Apply the pacing electrodes in the anterior-posterior or anterior-anterior position
Connect the electrode cables to the pacing electrodes
Set the desired heart rate on the pacemaker (70–80 beats per minute)
Turn the voltage setting to 0 mA.
Slowly increase the current (5–20 mA increments) until ventricular capture is observed
Assess the pulse and blood pressure and monitor the patient's response

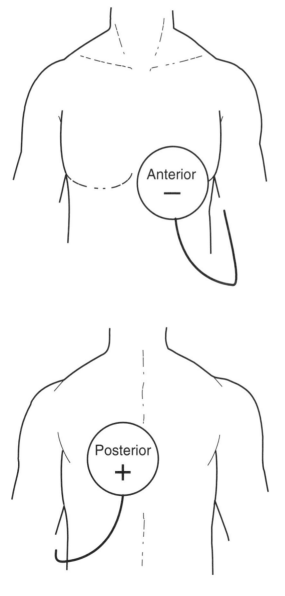

Figure 9–1.

Anterior-posterior pacing electrode placement.
The negative electrode is placed on the left anterior chest, halfway between the xiphoid process and left nipple, with the upper edge of the electrode below the nipple line. The positive electrode is placed on the left posterior chest beneath the scapula and lateral to the spine.

rameters (e.g., pacing rate and current output) are set, the unit is activated, and the ECG is observed for appropriate sensing. A pacing rate of 70 to 80 beats per minute is typically employed and the current output (mA) is initially set to nominal levels and slowly increased until evidence of capture is achieved (spike followed by wide QRS complex). Finally, in the setting of bradyasystolic arrest, set the current to maximal output (200 mA), then decrease the current if capture (pulse) is achieved.

SUMMARY

The prehospital evaluation and therapeutic intervention for myocardial ischemia or infarction represents a significant challenge. The paramedic must first evaluate a tremendous variety of presentations, some classic for myocardial ischemia but many others quite atypical, to recognize those patients likely to be experiencing cardiac injury. Attentive history, physical exam, and electrocardiographic evaluation will allow a tentative diagnosis of acute myocardial ischemia or infarction. Therapeutic interventions should all attempt to reduce myocardial oxygen demand while increasing oxygen delivery to cardiac tissue. The degree of prehospital therapy will depend on patient stability, transport time, and the various treatment modalities available. With appropriate recognition and thoughtful, carefully applied intervention, prehospital therapy of acute myocardial ischemia and infarction can reduce both the morbidity and mortality of this disease.

KEY POINTS SUMMARY

Pathophysiology of Myocardial Ischemia and Infarction

1. Cardiac ischemia develops when there is an imbalance such that myocardial oxygen supply is inadequate for the heart's metabolic demand. Myocardial infarction occurs as a result of unrelieved myocardial ischemia. Both myocardial ischemia and infarction represent a continuum of the same disease process and most often result from coronary atherosclerosis.

Origin of Ischemic Chest Pain

2. The chest discomfort of myocardial ischemia is due to the accumulation of lactic acid and carbon dioxide in ischemic myocardial tissue. The accumulation of such wastes creates changes in the myocardium that stimulates pain transmission in sympathetic nerves of the autonomic nervous system. The pain is transmitted to the lower cervical and upper five thoracic roots of the spinal cord, eventually connecting with the cerebral cortex. The cortex then interprets the incoming impulse as chest discomfort.

Historical Description of Chest Pain

3. The historical description of chest pain is an important diagnostic feature of infarction. Usually the chest discomfort of myocardial ischemia/infarction is described as crushing, pressure, tightness, or heaviness. Atypical descriptions of chest pain, such as burning or indigestion or sharp stabbing pain are not uncommon findings and should always be considered for the diagnosis of infarction.

The Physical Exam

4. The physical exam is often deceptively normal and rarely contributes to the diagnosis of myocardial infarction. There may be an increased or decreased heart rate with an increase or decrease in blood pressure. An S_3 or S_4 heart sound is occasionally heard, as well as the presence of a new systolic murmur and respiratory crackles.

ECG Evaluation of Myocardial Infarction

5. The electrocardiogram is the most time-honored test for the evaluation of acute myocardial ischemia. It is used to screen chest pain patients with atypical complaints not clearly suggestive of ischemia, to evaluate nonischemic causes of chest pain, to stratify the risk of acute myocardial ischemia in patients with suggestive chest pain, and to evaluate therapeutic interventions.

Treatment of Myocardial Ischemia and Infarction

6. The treatment of myocardial ischemia and infarction involves improving myocardial oxygen supply in relation to demand and preventing or treating complications. The following describes the prehospital management of AMI:
   - Ensure adequate airway, ventilation, and circulation
   - Administer oxygen and monitor its delivery with pulse oximetry
   - Evaluate vital signs
   - Apply the cardiac monitor, identify and treat dysrhythmias
   - Establish intravenous access and suppress dysrhythmias
   - Administer aspirin, nitroglycerin, and provide pain relief with narcotics
   - Acquire a 12-lead ECG
   - Prescreen for thrombolytic therapy
   - Initiate a cardiac alert
   - Initiate thrombolytics (prehospital or emergency department)

Special Patient Considerations

7. The hypotensive, hypoperfusing patient suffering from bradycardia requires the administration of atropine and/or early transcutaneous pacing to increase heart rate. If hypotension occurs in the setting of acute myocardial infarction and bradycardia is not the problem, then aggressive fluid challenge with isotonic crystalloid solutions is necessary. Tachydysrhythmias in the setting of AMI are treated as either ventricular or supraventricular in origin.

Pharmacologic Interventions

8. The following medications are used to treat acute myocardial infarction and its complications: oxygen, aspirin, nitroglycerin, morphine sulfate, nalbuphine, lidocaine, procainamide, bretylium, adenosine, verapamil, diltiazem, epinephrine, dopamine, dobutamine, nifedipine, nitroprusside, furosemide, magnesium, and thrombolytics.

BIBLIOGRAPHY

American Heart Association. *Textbook of Advanced Cardiac Life Support*. Dallas, TX; 1992.

Aufderheide TP, Haselow WC, Hendley GE, et al. Feasibility of prehospital r-TPA therapy in chest pain patients. *Ann Emerg Med*. 1992;21:379–373.

Aufderheide TP, Hendley GE, Thakur RK, et al. The diagnostic impact of prehospital 12-lead electrocardiography. *Ann Emerg Med*. 1990;19:1280–1287.

Bean WB. Masquerades of myocardial infarction. *Lancet*. 1977;1:1044–1046.

Beck RK. *Pharmacology for Prehospital Emergency Care*. Philadelphia, PA: FA Davis Company; 1992.

Behar S, Scher S, Karix L. Evaluation of the electrocardiogram in the emergency room as a decision-making tool. *Chest*. 1977;71:486–491.

Bruns BM, Dieckmann R, Shagoury C, et al. Safety of pre-hospital therapy with morphine sulfate. *Am J Emerg Med*. 1992;10:53–57.

Craddock LD. The physical examination in the acute cardiac ischemic syndromes. *J Emerg Med*. 1991;9:55–60.

Dillon MC, Calbreath DF, Dixon AM. Diagnostic problem in acute myocardial infarction. *Arch Intern Med*. 1982;142:33.

Donovan PJ, Cline DM, Whitley TW, et al. Prehospital care by EMTs and EMT-Is in a rural setting: Prolongation of scene times by ALS procedures. *Ann Emerg Med*. 1989;18:495–500.

Grim PS, Feldman T, Childers RW, et al. Evaluation of patients for the need of thrombolytic therapy in the prehospital setting. *Ann Emerg Med*. 1989;18:483–488.

Hargarten K, Chapman PD, Stueven HA, et al. Prehospital prophylactic lidocaine does not favorably affect outcome in patients with chest pain. *Ann Emerg Med*. 1990;19:1274–1279.

Hargarten KM, Aprahamian C, Stueven H, et al. Limitations of prehospital predictors of acute myocardial infarction and unstable angina. *Ann Emerg Med*. 1987;16:1325–1329.

Hedges JR, Kobernick MS. Detection of myocardial ischemia/infarction in the emergency department patient with chest discomfort. *Emerg Med Cl North Am*. 1988;6:317–340.

Herlitz J, Karlson BW, Liljeqvist JA, et al. Early identification of acute myocardial infarction and prognosis in relation to mode of transport to hospital. *Am J Emerg Med*. 1992;10:406–412.

Lee TH, Cook FE, Weisberg M. Acute chest pain in the emergency room: Identification and examination of low-risk patients. *Arch Intern Med*. 1985;145:65–69.

Oates JA, Wood AJJ. Adenosine and supraventricular tachycardia. *New Engl J Med*. 1991;325:1621–1629.

Pozen MW, D'Agostino RB, Mitchell JB. The usefulness of predictive instrument to reduce inappropriate admissions to the coronary care unit. *Ann Intern Med*. 1980;92:238–242.

Rouan GW, Lee TH, Cook EF. Clinical characteristics and outcome of acute myocardial infarction in patients with initially normal or nonspecific electrocardiograms: A report from the Multicenter Chest Pain Study. *Cardiol*. 1989;64:1087–1092.

Schroeder JS, Lamb IH, Hu M. The prehospital course of patients with chest pain: Analysis of the prodromal, symptomatic, decision-making, transportation and emergency room periods. *Am J Med*. 1978;65:742–748.

Thaulow E, Erikssen J, Sandvik L, et al. Initial clinical presentation of cardiac disease in asymptomatic men with silent myocardial ischemia and angiographically documented coronary artery disease (the Oslo Ischemia Study). *Am J Cardiol*. 1993;72:629–633.

Tierney WM, Fitzgerald J, McHenry R. Physicians' estimates of the probability of myocardial infarction in emergency room patients with chest pain. *Med Decis Making*. 1986;6:12–17.

Tierney WM, Roth BJ, Psaty B. Predictors of myocardial infarction in emergency room patients. *Crit Care Med*. 1985;13:526–530.

Uretsky BF, Farquhar DS, Berezin AF. Symptomatic myocardial infarction without chest pain: Prevalence and clinical course. *Am J Cardiol*. 1977;40:498–503.

10

Thrombolytic Therapy

LEARNING OBJECTIVES

1. Discuss the pathophysiology of myocardial infarction and the role of thrombolytic therapy.

2. Explain the physiological mechanism of thrombolytic agents.

3. Name, describe, and state the dosing regimens of streptokinase, eminase, and t-PA.

4. List the clinical indications for thrombolytic therapy.

5. Describe the appropriate history and physical assessment goals for the cardiac patient.

6. Discuss the assessment parameters and 12-lead ECG findings diagnostic of infarction.

7. List and describe the absolute and relative contraindications for thrombolytic therapy.

8. List and describe the complications of thrombolytic therapy.

9. Discuss the current evidence relative to the out-of-hospital administration of thrombolytic therapy.

10. Describe the cardiac alert and discuss the current statistics supporting its use.

INTRODUCTION

Roughly 1.5 million acute myocardial infarctions occur each year in the United States. One-third (500,000) of these patients die each year. The recent introduction of thrombolytic agents has reduced the mortality rate by 25 to 30% for patients who are treated in a timely manner. Unfortunately, a large number of myocardial infarction patients never receive this potentially lifesaving therapy or receive it late in the course of their infarction. Many large-scale studies have clearly demonstrated the benefits of thrombolytic therapy.

Because thrombolytic agents are most beneficial when administered early, rapid out-of-hospital identification of potential acute myocardial infarction is important. Recently studies have examined the role of thrombolytic agents in the out-of-hospital setting. Though most EMS systems consider thrombolytic therapy experimental, out-of-hospital identification and care for patients suffering acute myocardial infarction is increasingly important. Paramedics must thus be familiar with the pharmacology, indications, contraindications, significant complications, advantages, and disadvantages of out-of-hospital thrombolysis.

MYOCARDIAL INFARCTION

Acute myocardial infarction occurs when blood flow to the myocardium is abruptly decreased, resulting in insufficient delivery of oxygen and other metabolic substrates to the heart muscle (myocardium). Reduced blood flow usually occurs following thrombosis (a blood clot) of a coronary artery which supplies blood to the myocardium. Blood clots form in coronary arteries when atherosclerotic plaques rupture and expose surfaces of the coronary artery wall that induce thrombosis. The entire process of clot formation and interruption of coronary artery flow is complex, involving platelets and natural clot-forming mechanisms. Eventually, if blood flow to the myocardium is not reestablished, the heart muscle infarcts (dies).

If the clot occluding the coronary artery is dissolved, blood flow is returned to the heart, thereby preventing infarction. Thrombolytic agents work by dissolving these coronary artery clots and restoring blood flow to the myocardium. Thrombolytics are most effective when used early in the course of infarction, preferably within 6 or less hours of the onset of chest pain. The very early use of thrombolytics produces the best survival rates.

PHARMACOLOGY

All thrombolytic agents work by converting plasminogen to plasmin, which is the active agent that lyses (dissolves) clots (Figure 10–1). Clots are composed of fibrin, which is the substance that plasmin lyses. Plasmin not only lyses fibrin clots, it lyses the precursor of fibrin, fibrinogen, and inactivates certain clotting factors. Four thrombolytic agents are currently available: streptokinase, anisoylated streptokinase-plasminogen activator complex (APSAC), human recombinant tissue plasminogen activator (t-PA), and urokinase. Urokinase is available only for intracoronary administration and will not be discussed here. It is important to note that thrombolytic therapy will lyse blood clots in coronary arteries but it does not reverse the underlying atherosclerotic plaque. It is the atherosclerotic plaque which causes the clot in the first place.

Streptokinase

Streptokinase is produced by the bacteria streptococcus. It forms a complex by binding to plasminogen. This complex is able to convert free plasminogen into plasmin, which is the agent that actually dissolves or lyses the clots. Streptokinase is usually given in-

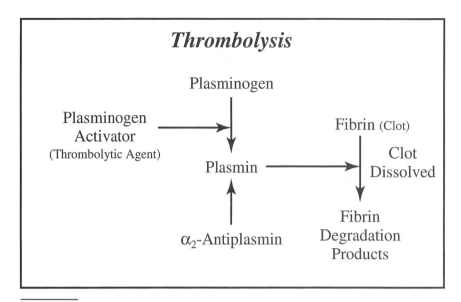

Figure 10–1.
Thrombolysis.

travenously over one hour as a dose of 1.5 million units. Of all the thrombolytic agents streptokinase is the cheapest, costing about $400 per patient.

Eminase (APSAC)

APSAC is a combination of streptokinase and plasminogen bound together. When AP-SAC is placed in water it becomes active and is able to convert plasminogen in the blood into plasmin. It is given as a single dose of 30 units over 5 minutes. Because APSAC is easy to administer it is attractive for out-of-hospital use. APSAC is somewhat more expensive than streptokinase, costing about $2000 per patient.

t-PA

Recombinant t-PA is a human protein which is made using recombinant genetic engineering technology and is therefore not derived from human blood. Human genes which code for t-PA are placed in bacteria which then produce the human t-PA.

Recombinant t-PA does not convert free plasminogen to plasmin very well, but it does convert plasminogen bound to fibrin at the site of a clot to plasmin. The idea here is to only convert plasminogen to plasmin at the site of a clot and leave the unbound plasminogen alone. Unbound plasmin, which has been converted from plasminogen, causes dysfunction of the clotting mechanisms. This can lead to increased bleeding problems during thrombolytic use. While this is good in theory, most studies have not shown any advantage for t-PA over other thrombolytic agents. In fact, some studies show that patients treated with t-PA are more likely to have a recurrence of the clot which was originally dissolved by the t-PA. Recently, one study (GUSTO, 1993) has suggested that t-PA may have a small advantage over streptokinase especially for anterior myocardial infarctions.

Traditional dosing for t-PA is usually a 6 to 10 mg bolus followed by an infusion of 44 to 50 mg over the first hour. During the following 2 hours the patient receives an additional 20 mg per hour infusion. Newer regimens for t-PA administration are now being used. A bolus of 15 mg is given followed by 0.75 mg/kg (maximum 50 mg) over 30 minutes, then 0.5 mg/kg (maximum 35 mg) over one hour. This is the so-called acceler-ated dosing for t-PA. At a cost of $2800 per patient, t-PA is the most expensive of the thrombolytics.

Much debate has centered around the benefit of one thrombolytic over the other. However, the minor differences in complication rates and utility are far overshadowed by the importance of simply giving one of these agents as early as possible during the course of an acute myocardial infarction.

CLINICAL APPLICATION

Indications

Thrombolytic therapy is indicated when the patient is having an acute myocardial in-farction within 6 to 12 hours of the onset of chest pain. Thrombolytics are also indicated within 24 hours of the onset of pain if the pain is intermittent in nature. Patients who are treated 6 to 12 hours after the onset of pain benefit less than patients treated within 6 hours of pain. Because the benefit of thrombolytic agents given 6 to 12 hours after the onset of symptoms is less, the risk-to-benefit ratio is worse. Age greater than 75 years was previously considered a contraindication. Recent studies indicate, however, that age is not a contraindication. The chest pain should be consistent with acute myocardial infarction and at least 0.1 mV (1 mm) of ST-segment elevation should be present in at least two contiguous ECG leads (Table 10-1).

Chest Pain

The evaluation of chest pain includes location, quality, duration, speed of onset, radia-tion, precipitating factors, associated symptoms, aggravating factors, and relieving fac-tors (Table 10-2).

Most patients with cardiac pain will have an sudden onset of pain at rest. Discom-fort as a result of acute MI is often described as crushing, squeezing, tightness, or pres-sure. The pain is usually substernal or left-sided and may radiate to one or both arms, the neck, jaw, or back. At least 15 to 30 minutes of pain is typical of myocardial infarc-tion. MI pain is usually not affected by position, activity, or deep breathing and is not re-lieved by sublingual nitroglycerin or rest. The use of a scale from 1 to 10, with 1 being no pain and 10 being the worst pain the patient has ever experienced, facilitates com-munication of the pain and assessment of the effectiveness of therapy. However, the severity of a patient's pain does not necessarily correlate with actual myocardial infarc-tion. Patients often have little chest pain despite significant myocardial infarction.

Associated symptoms may include nausea, vomiting, weakness, dizziness, and di-aphoresis. Elderly patients, especially those older than 85, often do not have classic symptoms. They commonly present with only shortness of breath as a symptom of their

---

TABLE 10–1   •   Indications for Thrombolytic Therapy

Clinical history consistent with myocardial infarction
Duration of symptoms < 6–12 hours or < 24 hours with stuttering pain
EKG criteria
  ST elevation > 1 mm in two contiguous limb leads
  ST elevation > 2 mm in two contiguous precordial leads
Consider thrombolysis for strong clinical history associated with
  ST elevation > 1 mm in any two contiguous leads
  Left bundle branch block
  Pathologic Q waves > 2 mm
  T wave inversion

TABLE 10–2 • **Chest Pain Evaluation (O-X Format)**

SIGNS OF CARDIAC CHEST PAIN

Overall (Primary) Survey
  ABCs
  Age
  Vital signs
  Oxygen therapy
  Cardiac monitoring
  History of previous heart conditions
  Diabetes
  Hypertension
  Stroke
  Medications
Position
  Left chest
  Right chest
  Substernal
  Epigastric
  Mid-back
  Generalized
Quality
  Pressure/squeezing
  Discomfort
  Burning
  Sharp
  Aching
Radiation
  Left or right arm
  Neck
  Back
  Jaw
  Anywhere at all
Signs/Symptoms
  Nausea
  Vomiting
  Diaphoresis
  Anxiety
  Shortness of breath
  Dizziness
Timing/Duration
  When did the pain begin?
  When did the pain end?
  Does it come and go?
Uncomfortable feeling
  Pain scale from 0 to 10
    0 = no pain/discomfort
    10 = worst pain/discomfort

SIGNS OF NONCARDIAC PAIN

Variation
  Variation with deep inspiration
  Pain increased or changed with body position
Worse
  Pain reproduced or worse with palpation
e**X**iting
  Pain lasts a few, fleeting seconds

Note: Many patients with chest pain of cardiac origin have atypical pain. Atypical characteristics of the patient's chest pain *does not rule out myocardial ischemia/infarction.*

cardiac ischemia. It is significant that aortic dissection can produce pain which closely resembles heart pain.

Past Medical History

Important historical features for myocardial infarction include past history of MI and family history of MI. Past history of coronary artery bypass or balloon angioplasty (percutaneous transluminal balloon angioplasty, PTCA) confirms a history of coronary artery disease for the patient. Other underlying medical problems are also important risk factors for coronary artery disease, such as diabetes, high cholesterol, smoking, and high blood pressure (hypertension). Patients who use cocaine or crack are also at risk for myocardial infarction. The role of thrombolytic therapy for infarction due to cocaine use is controversial.

Physical Examination

The physical examination is often deceptively normal in patients suffering acute myocardial infarction. There may be an increased heart rate (due to increased circulating epinephrine and sympathetic tone) or decreased heart rate (due to conduction disturbances or increased vagal tone). Similarly, blood pressure may be either elevated or decreased. An S_3 or S_4 heart sound is occasionally heard due to heart failure or decreased myocardial compliance. Rales suggest left-sided heart failure while jugular venous distention, hepatojugular reflux, and peripheral edema suggest right-heart failure. It is important to note that left-sided heart failure is the most common cause of right-sided heart failure. New systolic or diastolic heart murmurs are sometimes present when the papillary muscles (muscles which stabilize the heart valves) are injured or ruptured or when there is rupture of the septum separating the right and left ventricles. Pericardial rubs suggest pericarditis which can cause chest pain that is easily confused with myocardial infarction.

Pulses should be palpated in each arm and a blood pressure obtained from each arm. Unequal pulses or a blood pressure difference greater than 20 mmHg from one arm to the other is suggestive of aortic dissection.

12-Lead ECG

The ECG changes associated with myocardial infarction are ST segment elevation of at least 0.1 mV (1 mm), Q waves, and T wave inversions. The first change seen during myocardial infarction is elevation of the ST segment. When Q waves are present these indicate myocardial necrosis (death). T wave inversion does not usually occur until 6 to 24 hours after the onset of pain. Early repolarization, a normal variation, can cause ST segment elevation or J-point elevation in all or most leads on the ECG. Pericarditis is also associated with ST elevation. These conditions mimic the changes of myocardial infarction on the ECG and must therefore be differentiated from actual myocardial infarction.

Contraindications

There are absolute and relative contraindications to thrombolytic therapy (Table 10–3). Absolute contraindications include active internal bleeding, suspected aortic dissection, prolonged CPR, recent head trauma or intracranial neoplasm or history of hemorrhagic cerebrovascular accident (CVA), any hemorrhagic ophthalmologic condition, pregnancy, recorded blood pressure > 200/120 mmHg and previous allergic reaction to the thrombolytic agent.

TABLE 10–3 • **Contraindications for Thrombolytic Therapy**

ABSOLUTE

Active internal bleeding (GI bleed, etc.)
Suspected aortic dissection
   Right arm systolic BP vs. left arm BP < 20 mmHg
Prolonged CPR (> 10 min)
Recent head trauma
Brain tumor
Recent stroke (within 6 months)
Atrioventricular malformation or aneurysm
Hemorrhagic ophthalmologic conditions
Pregnancy
BP greater than 200/110
Previous allergic reaction to the thrombolytic agent
Pulmonary edema or cardiogenic shock

RELATIVE

Surgery within the past 2 weeks
Severe hypertension by history
Active peptic ulcer disease
History of stroke
Known bleeding disorder or use of anticoagulants (Coumadin/warfarin)
Significant liver disease
Previous exposure to thrombolytics (streptokinase or APSAC)
Pericarditis

Surgery within the past two weeks, history of severe hypertension (with or without drug therapy), active peptic ulcer disease, history of CVA, known bleeding disorder (e.g., hemophilia), current use of Coumadin or heparin (anticoagulants), significant liver dysfunction, and prior exposure to streptokinase or APSAC (especially within the last nine months) are relative contraindications to thrombolytic therapy.

Patients who are incorrectly diagnosed with an acute myocardial infarction and given thrombolytics are at additional risk for complications. The symptoms of aortic dissection can mimic acute myocardial infarction, therefore aortic dissection must be differentiated from acute myocardial infarction. Administration of thrombolytics during acute aortic dissection will produce catastrophic results.

Elderly

The risk of complications from thrombolytic therapy increases with age. Patients older than 70 are two times more likely than patients less than 70 years old to have intracerebral hemorrhage as a result of thrombolytic therapy. Severe bleeding requiring transfusion is also more common in the elderly. Thus, another relative contraindication to therapy is patient age greater than 70 years. Patients with advanced age require very careful evaluation of risk factors for CVA and bleeding. It is especially important to note any past history of CVA, bleeding problems, recent surgery, gastrointestinal bleeding, peptic ulcer disease, and hypertension.

Though the risk of complications is greater for the elderly patient, the potential benefit is also greater. Thrombolytic therapy can decrease overall mortality by up to two times more than seen with younger age groups also treated with thrombolytics. At this time, advanced age is no longer a contraindication for thrombolytic therapy.

Late Treatment

Several recent studies indicate that patients treated with thrombolytics within 12 hours of the onset of pain may receive some benefit, though less than the benefit if given within

6 hours. The evidence for treatment after 12 hours of pain is less convincing. Patients who present with a stuttering pattern of pain or are elderly or are having large anterior infarctions may benefit more from therapy in the 6 to 12 hour range. Some physicians think that these patients may even benefit from treatment up to 24 hours after the onset of pain, especially if the pain pattern is intermittent.

Hypertension

Patients with long-standing histories of high blood pressure are at increased risk for intracerebral bleeds when treated with thrombolytics. Therefore, they are often not given thrombolytic therapy. Those patients with acute elevation of their blood pressure have a somewhat smaller risk of CVA when treated with thrombolytics. Thrombolytic therapy may be indicated in these patients along with aggressive efforts at blood pressure reduction. Because such aggressive therapy for blood pressure reduction is usually only possible in the hospital setting, field use of thrombolytic agents in hypertensive patients is usually not possible.

Cardiogenic Shock and Pulmonary Edema

Patients who are in pulmonary edema or cardiogenic shock as a result of an acute myocardial infarction do not seem to benefit from thrombolytic therapy. Two different studies have demonstrated no decrease in mortality for patients treated with thrombolytic therapy if they are in cardiogenic shock or severe pulmonary edema. The treatment of choice for patients in cardiogenic shock during acute myocardial infarction is percutaneous transluminal coronary angioplasty (PTCA, opening the closed artery with a balloon inserted into the artery during coronary catheterization). If severe pulmonary edema or cardiogenic shock is present during acute myocardial infarction, rapid transport to a facility capable of performing PTCA is indicated.

Nondiagnostic 12-Lead ECG

Several studies have looked at the issue of patients who are probably having an acute myocardial infarction and do not demonstrate ST segment elevation on ECG. These patients may demonstrate ST segment depression, a new left bundle branch block, or other abnormalities. Patients who have only ST segment depression on the 12-lead ECG do not benefit from thrombolytic therapy. Those with new left bundle branch block, pathologic Q waves greater than 2 mm, T wave inversion, second- or third-degree heart block, or other arrhythmias and who have other clinical characteristics of acute MI do benefit from thrombolytics. In the out-of-hospital setting old 12-lead ECGs are not usually available, making it difficult to determine if a left bundle branch block or other abnormality is new. The conclusion is, if there is no ST elevation by electrocardiogram, thrombolytics are usually not indicated in the field.

Prior Surgery

A history of recent surgery raises concerns that thrombolytic therapy will disrupt the hemostatic plugs that form after the surgery to stop bleeding. Most physicians believe that patients who have undergone surgery within the last two weeks should not be given thrombolytic therapy. There has not been any clinically proven safe interval established for thrombolytic therapy. A two-week interval, however, seems to be reasonable.

TABLE 10–4 • **Complications of Thrombolytic Therapy**

Systemic bleeding (GI, GU, from IV sites)
Intracranial bleeding
Anaphylactic shock/allergic reactions
Immune complex disease
Hypotension

COMPLICATIONS

One percent of patients treated with thrombolytics develop intracerebral bleeding. Intracerebral hemorrhage is associated with a 40 to 50% mortality rate and severe morbidity in those who survive. Another 1% of all patients receiving thrombolytic therapy develop major bleeding, requiring transfusion. Common sites for bleeding include arterial and central venous puncture sites, gastrointestinal tract, and the genitourinary tract (Table 10–4).

Hypotension occurs more frequently in patients receiving streptokinase or APSAC. The hypotension associated with streptokinase or APSAC is usually brief and responds to intravenous fluid administration and slowing the rate of the thrombolytic infusion. Hypotension is also a complication of acute myocardial infarction and this must be recognized as different from the hypotension of thrombolytic therapy. Intravenous fluid may also be used to treat hypotension from acute MI. However, hypotension as a result of MI will usually not respond as quickly and may require pressor support.

Anaphylactic shock occurs in 0.2% of patients undergoing thrombolytic therapy. Delayed immune complex disease has also been observed in patients treated with thrombolytics. Those patients who have previously been treated with streptokinase or APSAC are at a much higher risk for anaphylaxis. Because of the risk for anaphylaxis, patients who have previously received streptokinase or APSAC should probably not be treated with these agents a second time. Previous anaphylactic reaction to streptokinase or APSAC is an absolute contraindication to administration of these agents.

OUT-OF-HOSPITAL ADMINISTRATION OF THROMBOLYTIC THERAPY: THE EVIDENCE

Most large clinical trials of thrombolytics demonstrate an improvement in mortality with early treatment. Theoretically, thrombolytics given in the out-of-hospital setting may improve mortality by decreasing the time from the onset of pain to delivery of the drug. However, there are two questions to be answered prior to large scale out-of-hospital administration of thrombolytic therapy. First, is thrombolytic therapy given in the field safe? Second, is there an improvement in mortality with thrombolytic therapy in the field?

A number of trials have addressed these issues (e.g., Aufderheide et al., 1992; Bibbus et al., 1987; Weaver et al., 1993). The first trials assessed the possibility of giving thrombolytics in the field by grading if therapy would be instituted based on the clinical presentation of the patient and the results of a 12-lead ECG. These trials did not actually give the drugs in the field. The largest studies that actually gave thrombolytic agents in the out-of-hospital setting involved physicians who were present at the scene. These studies were conducted in Europe and Israel, where physicians provide out-of-hospital care on a routine basis. Recently a large American study has been completed in western Washington state called MITI, which involved the out-of-hospital administration of thrombolytics by paramedics.

The studies to date seem to indicate that it is safe to give thrombolytics in the field. None of the out-of-hospital trials of thrombolytic agents have experienced any increase in the rate of complications from thrombolytic therapy. These studies used strict checklists of indications and contraindications which had to be met before thrombolytic therapy could be considered (Figure 10–2). In addition, the history and a 12-lead ECG were transmitted to a physician at the base station who made the actual decisions regarding the use of thrombolytics after discussion with the paramedics. All of the paramedics involved in these trials underwent additional intensive training for the evaluation of patients with suspected acute myocardial infarction.

Two larger studies have been completed in which thrombolytic therapy was administered in the field. The largest, by far, was conducted in Europe and Canada by the European Myocardial Infarction Project Group (EMIP). They enrolled over 5000 patients and treated them with either a placebo or APSAC prior to hospital arrival. Once the patients arrived at the hospital, those who received a placebo in the field were given APSAC. They were unable to demonstrate any reduction in either morbidity or mortality when the thrombolytic and placebo groups were compared.

Figure 10–2.
Checklist used by paramedics during the MITI trial.

(Modified from Kennedy JW et al. The potential for prehospital thrombolytic therapy. *Clin. Cardiol.* 12, VIII: 23–26, 1990. Copyrighted and reprinted with the permission of Clinical Cardiology Publishing Company, Inc., and/or the Foundation for Advances in Medicine and Science, Inc. Mahwah, NJ 07430-0823, USA.)

HEART PAIN CHECKLIST (For Paramedic Use)

Yes	(☒ = meets criteria)	No
☐	Oriented, can cooperate	—
☐	Heart pain	—
☐	Pain for more than 15 min and less than 6 hr	—
☐	Age (35-74)	—
☐	BP Right arm _____ / _____	—
☐	BP Left arm _____ / _____	—
☐	Systolic is more than 80 and less than 180	—
☐	Systolic right arm versus left arm less than 20	—
☐	Diastolic is less than 120	—
—	Stroke, seizures, brain surgery	☐
—	Central lines or trauma	☐
—	Takes Warfarin, Coumadin	☐
—	Known bleeding problems	☐
—	GI bleed in last 12 months	☐
—	Surgery in last 2 months	☐
—	Cancer, terminal	☐
—	Kidney, liver problems, diabetes	☐
—	Colitis, Crohn's Enteritis	☐

If above boxes are checked, proceed with ECG

☐	ECG done	—
☐	ECG received by doctor	—
☐	Meets criteria for pre-hosp t-PA	—
☐	Patient informed	—
	Kit ID#_____	
☐	t-PA given, AMT incl bolus	—
☐	ASA (5gr) given	—

TIMES

Pain began	_____ : _____
Decision time	_____ : _____
t-PA bolus	_____ : _____
Began transport	_____ : _____
Hospital arrival	_____ : _____

The second study was the MITI study in western Washington state. They studied 360 patients who were given either a placebo or APSAC. Paramedics took a history and did a brief physical examination, including a blood pressure in each arm. They filled out a checklist to evaluate patients as candidates for thrombolytic therapy (Figure 10–2). If the patient met the criteria, a 12-lead ECG was done and the history, physical findings, and ECG were transmitted to the hospital where a physician decided if the thrombolytic therapy was to be given. Those who received a placebo were again given APSAC on arrival at the hospital.

Again they were unable to demonstrate any reduction in either morbidity or mortality by giving thrombolytics in the out-of-hospital setting. The MITI group then looked at a small portion of their patients (82) who received thrombolytics both in the field and in the hospital within 70 minutes after the onset of the chest pain. These patients had a mortality rate of 1.2% compared to an 8.7% mortality for patients treated after 90 minutes of chest pain. Because this data was analyzed retrospectively and is a secondary analysis of a subgroup, caution must be used when interpreting these data.

The EMIP group combined the data from their study, MITI, and three other smaller studies. They found a 17% reduction in mortality for the combined out-of-hospital group over the combined group given in hospital thrombolytics. This meta-analysis suggests that there may be a benefit from out-of-hospital thrombolytic therapy. Data produced by meta-analysis is, however, not as reliable as data produced by prospective randomized-blinded studies such as EMIP and MITI. Therefore, the 17% improvement in mortality with out-of-hospital administration of thrombolytics observed by meta-analysis needs conformation with a prospective study.

Intracranial bleeding is a very serious complication of thrombolytic therapy which occurs in about 1% of patients treated. This is a catastrophic event for those patients. Serious questions have been raised about the paramedic's liability in such situations, given the litigious society in which we currently live. Questions have also been raised about the ability of anyone to evaluate the risk/benefit ratio of such therapy in the uncontrolled environment outside the hospital.

MITI and the experience of paramedics in Cincinnati have demonstrated that only about 4% of patients with chest pain in the field meet eligibility requirements for thrombolytic therapy. Given the low numbers of patients who may receive thrombolytic therapy in the field and the high cost of such programs, another question arises: Is the cost-to-benefit ratio good enough to support thrombolytic therapy in the out-of-hospital setting?

The Cardiac Alert

Once a patient who is eligible for thrombolytic therapy presents to an emergency department, the average delay to beginning of therapy is 60 minutes (even in many of the best hospitals). It is possible that out-of-hospital diagnosis of myocardial infarction with a 12-lead ECG transmitted to the hospital may reduce the time to thrombolytic therapy in the hospital. A cardiac alert similar to current trauma alerts could be called, allowing the emergency department to prepare for thrombolytic therapy. This would represent an additional benefit to patients even if thrombolytics are not actually given in the field. A study done in Salt Lake City showed that time to thrombolysis in the hospital was reduced by 48 minutes on the average for patients who had in-field ECGs demonstrating acute myocardial infarction (Karagounis et al., 1990).

The bottom line is that not enough evidence is currently available to justify out-of-hospital administration of thrombolytic therapy. Califf and Harrelson-Woodlief state: "Until the evidence is available, communities should be cautious about instituting major programs for at-home treatment [with thrombolytics] as a routine practice" (*JACC* 1990;15:938). Recent studies do suggest that further evaluation is needed to define the final role for out-of-hospital thrombolysis. The American College of Emergency Physicians (ACEP) recently published their guidelines for the out-of-hospital use of thrombolytic agents. Their summary states:

> Recognizing that prehospital thrombolytic therapy may provide benefit to certain subsets of patients, the routine prehospital use of thrombolytic agents should be discouraged pending further scientific delineation and documentation of those subgroups. ACEP encourages further investigation to document feasibility, efficacy, cost-effectiveness, and safety of use of these agents in this environment. Detailed education is needed in such areas as contraindications and the mechanics of drug administration. On-line medical direction is paramount to the successful use of these agents in the prehospital setting. (Benson NH, et al.: *Annals of Emergency Medicine* 1994;23:1047–8.)

SUMMARY

Thrombolytics have the potential to significantly improve the outcome of patients suffering from acute myocardial infarction. However, these drugs are not without serious side effects. Patients who receive thrombolytics are prone to develop systemic bleeding, intracranial bleeding, anaphylactic shock, immune complex disease, and hypotension. Thrombolytics should be used with patients undergoing an acute myocardial infarction with diagnostic ECG changes and no contraindications. When used correctly, a 25 to 30% reduction in mortality can be expected. About 1% of treated patients will experience major bleeding (requiring transfusion) and between 0.5 and 1.0% of patients will have strokes.

Knowledge about thrombolytic therapy will enhance the paramedic's ability to evaluate and treat the patient with suspected myocardial infarction (Table 10–5). Out-of-hospital acquisition of 12-lead EKGs reduces the time required for the patient to receive thrombolytic therapy in the emergency department. An exciting new era of the cardiac alert will likely soon be here, allowing better patient care because of paramedic input.

TABLE 10–5 • **Chest Pain Guidelines**

INCLUSION CRITERIA
At least 30 years of age
Systolic blood pressure > 90 mmHg
Assess chest pain (see Table 2)
No atypical chest pain (see Table 2 **V-X**)

TREATMENT
Appropriate oxygen therapy*
Obtain 12-lead ECG
IV D_5W or NS (TKO rate)
Nitroglycerin (NTG, 0.4 mg tablet, or spray)
Repeat NTG every 5 minutes
   Systolic pressure > 90 mmHg
   Chest pain continues
   3 doses max. (total 1.2 mg)
Administer aspirin (ASA, 160 mg by mouth)
Repeat vital signs (BP, P, RR)
Note relief or change in chest pain (scale 1–10)
Monitor vital signs every 5 minutes

Note: Appropriate oxygen therapy for patients with chest pain is usually 10–15 LPM by non-rebreather mask. Two (2) liters of oxygen per minute by nasal cannula is often better tolerated and therefore advisable in alert patients who have no dyspnea or other indications for high-flow oxygen.

KEY POINTS SUMMARY

Myocardial Infarction and Thrombolytic Therapy

1. Acute myocardial infarction is caused by complete occlusion of one or more of the coronary arteries. This results in the insufficient delivery of oxygen and other metabolic substrates to the heart muscle. Reduced coronary blood flow is almost always due to coronary thrombosis (a blood clot) and if not resolved, the heart muscle will die.

2. Thrombolytic therapy is one of the most important advances in the treatment of acute myocardial infarction. Thrombolytic agents function by dissolving coronary artery clots and restoring blood flow+ to areas of jeopardized myocardium. Thrombolytics are most effective when used early in the course of infarction (< 6 hours following the onset of symptoms).

Pharmacology and Mechanism of Action

3. Thrombolytic agents work by converting plasminogen to plasmin. Plasmin is the active agent that lyses fibrin clots. Furthermore, plasmin not only lyses clots, but it lyses the precursor of fibrin (fibrinogen) and inactivates clotting factors. Three thrombolytic agents are currently available for emergency use. They are streptokinase, eminase, and tissue plasminogen activator.

4. Streptokinase
   - Origin: Produced from streptococci bacteria
   - Mechanism: Forms a complex by binding to circulating and blood clot plasminogen, thereby stimulating the production of plasmin
   - Dose: 1.5 million units IV over 1 hour
   - Cost: about $400 per patient

5. Eminase (APSAC)
   - Origin: Combination of streptokinase and plasminogen bound together
   - Mechanism: Directly acts to convert circulating plasminogen to plasmin
   - Dose: Single dose of 30 units IV over 5 minutes.
   - Cost: about $2000 per patient

6. Tissue Plasminogen Activator (t-PA)
   - Origin: Recombinant genetic engineering
   - Mechanism: Converts clot bound plasminogen to plasmin
   - Traditional Dose: 6 to 10 mg IV bolus followed by an infusion of 50 mg over the first hour. An additional 20 mg/hr is administered over the next 2 hours.
   - Accelerated Dose: 15 mg IV followed by 0.75 mg/kg over 30 minutes. An additional 0.5 mg/kg is administered over 1 hour.
   - Cost: about $2800 per patient

Indications for Thrombolytic Therapy

7. Thrombolytic therapy is indicated for an evolving MI within 6 to 12 hours following the onset of symptoms (chest pain, etc.). The chest pain and other symptoms should be consistent with acute myocardial infarction and at least 1 mm of ST segment elevation should be present in at least two anatomically contiguous ECG leads.

Contraindications for Thrombolytic Therapy

8. Two classifications of contraindications exist for thrombolytics, absolute and relative.

9. Absolute contraindications include active internal bleeding, suspected aortic dissection, prolonged CPR, recent head trauma or intracranial neoplasm, history of hemorrhagic CVA, blood pressure greater than 200/120 mmHg, and previous allergies to thrombolytics

10. Relative contraindications include surgery within the past 2 weeks, history of severe hypertension, active peptic ulcer, history of CVA, known bleeding (hemophilia), use of anticoagulants (Coumadin or heparin), significant liver dysfunction, and prior exposure to streptokinase or eminase within the last 9 months.

Complications of Thrombolytic Therapy

11. The most significant complication associated with the use of thrombolytics is intracerebral bleeding. Although only 1% of patients treated with thrombolytic agents develop intracerebral bleeding, the mortality rate is 40 to 50%. Other complications include systemic bleeding, hypotension, anaphylactic shock, and immune complex disease.

Out-Of-Hospital Administration of Thrombolytic Therapy

12. Most large clinical trials of thrombolytics demonstrate an improvement in mortality with early administration. To date, four trials have addressed the issue of delivering thrombolytic agents in the field. These include studies in Europe, Israel, Canada, and Seattle, Washington. All four indicate that it is safe to administer thrombolytic agents in the field for the treatment of acute myocardial infarction, but each failed to demonstrate a reduction in either morbidity or mortality.

The Cardiac Alert

13. Currently, not enough evidence exists to justify the out-of-hospital administration of thrombolytics. However, the acquisition of an out-of-hospital 12-lead ECG combined with the use of a cardiac alert has clearly demonstrated the ability to reduce the door-to-drug time for thrombolytic therapy in the emergency department. Cardiac alerts, similar to current trauma alerts, allow for the early notification of patients experiencing acute myocardial infarction in the field. This in turn enables the receiving hospital to prepare in advance for the early delivery of thrombolytic therapy.

BIBLIOGRAPHY

Albrich JM, Rothrock S, Salluzzo R. Acute myocardial infarction: Comprehensive guidelines for diagnosis, stabilization, and mortality reduction. *Emergency Medicine Reports.* 1994;15(6):51–62.

Anderson JL, Karagounis L, Allen A, Bradford MJ, Menlove RL, Pryor TA. Older age and elevated blood pressure are risk factors for intracerebral hemorrhage after thrombolysis. *American Journal of Cardiology.* 1991;68:166–170.

Aufderheide TP, Haselow WC, Hendley GE, et al. Feasibility of prehospital r-TPA therapy in chest pain patients. *Annals of Emergency Medicine.* 1992;21:379–383.

Aufderheide TP, Hendley GE, Thakur RK, et al. The diagnostic impact of prehospital 12-lead electrocardiography. *Annals of Emergency Medicine.* 1990;19:1280–1287.

Aufderheide TP, Keelan MH, Hendley GE, et al. Milwaukee prehospital chest pain project—Phase I: Feasibility and accuracy of prehospital thrombolytic candidate selection. *American Journal of Cardiology.* 1992;69:991–996.

Benson NH, Maningas PA, Krohmer JR, Balcombe DJ, Swor R. Guidelines for the prehospital use of thrombolytic agents. *Annals of Emergency Medicine.* 1994;23:1047–1048.

Bertini G, Rostagno C, Taddei T, et al. Evaluation of a mobile coronary care unit protocol in patients with acute onset chest pain. *Journal of Emergency Medicine.* 1991;9:57–63.

Bippus P, Storch W, Andersen D, Schröder R. Thrombolysis started at home in acute myocardial infarction: Feasibility and time-gain. *Circulation.* 1987;76(suppl. IV, October):IV–122.

Bossaert LL, Demey HE, Colemont LJ, et al. Prehospital thrombolytic treatment of acute myocardial infarction with anisoylated plasminogen streptokinase activator complex. *Critical Care Medicine.* 1988;16:823–830.

Califf RM, Harrelson-Woodlief SL. At home thrombolysis. *Journal of the American College of Cardiology.* 1990;15:937–939.

Castaigne AD, Christian H, Duval-Moulin AM, et al. Prehospital use of APSAC: Results of a placebo-controlled study. *American Journal of Cardiology.* 1989;64:30A–33A.

Cayten CG, Oler J, Walker K, Murphy J, Morganroth J, Staroscik R. The effect of telemetry on urban prehospital cardiac care. *Annals of Emergency Medicine.* 1985;14:976–981.

Cummins RO, Eisenberg MS. From pain to reperfusion: What role for the prehospital 12-lead ECG? *Annals of Emergency Medicine.* 1990;19:1343–1346.

EMIP Group. Prehospital thrombolytic therapy in patients with suspected acute myocardial infarction. *New England Journal of Medicine.* 1993;329:383–389.

Foster DB, Dufendach JH, Barkdoll CM, Mitchell BK. Prehospital recognition of AMI using independent nurse/paramedic 12-lead ECG evaluation: Impact on in-hospital times to thrombolysis in a rural community hospital. *American Journal of Emergency Medicine.* 1994;12(1):25–31.

Gibler WB, Kereiakes DJ, Dean EN, et al. Prehospital diagnosis and treatment of acute myocardial infarction: A north-south perspective. *American Heart Journal.* 1991;121(1):1–11.

GISSI. Long-term effects of intravenous thrombolysis in acute myocardial infarction: Final report of the GISSI study. *Lancet.* 1987;2:871–874.

Gokli AR, Kovar JL, Kowalenko T, Nowak RM. Prehospital care of acute myocardial infarction: A review. *Henry Ford Hospital Medical Journal.* 1991;39(3–4):170–175.

GREAT Group. Feasibility, safety, and efficacy of domiciliary thrombolysis by general practitioners: Grampian region early anistreplase trial. *British Medical Journal.* 1992;305:548–553.

Greenberg H, Sherrid M, Lynn S, et al. Out-of-hospital paramedic administered streptokinase for acute myocardial infarction. *Lancet.* 1988;2:1187.

Grim P, Feldman T, Martin M, Donovan R, Nevins V, Childers R. Cellular telephone transmission of 12-lead electrocardiograms from ambulance to hospital. *American Journal of Cardiology.* 1987;60:715–720.

GUSTO Investigators. An international randomized trial comparing four thrombolytic strategies for acute myocardial infarction. *New England Journal of Medicine.* 1993;329:673–680.

Hargarten KM, Aprahamian C, Stueven H, Olson DW, Aufderheide TP, Mateer JR. Limitations of prehospital predictors of acute myocardial infarction and unstable angina. *Annals of Emergency Medicine.* 1987;16:1325–1329.

Karagounis L, Ipsen SK, Jessop MR, et al. Impact of field-transmitted electrocardiography on time to in-hospital thrombolytic therapy in acute myocardial infarction. *American Journal of Cardiology.* 1990;66:786–791.

Kennedy JW, Weaver WD. The potential for prehospital thrombolytic therapy. *Clinical Cardiology.* 1990;13(VIII):23–26.

Kereiakes DJ, Weaver DW, Anderson JL, et al. Time delays in the diagnosis and treatment of acute myocardial infarction: A tale of eight cities. Report from the prehospital study group and the Cincinnati heart project. *American Heart Journal.* 1990;120:773–780.

Koren G, Weiss A, Hasin Y, et al. Prevention of myocardial damage in acute myocardial ischemia by early treatment with intravenous streptokinase. *New England Journal of Medicine.* 1985;313:1384–1389.

Kowalenko T, Kereiakes DJ, Gibler WB. Prehospital diagnosis and treatment of acute myocardial infarction: A critical review. *American Heart Journal.* 1992;123(1):181–190.

Otto LA, Aufderheide TP. Evaluation of ST segment elevation criteria for the prehospital electrocardiographic diagnosis of acute myocardial infarction. *Annals of Emergency Medicine.* 1994;23(1):17–24.

Roth A, Barbash GI, Hod H, et al. Should thrombolytic therapy be administered in the mobile intensive care unit in patients with evolving myocardial infarction? A pilot study. *Journal of the American College of Cardiology.* 1990;15:932–936.

Scott JL, Pigman EC, Gordon GG, Silverstein S. Ischemic heart disease. In: Rosen P, Barkin RM, eds. *Emergency Medicine Concepts and Clinical Practice.* St. Louis, MO: Mosby Year Book, 1992, pp. 1361–1364.

Setaro JF, Cabin HS. Right ventricular infarction. *Cardiology Clinics.* 1992;10(1):69–90.

Sharkey SW, Brunette DD, Ruiz E, et al. An analysis of time delays preceding thrombolysis for acute myocardial infarction. *Journal of the American Medical Association.* 1989;262:3171–3174.

Weaver WD, Cerqueira M, Hallstrom AP, et

al. Prehospital-initiated vs hospital-initiated thrombolytic therapy: The myocardial infarction triage and intervention trial. *Journal of the American Medical Association.* 1993;270:1211–1216.

Weaver WD, Eisenberg MS, Martin JS, et al.

Myocardial infarction triage and intervention project—Phase I: Patient characteristics and feasibility of prehospital initiation of thrombolytic therapy. *Journal of the American College of Cardiology.* 1990;15:925–931.

Page numbers followed by *t* indicate tables; those followed by *f* indicate figure.